Manual of Psychiatric Emergencies

Third Edition

Steven E. Hyman, M.D.
Associate Professor of Psychiatry, Harvard Medical School; Director of Research, Department of Psychiatry, Massachusetts General Hospital, Boston

George E. Tesar, M.D.
Chairman, Department of Psychiatry and Psychology, Cleveland Clinic Foundation, Cleveland

Little, Brown and Company
Boston/New York/Toronto/London

Third Edition

Library of Congress Cataloging-in-Publication Data

Manual of psychiatric emergencies / [edited by] Steven E. Hyman, George E. Tesar. — 3rd ed.
p. cm.
Includes bibliographical references and index.
ISBN 0-316-38728-2
1. Psychiatric emergencies—Handbooks, manuals, etc. I. Hyman, Steven E. II. Tesar, George E.
[DNLM: 1. Crisis Intervention—handbooks. 2. Mental Disorders—handbooks. 3. Emergency Services, Psychiatric—handbooks. 4. Mental Health Services—handbooks. WM 34 M294 1994]
RC480.6.M354 1994
616.89'025—dc20
DNLM/DLC
for Library of Congress 93-1834
CIP

Printed in the United States of America

SEM

Second Printing

Sponsoring Editor: Kristin Odmark
Production Editor: Marie A. Salter
Copyeditor: Debra Corman
Indexer: Nancy Newman
Production Supervisor: Michael A. Granger
Cover Designer: Linda Dana Willis

To Barbara, Emily, and Julia
and
to Kristine and Thomas

Contents

Preface

In recent years psychiatry has been moving closer to the mainstream of American medicine. This development means only good things for clinical care as long as psychiatrists do not lose their traditional interpersonal skills while attaining new ones. The successful evaluation and management of psychiatric emergencies requires that physicians be able to use a great variety of skills, both psychological and medical, confidently and flexibly.

This manual is meant not only for psychiatrists, but for all physicians called on to evaluate and treat patients with acute mental and behavioral symptoms. It is hoped that the manual will prove useful in a variety of settings, including emergency departments, general hospitals, and psychiatric hospitals. The emphasis is on differential diagnosis and emergency management, not long-term treatment. Particular strategies for management are recommended throughout, but in any particular case, the best therapy will depend on the exact clinical circumstances and will require the judgment of the physician.

Since its first edition this manual has evolved due to the efforts of its many contributors. However, much of the material has been honed in interactions with the excellent psychiatric residents of the Massachusetts General Hospital, especially during their tours of duty in the Acute Psychiatry Service. We owe these residents a tremendous debt of gratitude for their stimulating questions, comments, and level of interest. We also thank in particular Dr. Ned Cassem, Chief of the Psychiatry Service at Massachusetts General Hospital, who has supported us and throughout his career has stood as an exemplar of clinical excellence. We also thank Crystal Moore, who has been the administrative backbone of the Acute Psychiatry Service. Kristin Odmark, our editor at Little, Brown, struggled constantly against our recalcitrance; without her this third edition would not have become a reality.

S. E. H.
G. E. T.

Contributing Authors

Paul J. Barreira, M.D.	Associate Professor of Psychiatry, University of Massachusetts Medical School; Director, Residency Training in Psychiatry, University of Massachusetts Medical Center, Worcester, Massachusetts
Eugene V. Beresin, M.D.	Assistant Professor of Psychiatry, Harvard Medical School; Director, Child and Adolescent Psychiatry Residency Training, Massachusetts General Hospital, Boston
Barbara E. Bierer, M.D.	Associate Professor of Medicine, Harvard Medical School; Associate Physician, Hematology-Oncology Division, Brigham and Women's Hospital, Boston
Michael F. Bierer, M.D., M.P.H.	Instructor in Medicine, Harvard Medical School; Assistant Physician, Massachusetts General Hospital, Boston
M. Cornelia Cremens, M.D., M.P.H.	Instructor in Psychiatry, Harvard Medical School; Director, Medical Student Education, Massachusetts General Hospital, Boston
William E. Falk, M.D.	Assistant Professor of Psychiatry, Harvard Medical School; Deputy Chief, Psychopharmacology Unit, Psychiatry Service, Massachusetts General Hospital, Boston
Anne Fishel, Ph.D.	Instructor in Psychology, Harvard Medical School; Clinical Associate in Psychology, Massachusetts General Hospital, Boston
Donald C. Goff, M.D.	Assistant Professor of Psychiatry, Harvard Medical School; Associate Psychiatrist, Massachusetts General Hospital, Boston

Christopher Gordon, M.D.	Assistant Psychiatrist, Massachusetts General Hospital, Boston; Medical Director, Human Resource Institute, Brookline, Massachusetts
Shelly F. Greenfield, M.D., M.P.H.	Research Fellow, Alcohol and Drug Abuse Research Center, Harvard Medical School, Boston; Assistant Psychiatrist, McLean Hospital, Belmont, Massachusetts
Mark J. Hauser, M.D.	Clinical Instructor in Psychiatry, Harvard Medical School; Forensic Psychiatrist and Research Associate, Program in Psychiatry and the Law, Massachusetts Mental Health Center, Boston
Steven K. Hoge, M.D.	Associate Professor of Psychiatry and Law, University of Virginia Schools of Law and Medicine; Medical Director, Institute of Law, Psychiatry, and Public Policy, University of Virginia, Charlottesville, Virginia
Steven E. Hyman, M.D.	Associate Professor of Psychiatry, Harvard Medical School; Director of Research, Department of Psychiatry, Massachusetts General Hospital, Boston
Michael A. Jenike, M.D.	Associate Professor of Psychiatry, Harvard Medical School; Associate Chief for Research, Department of Psychiatry, Massachusetts General Hospital, Boston
Patricia Mian, R.N., M.S., C.S.	Psychiatric Clinical Nurse Specialist, Massachusetts General Hospital, Boston
Steven M. Mirin, M.D.	Professor of Psychiatry, Harvard Medical School, Boston; Psychiatrist-in-Chief and General Director, McLean Hospital, Belmont, Massachusetts
Abigail R. Ostow, M.D.	Staff Psychiatrist, Harvard Community Health Plan, Kenmore Center, Boston, Massachusetts
Nancy Rappaport, M.D.	Clinical Fellow, Harvard Medical School, Boston; Child Psychiatrist and Child Fellow, Cambridge Hospital, Cambridge, Massachusetts
John J. Ratey, M.D.	Assistant Professor of Psychiatry, Harvard Medical School, Boston; Director of Research, Medfield State Hospital, Medfield, Massachusetts

Paula K. Rauch, M.D.	Clinical Instructor in Psychiatry, Harvard Medical School; Associate Director, Child Psychiatry Consultation-Liaison Service, Massachusetts General Hospital, Boston
Julia M. Reade, M.D.	Instructor in Psychiatry, Harvard Medical School; Clinical Assistant in Psychiatry, Massachusetts General Hospital, Boston
Jerrold F. Rosenbaum, M.D.	Associate Professor of Psychiatry, Harvard Medical School; Chief, Clinical Psychopharmacology, Massachusetts General Hospital, Boston
M. Elizabeth Ross, M.D., Ph.D.	Assistant Professor of Neurology, University of Minnesota Medical School—Minneapolis; Attending Neurologist, University of Minnesota Hospital and Clinics, Minneapolis
Anthony J. Rothschild, M.D.	Associate Professor of Psychiatry, Harvard Medical School, Boston; Clinical Director, Affective Disease Program, McLean Hospital, Belmont, Massachusetts
Ronald Schouten, J.D., M.D.	Instructor in Psychiatry, Harvard Medical School; Director, Law and Psychiatry Service, Massachusetts General Hospital, Boston
Theodore A. Stern, M.D.	Associate Professor of Psychiatry, Harvard Medical School; Psychiatrist and Director, Resident Psychiatric Consultation Service, Massachusetts General Hospital, Boston
Paul Summergrad, M.D.	Assistant Professor of Psychiatry, Harvard Medical School; Director, Inpatient Psychiatric Service, Massachusetts General Hospital, Boston
George E. Tesar, M.D.	Chairman, Department of Psychiatry and Psychology, Cleveland Clinic Foundation, Cleveland
Adele C. Viguera, M.D.	Clinical Fellow in Psychiatry, Harvard Medical School, Boston; McLean Hospital, Belmont, Massachusetts
Roger D. Weiss, M.D.	Associate Professor of Psychiatry, Harvard Medical School, Boston; Clinical Director, Alcohol and Drug Abuse Program, McLean Hospital, Belmont, Massachusetts

Fundamental Topics in Emergency Psychiatry

Notice. The indications and dosages of all drugs in this book have been recommended in the medical literature and conform to the practices of the general medical community. The medications described do not necessarily have specific approval by the Food and Drug Administration for use in the diseases and dosages for which they are recommended. The package insert for each drug should be consulted for use and dosage as approved by the FDA. Because standards for usage change, it is advisable to keep abreast of revised recommendations, particularly those concerning new drugs.

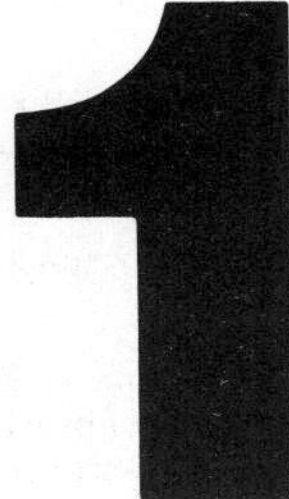

The Emergency Psychiatric Evaluation, Including the Mental Status Examination

Steven E. Hyman
George E. Tesar

I. Initial approach. Symptoms and signs of mental disturbance may be the presenting features of a psychiatric, neurologic, or medical problem; thus, the clinician must be open-minded and thorough in evaluating patients with apparent psychiatric emergencies. The initial approach to the patient should be direct, warm, and concerned; as the evaluation proceeds and the physician develops hypotheses as to what the problem is, he or she can modify the interview and examination to fit the situation. To deal effectively with the range of psychiatric emergencies, a physician needs the skill to make a rapid assessment of the patient and a mental triage so that the evaluation moves in the right direction. It is wrong to sit and listen passively if the patient appears to have an acute psychosis or organic brain syndrome, just as it is inappropriate to intervene too rapidly if the patient appears to be personality disordered and seeking hospitalization in order to regress. In general, the emergency assessment includes an interview, a mental status examination, a general physical and neurologic examination, and relevant laboratory tests, with additions or omissions as clinically indicated.

II. The interview is often limited by time pressures and by the severity and nature of the patient's symptoms.

A. The physician should introduce himself or herself and address the patient by his or her last name to show respect and to maintain an appropriate interpersonal distance.

B. If the patient is able to tell a coherent story, it is best to let the patient tell it in his or her own words, but as the interview progresses the physician must be sure to obtain all necessary data in a reasonable amount of time.

C. In emergency situations, the physician must **take all suicidal and homicidal threats, gestures, and attempts seriously,** even if at first glance the patient appears to be manipulative.

D. At the end of the evaluation the physician must be forthright and clear in discussing his or her recommendations. It is useful to ask the patient how he or she feels about the recommended treatment or disposition in order to identify any immediate compliance problems. Occasionally the disposition will involve involuntary treatment; every attempt should be made to improve the patient's compliance by clearly explaining the reasons why treatment is necessary.

E. Special situations arise if the patient is violent or is psychotic or delirious to the point that he or she is unable to carry on a conversation. Depending on the situation, restraint or rapid medical treatment may be necessary before any further assessment is possible.

F. Content of the interview

1. Presenting problem

a. Insofar as it is possible, the patient should be allowed to tell his or her story but should not be allowed to ramble. Time limitations require that the current problem be focused on, although it is necessary to get some idea of more chronic problems and lifelong coping mechanisms. With some patients corroborating data will be needed from those who accompanied them or from the patient's current therapist, if any.

b. Symptoms, their nature of onset (including precipitating circumstances, if any), severity, and duration should be clarified.

2. Past history of psychiatric illness and response to treatments should be obtained. Patients should be asked directly about any history of psychiatric hospitalization, because many individuals fail to mention hospitalizations spontaneously.

3. Patients should be asked about **alcohol and illicit drug use.** If there is a pattern of abuse it should be determined whether it is continuing and whether there is evidence that the patient is addicted.

4. A history of medical illness and any current medical symptoms should be obtained. Patients should be asked about **all medications** they use, both prescribed and over-the-counter. If not already reported, patients should be asked about sleep problems, appetite, ability to concentrate, energy level, and sexual function.

5. Family history of psychiatric and neurologic disorders should be obtained. It is often misleading, however, to accept psychiatric diagnoses of family members at face value. Given recent improvements in psychiatric diagnosis, it is worth asking briefly about the family member's symptoms and treatment response to decide whether the reported diagnosis is likely to be correct (e.g., many patients diagnosed as having paranoid schizophrenia in past years actually had manic-depressive illness).

6. Personal and social history

a. The patient's current level of functioning and best prior level of functioning should be ascertained. Determination of the patient's highest level of education, work history, military history, legal history, and history of seeking disability is helpful in interpreting his or her current level of functioning.

b. To reach a disposition, the physician must know whether the patient comes from an environment where he or she can be supported, watched, and supervised or from a chaotic and disruptive environment, or whether the patient lives alone.

c. It is important to find out whether there is a history of legal difficulties and whether there are any criminal charges pending.

d. A detailed developmental history is beyond the scope of an emergency evaluation, although a brief history may help uncover typical patterns of behavior in personality disordered patients (see Chap. 22).

III. The mental status examination. A careful and systematic mental status examination is critical to the workup of patients presenting with psychiatric emergencies. The mental status examination cannot be approached haphazardly because it is a hierarchical examination. (For example, if inattention is missed early in the examination, memory and higher cognitive functions will be improperly judged later; if aphasia is missed, the thought content might be misinterpreted as representing a psychosis.) A brief, screening cognitive mental status examination is given in Fig. 1.1. This Mini-Mental State Examination is currently in wide use but *does not replace* a full examination. A full mental status examination includes the following:

A. Level of consciousness

1. Patients may be described as alert, lethargic, stuporous, or comatose; however, specific descriptions should be provided when the mental status is

Orientation

1. What is the (year) (season) (month) (day) (date)? Ask specifically for parts omitted, e.g., "Can you also tell me what season it is?" (One point for each correct; maximum score is 5)
2. Where are we: (state) (county) (town) (hospital) (floor)? (One point for each correct; maximum score is 5)

Registration

Ask the patient if you may test his or her memory. Then say the names of three unrelated objects, clearly and slowly, about one second each. After you have said all three, ask the patient to repeat them. Give one point for each correct answer. This first repetition determines his or her score (0–3), but keep saying them until the patient can repeat all three, up to 6 trials. Count trials and record. If the patient does not eventually learn all three, recall cannot be meaningfully tested.

Attention and Calculation

Ask the patient to begin with 100 and count backwards by 7. Stop after five subtractions (93, 86, 79, 72, 65). Score the total number of correct answers. If the patient cannot or will not perform this task, ask him or her to spell the word *world* backwards. The score is the number of letters in correct order, e.g., dlrow = 5, dlorw = 3. (Maximum score is 5)

Recall

Ask the patient if he or she can recall the three words you previously asked him or her to remember. Score 0–3.

Language

1. Naming: Show the patient a wristwatch and ask him or her what it is. Repeat for a pencil. Score 0–2.
2. Repetition: Ask the patient to repeat the following sentence after you. "No ifs, ands, or buts." Allow only one trial. Score 0 or 1.
3. Three-stage command: Give the patient a piece of blank paper and the following command: "Take this piece of paper in your right hand, fold it in half, and put in on the floor." Score one point for each part correctly executed (0–3).
4. Reading: On a blank piece of paper print the sentence "Close your eyes" in letters large enough for the patient to see clearly. Ask him or her to read it and do what it says. Score one point only if the patient actually closes his or her eyes.
5. Writing: Give the patient a blank piece of paper and ask him or her to write a sentence for you. Do not dictate the sentence; it is to be written spontaneously. It must contain a subject and verb and be sensible. Correct grammar and punctuation are not necessary. (One point)
6. Copying: On a blank piece of paper, draw intersecting pentagons, each side about 1 in., and ask the patient to copy it exactly as it is. All 10 angles must be present, and two must intersect to score one point. Tremor and rotation are ignored.

Total score ______

Estimate the patient's level of consciousness along a continuum:

____

Alert Drowsy Stupor Coma

Fig. 1-1. A version of the Mini-Mental State Examination. (Adapted from *Journal of Psychiatric Research* 12:189, M. F. Folstein, S. E. Folstein, and P. R. McHugh. Mini-mental state: A practical method for grading the cognitive state of patients for the clinician. Copyright 1975, Pergamon Press, Ltd.)

abnormal—for example, whether the patient's eyes are open or closed and the normalcy of spontaneous eye movements; the amount of spontaneous speech or if there is none, the stimulus needed to evoke vocalization; and the speed and coordination of voluntary motor movements, or if there are none, the stimulus needed to evoke movement and description of the response.

2. Disorders of consciousness seen in the emergency department include stupor and coma, delirium (in which the level of consciousness may be abnormal or fluctuate), dreamy states accompanying partial complex seizures, and dissociated states accompanying some psychiatric disorders.

3. The maintenance of consciousness depends on the cerebral cortex, the thalamic intralaminar nuclei, and the brainstem reticular formation, particularly the mesencephalic and rostral pontine tegmentum. To impair consciousness, cortical lesions have to be diffuse (which includes toxic-metabolic causes) or bilateral. Focal pathology in one hemisphere can impair consciousness if swelling affects the other hemisphere.

B. **Appearance and behavior** should be described, including the patient's overall appearance, dress, and grooming. The degree of cooperation with the interviewer and eye contact should be noted. Motor activity should be assessed, including the level of activity (e.g., psychomotor agitation or retardation), as should any posturing, tics, or involuntary movements. Asymmetries of grooming or dress, which could be due to unilateral neglect, for example, should be noted.

C. **Attention** is a term used to refer to two different mental functions:

1. The first meaning of attention is comprised of:

   a. **Vigilance,** the degree to which the patient can select appropriate stimuli to perceive and process, and

   b. **Concentration,** the degree to which the patient is able to maintain that attention.

   c. A patient's ability to attend must be assessed before other cognitive functions can be evaluated. Inattention will, for example, make it impossible to accurately test a patient's memory. Attention may be judged by asking the patient to repeat a series of random digits. The examiner should begin with two digits and increase the number as the patient succeeds. Normal individuals should be able to repeat five to seven digits. Inattention may be caused by anxiety, mania, depression, or diffuse brain dysfunction resulting, for example, from drugs, delirium, head injuries, or cortical (especially frontal) damage. The patient's level of consciousness (overall alertness) and other findings should help differentiate among these states. If abnormalities of alertness and attention are both present, an organic brain syndrome is the most likely diagnosis.

2. The other meaning of attention is the patient's ability to notice (as opposed to neglect) stimuli in all sensory spheres. Neglect can be tested for by performing a sensory examination. Subtle cases can be detected by noting extinction of a response on one side with simultaneous bilateral sensory stimulation. Neglect is most often due to a stroke of the nondominant cerebral hemisphere producing contralateral symptoms.

D. **Mood and affect**

1. Mood describes a patient's pervasive and sustained emotion (e.g., depressed, anxious, elated, irritable).

2. Affect is the observable pattern of behaviors that are the outward expression of the patient's current feeling state. Affect is more variable over time than mood.

a. During the course of the interview the patient's range of affects and their amplitude should be noted.

(1) The range of affect may be described as normal (or broad), restricted, or flat (no affective expression). The range of affect deemed normal depends on the context and the patient's cultural background.

(2) The amplitude of affects should be described as excessive (e.g., excessive anger), normal, or blunted (reduction in the intensity of affective expression).

b. Affect is said to be **inappropriate** when clearly discordant with the content of the person's speech. Affect is **labile** when abruptly and rapidly shifting.

c. Special attention must be paid in trying to distinguish apathy, suggestive of frontal lobe disease, from depressed or blunted affect. It may be difficult to do so with certainty; thus, it is important to look for other mental status findings that would confirm the presence of one syndrome or another (e.g., perseveration for frontal disease, guilt or diminished self-esteem for depression).

E. Language testing can suggest the presence of specific anatomic lesions and is a necessary prerequisite to the examination of thought content. Examination of speech can also be useful in differentiating specific psychiatric disorders. Testing of language includes the following:

1. Listening to the patient's **spontaneous speech,** or if there is none, asking open-ended questions. This will allow the examiner to judge the fluency, articulation, prosody, rate, and pressure of the patient's speech.

2. Comprehension can be tested by asking direct questions and asking the patient to follow commands.

3. Naming should be tested by pointing out body parts, objects, and parts of objects.

4. The patient's abilty to **repeat** short phrases and neologisms should be tested.

5. The patient should be asked to read and produce a writing sample; the test of writing can be used to test orientation by asking the patient to write his or her name, the date, and place. The patient should also be asked to write a short sentence.

6. Abnormalities of speech and language functions include the following:

a. Dysarthria, or distorted articulation, suggests either metabolic brain disease, intoxication, or a focal lesion of the brain regions necessary for the motor aspects of speaking.

b. Dysprosody, or abnormal speech inflection and rhythm, suggests a lesion of the right (nondominant) hemisphere. It is important not to mistake the inflectionless speech of dysprosody for depression.

c. Aphasia is the loss of language function caused by brain dysfunction. There are different types depending on the region of the brain that has been injured. The following descriptions are clinically useful oversimplifications:

(1) Aphasias due to lesions of **Broca's area** (the anterior speech area) produce effortful, sparse, agrammatic speech (nonfluent aphasia). These aphasias are most commonly due to left middle cerebral artery infarcts. Most patients have associated dysarthria and other motor deficits. Affectively many of these patients are agitated and depressed.

(2) **Wernicke's aphasia** produces fluent speech with a paucity of nominatives and many paraphasic errors (word substitutions), which may include neologisms. Comprehension, naming, and repetition are also impaired. The lesion is usually in the superior temporal gyrus and posterior sylvian region. Perisylvian infarctions may produce Wernicke's aphasia with no additional evidence of focal neurologic disease. If comprehension and other aspects of language are not tested, the resulting speech, which is often nonsensical and full of neologisms, may be mistaken for a psychotic process or a confusional state, with potentially disastrous consequences. Patients with Wernicke's aphasia may have affective abnormalities; some are euphoric, but others appear paranoid and may be combative.

(3) **Conduction aphasia** is fluent, paraphasic speech with good comprehension but very poor repetition. It can result from a small cortical infarct of the parietal operculum or supramarginal gyrus or may be the result of a resolving Wernicke's aphasia.

(4) **Anomic aphasia** is a term used when naming is impaired out of proportion to other language functions. There may also be word-finding difficulties in spontaneous speech.

(5) **Global aphasia** refers to sparse, nonfluent speech with impairment of all language functions. It is due to large dominant hemisphere lesions.

d. **Agraphia** is a disturbance in writing; it refers to errors in language, not to motor difficulties.

e. **Alexia** is an acquired reading disturbance not due to visual problems.

f. Abnormalities of **rate, loudness, and pressure of speech.** The rate of speech is often abnormal in patients with affective disorders or anxiety. Depression or the apathy of frontal lobe disease may result in a paucity of spontaneous speech with long latencies before questions are answered. In addition, depression and some mixed affective states may cause speech to be slow. Mania may result in speech that is loud, rapid, and pressured. Pressured speech should not be confused with rapidity; it represents the difficulty that one has interrupting the flow of speech. Speech may be slow but extremely difficult to interrupt if the patient is controlling and obsessional.

g. **The form of the speech** may be abnormal even in the absence of aphasia. Vague, overelaborate, digressive, and neologistic speech is suggestive of a psychosis.

F. **Orientation and memory.** Tests of memory and cognition are often threatening to patients; thus, their necessity should be carefully and politely explained. Every attempt should be made to preserve the dignity of patients during cognitive testing.

1. **Orientation.** The patient should be asked his or her name and age; the present place, address, and city; and the day of the week and date. Some of these questions can be combined with the test of writing. Orientation requires attention and memory. The often-made generalization that disorientation (confusion) is pathognomonic of organic mental disorders is wrong. In fact, many patients with acute psychoses, especially acute mania, are not oriented to time or place based on failure to attend to or register such data.

2. **Memory.** Although different terminology is often applied, there are at least three types of memory that are relevant in the emergency examination and that depend on different cerebral structures.

a. **Immediate recall** or **primary memory.** When sensory information is perceived and attended to, it is transferred to primary memory. This type of memory has a limited capacity and lasts no longer than a few minutes or until the individual is distracted. Indeed, information must be actively rehearsed to be retained in primary memory. This type of memory can be tested by naming three unrelated objects and asking the patient to repeat them immediately.

b. **Recent** or **secondary memory.** Information that is retained for any significant length of time requires recent memory. This type of memory can store a relatively unlimited amount of information from minutes to months. The distinguishing clinical feature of this type of memory is that it requires intact midline diencephalic structures (including the dorsomedial nucleus of the thalamus and the mamillary bodies of the hypothalamus) and temporal structures (including the hippocampus and adjacent regions of cerebral cortex and the amygdala). Assuming that the patient is able to pay attention and register the three objects in the test described above, secondary memory can be tested by asking the patient to remember the objects and then asking to recall them five minutes later. The normal patient should recall all three. Knowledge of the date and place on tests of orientation also require recent memory.

c. **Remote** or **tertiary memory.** When information has been retained for many months or years, it becomes extremely resistant to disruption, a process known as consolidation. This type of memory appears to be stored in distributed fashion throughout the cerebral cortex. It is distinguished from recent memory in that it no longer requires diencephalic or temporal structures for recall. An adequate assessment of remote memory requires a verifiable external source of information. Historical facts can be used as long as the examiner considers the patient's education level and cultural background.

d. **The amnesia syndrome.** In clinical practice, true deficits of memory (i.e., not apparent deficits actually due to inattention) most commonly represent what may be called the **amnesia syndrome.** This syndrome is limited to recent or secondary memory and consists of a degree of retrograde amnesia (failure to recall past events), most pronounced for the most recent events and sparing older memories, combined with anterograde amnesia (diminished ability to learn new information). The amnesia syndrome is due to bilateral insults to the diencephalic or temporal structures (see sec. **III.F.2.b**). The syndrome can be transient—for example, due to a seizure, bilateral electroconvulsive therapy, concussion, or transient global amnesia (see Chap. 26). Alternatively, it can be long-lasting or permanent—for example, due to Korsakoff's syndrome (which causes lesions of the thalamus, fornix, and mamillary bodies), herpes simplex encephalitis (which frequently attacks the temporal lobes), or Alzheimer's disease (which most often destroys temporal cortex early in its course). Inattention and amnesia can also be produced by certain drugs, most notably high-potency benzodiazepines (e.g., triazolam) or anticholinergic drugs (e.g., scopolamine).

e. **Clinical implications.** Presence of the amnesia syndrome suggests an organic disorder and therefore requires an appropriate toxicologic, medical, and neurologic workup. In contrast, patients who are alert and readily learn new information (e.g., your name or the name of the hospital) but who cannot recollect their own name or address (assuming they have not gotten a new address in the last few weeks) do not have a "physiologic" memory disorder. One's own identity is a very old memory likely to be distributed throughout the cortex and is highly resistant to disruption. Thus, such patients are likely to have a dissociative disorder or may be malingering.

G. **Constructional ability.** Impairments of constructional ability suggest right parietal lobe dysfunction, which may be due, for example, to stroke or a dementing process. Patients may be asked to draw a cube or a house. Alternatively, the patient can be asked to copy a complex figure, such as two intersecting pentagons. Drawing a clock is useful because it may also reveal hemineglect or poor planning due to frontal lobe pathology.

H. **Calculation,** a complex task involving both attention and higher functions, may be tested by asking the patient simple arithmetic problems, such as serially subtracting 7, starting from 100. The ability to calculate depends on the patient's education level.

I. **Form and content of thought**

1. **The form** of the patient's thought processes is often abnormal in psychotic disorders. Patients should be able to give their history in a logical, chronological fashion. If interrupted, they should be able to pick up their train of thought again. Tangentiality and flight of ideas are common in mania. Rambling or incoherent thinking with loose associations suggests psychosis, delirium, or dementia.

2. **The content** of the patient's thought may be helpful in psychiatric diagnosis. The examiner should consider whether the content is impoverished and whether the patient's thought includes delusions (false beliefs firmly held despite what almost everyone else in the person's culture believes and despite obvious and incontrovertible proof to the contrary); ideas of reference (ideas, held less strongly than delusions, that events, objects, or other people have a particular and unusual significance relating to the patient); delusions of thought broadcasting, thought insertion, or other bizarre delusions; obsessions (ego-dystonic, intrusive ideas that the patient can reality-test); phobias; ideas of worthlessness, helplessness, or hopelessness; and suicidal or homicidal ideas. It may be difficult to distinguish obsessions from delusions in some cases, but it is important to do so because of the strikingly different diagnostic implications.

J. **Perception.** Sensory illusions (misinterpretations of external stimuli) may occur in psychoses but may be more common with organic brain syndromes or hallucinogen use. Hallucinations of any sensory modality may occur in psychosis or organic delirium, although visual, tactile, or olfactory hallucinations are more common with organic processes. Psychotic patients may be reticent about reporting hallucinations; the subject may be introduced by asking whether the patient has had any unusual experiences recently, such as hearing voices that other people could not hear. The presence of distortions (altered perceptions of external stimuli—e.g., macropsia) suggests organic brain pathology.

IV. **Quantifiable mental status examinations.** It may be helpful to follow the progress of patients with organic mental disorders with a standardized, quantifiable mental status examination that can be repeated daily. The most widely used is the Mini-Mental State Examination of Folstein, Folstein, and McHugh (see Fig. 1-1). Although the Mini-Mental State Examination is not a substitute for a full mental status examination, judiciously used it can improve clinical management of many patients.

V. **Physical and neurologic** examinations are important parts of the emergency psychiatric evaluation, although judgment is called for—that is, the examination should be particularly thorough for any patient with acute onset of mental symptoms and is an unnecessary invasion for a patient being seen for sudden bereavement. If the patient is too disturbed to comply with a full neurologic examination in the emergency room, a clear note should be made of it so that a full examination can be performed as soon as it is feasible.

VI. **Laboratory and other tests.** Throughout this manual relevant laboratory tests are outlined that are indicated for the workup of suspected disorders. **Computed**

tomographic (CT) scans should be obtained if focal neurologic deficits are discovered or if mass lesions, intracranial bleeding, or hydrocephalus are suspected to be the cause of a mental status abnormality. The CT scan should not be used as a general screening test. An electroencephalogram (EEG) is useful when complex partial seizures or other seizure types are suspected and may be helpful in working up metabolic encephalopathies. A lumbar puncture is indicated if there is a suspicion of a central nervous system infection.

Selected Readings

Damasio, A. R. Aphasia. *N. Engl. J. Med.* 326:531, 1992.

Folstein, M. F., Folstein, S. E., and McHugh, P. R. "Mini-mental state," a practical method for grading the cognitive state of patients for the clinician. *J. Psychiatr. Res.* 12:189, 1975.

Marin, R. S. Differential diagnosis and classification of apathy. *Am. J. Psychiatry* 147:22, 1990.

Mesulam, M. M. *Principles of Behavioral Neurology.* Philadelphia: F. A. Davis, 1985.

Strub, R. L., and Black, F. W. *The Mental Status Examination in Neurology* (2nd ed.). Philadelphia: F. A. Davis, 1985.

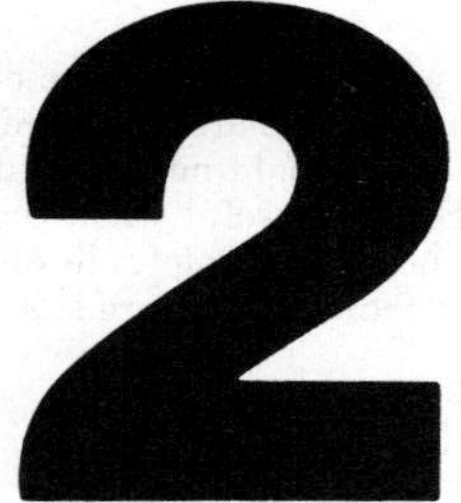

Crisis Intervention: A General Approach

Christopher Gordon

I. Serious life stresses may precipitate visits to an emergency department, even by individuals with no underlying psychiatric disorder.

A. Crisis intervention is a method of helpful involvement with patients and their families during such times of severe stress. The goals of crisis intervention are to succor the person who is in distress, to help him or her through a period of difficulty with dignity, to prevent lasting psychological scarring from the experience, and, if possible, to help the person garner some positive benefit from coping with the crisis.

B. Crisis intervention is not a substitute for a thorough psychiatric evaluation, nor should it be construed as a "quick fix" approach to care. Effective intervention in a crisis involves rapidly establishing rapport with the person under stress, ascertaining the nature of the problem at hand, and negotiating reasonable, practical treatment. For some patients crisis intervention is a prelude to more definitive treatment—for example, defusing a family crisis to the point that a troubled member may be willing to take psychotropic medications. In other cases, the crisis intervention is itself sufficient treatment—for example, in many cases of catastrophic loss, such as the sudden death of a child.

II. Crisis and intervention

A. Overview. Crisis is in the eye of the beholder. A relatively massive insult may be borne by some people without untoward consequences while seemingly mild stresses overwhelm others. Whatever its source, a crisis threatens to swamp the psychological resources of the person. Such a threat may result either from the magnitude of the danger or the fragility of the person experiencing it, or it may result from a special characteristic of the problem at hand that fits with a vulnerability of an individual in a particularly threatening way. For example, a child's first asthma attack would frighten nearly any parent, but if that parent's sibling had died of just such an attack, the event would be especially nightmarish. Most crises are self-limited and resolve naturally. However, occasionally the problem overwhelms the person's usual problem-solving strategies, producing a sense of helplessness and fright and a retreat to unaccustomed (and usually less effective) coping mechanisms—for example, projection, denial, or disorganization. It is often at this point that psychiatric assistance is sought, whether by the patient or by his or her primary physician.

B. As a way of keeping these ideas in focus, the physician approaching a patient in crisis should bear in mind the following questions (these are not questions to be asked of the patient, but a guide for the clinician):

1. What is distressing this person now? Even if the trauma is obvious, what is the meaning of the problem to the patient?
2. How does this person usually deal with stress? How has he or she dealt with severe stress in the past? What resources and liabilities do these experiences indicate?
3. What would appear to be helpful to this person, and how should help be

offered in a way that would be most acceptable? What might the person want that he or she may find it difficult to ask for?

4. What resources are available to both the patient and the clinician to deal with the current problem?

C. Speaking the patient's language. To be helpful in crisis intervention it is necessary for the physician to appreciate the patient's usual way of dealing with the world and to approach the patient using language and a perspective on the problem that feel right and familiar to the person under stress. It is crucial to make the patient feel, very rapidly, that his or her situation is understood by the physician, from the patient's perspective, in the patient's own terms, and in such a way that the patient's dignity is protected.

III. The crisis interview

A. Overview. An effective crisis interview may amount to nothing more than guaranteeing a family some dignified privacy, as may be needed in the case of a sudden and catastrophic loss, or it may require a complex set of interventions and maneuvers designed to create an atmosphere of alliance, comfort, and problem solving. Schematically the elements of such a complex encounter would include the following (which will be fully discussed below):

1. Establishing rapport with the patient.
2. Rapidly understanding the patient's perspective.
3. Obtaining a history.
4. Constructing a formulation about the patient and about the meaning of the stressful event to him or her.
5. Actively negotiating with the patient about the nature of the problem.
6. Actively negotiating with the patient about solutions to the problem.

B. The elements of crisis intervention

1. Establishing rapport

a. When a caregiver comes into contact with a patient or a family in crisis, it is often the simplest courtesies that offer the best way to make contact. Offering an apology if the family has been kept waiting, inquiring after their physical comfort, simply acknowledging the seriousness of what has transpired, or asking if the patient or family needs anything are ordinary kindnesses that can be an important first step toward demystifying the encounter between clinician and patient and establishing that the clinician means to help.

b. In most cases it is best for the clinician to be open and direct about the role he or she will play, explaining what he or she is doing, and why, in a simple and direct manner.

c. In these early moments with the patient or family, it is important not to assume that one understands the meaning of the crisis, but rather to listen carefully to the patient or family, with special focus on what has happened in the immediate past that may shed light on why the problem has occurred at this time and why it has taken the shape that it has.

2. Establishing the patient's or family's perspective

a. Particularly in the early stages of the crisis interview, it is important to attend to the person's exact words as the problem is described, listening for:

(1) How the person or family understands the current problem—for example, does the person or family feel victimized, threatened, or in need of support or information?

(2) How the main people in the current problem are portrayed—for example, does the person or family seem open to outside helpers or do outsiders seem distrusted; does the person or family seem to turn in toward its own resources or outward in search of help?

(3) How feelings are handled—for example, does the person or family seem to address the problem in affective terms, or do feelings seem to be avoided?

b. Once the clinician believes that he or she understands the patient's or family's perspective and what the problem appears to be, this understanding should be reflected back to the patient or family. The clinician should listen carefully for signs that he or she is mistaken and should negotiate a consensus with the patient or family about the nature of the problem.

c. As one listens, it is important to form hypotheses about what the patient or family wants. These desires are often not stated or even acknowledged until later in the interview, but a skillful clinician may recognize the unstated request and move more easily toward it.

d. As soon as possible, the clinician should express an appreciation of the problem and of the patient's attempts to cope with it, even if those attempts appear to have been largely maladaptive. For example, a crisis might emerge in a family where the father is refusing admission for an evolving myocardial infarct; the clinician called to help negotiate with such a patient must attend respectfully to the patient's experience, saying perhaps, "I gather that even if you are ill, you want to make your own decisions about your care, or at least participate in them, and not be dictated to by strangers. That seems reasonable, especially in something as important as this. Although I, too, am a stranger to you, I would like to help you and your family come to the best decision for you."

3. Obtaining a thorough history

a. In the opening moments of a crisis interview, it is important to let the person tell his or her story if he or she is willing. A common error is to jump in prematurely with closed-ended or "yes or no" questions, or lists of symptoms designed to clarify a differential diagnosis. An example of such an error would be to rapidly inquire of a bereaved widow a list of the neurovegetative signs of depression rather than listening to how she feels. Later it will be important to know these answers, but if asked too early in the interview, such questions tend to make it difficult for the patient to feel free to speak.

b. It is important to obtain a thorough history of the present problem, however, with special attention to why the patient or family has come for care now. This is particularly important if the patient has an extensive prior psychiatric history.

c. Depending on the circumstances, it is not always desirable to take a detailed psychiatric history during crisis intervention. For example, when called to see a grieving patient in the emergency room after the unexpected death of a spouse (see Chap. 6) or when asked to see a victim of violence, such as rape (see Chap. 13), taking a detailed psychiatric history may imply that the patient's crisis is in some way pathologic, which may alienate the patient. In these cases it is important that the clinician listen carefully for any evidence of underlying psychiatric disorder, in which case a more thorough evaluation will be necessary—for example, if the bereaved spouse mentions that he or she is contemplating an overdose. In addition, it can be tactfully asked toward the end of the interview whether the patient has ever had any kind of psychiatric trouble in the past.

d. If it appears that a thorough psychiatric and/or medical history is necessary, it is best to move through the history systematically, explaining what is being asked and why. If it is necessary to inquire about a potentially offensive topic, it may be wise to defer the question until late in the interview when there is more data and better rapport, but such questions should not be avoided. It is often best to precede a potentially painful question with a warning, such as, "I know this is a personal question, but would it be all right with you if I asked about . . . ?" Such introductions have the impact of warning a patient before a painful procedure, rather like warming a stethoscope before putting it on a patient's bare flesh.

e. Over the course of the interview be sure to establish:

(1) **Key people in the patient's life,** both present and past, being alert for changes in these relationships in the time immediately preceding the crisis, as well as possible anniversaries of important interactions with these people.

(2) **Current caregivers in the person's life,** since many patients who come for emergency psychiatric care are already in some form of treatment. If the patient has a personality disorder the ongoing treatment may be stormy; difficulties with the current therapist often precipitate crises, and consultations with that therapist often provide solutions (see Chap. 22).

(3) **Past crises and how they were handled;** what worked and what did not. When a person has weathered much strife in his or her life, yet seems swamped by a particular event, either that event has some particularly catastrophic meaning or, more commonly, the person has been made more susceptible to stress by an underlying primary psychiatric disorder, most often depression. When a patient seems uncharacteristically overwhelmed and an obvious and convincing reason cannot be found, the physician should search assiduously for evidence of depression or another primary psychiatric disorder.

(4) **Psychological strengths and resources.** Sometimes in a careful medical or psychiatric evaluation so much emphasis is placed on detecting and cataloguing the patient's pathology that little effort is expended noting the patient's strengths and capacities. In all clinical interactions, however, and especially in crisis intervention, the patient's strengths will be crucial in any successful outcome. It is necessary to note how the person solves problems, what he or she does well, and what interpersonal skills the person possesses, and to make these central to the negotiated plan.

4. **Constructing a formulation.** A psychologic formulation represents an attempt to understand why a person or family functions in a particular way over time and serves as a guide for how the person can best be helped in crisis. The formulation should capture the recurring pattern of feeling, defenses, and relationships that characterize a person's behavior and experience, and should illuminate how the person is dealing with the current crisis. In long-term psychotherapy, the formulation can be constructed over many hours; in crisis intervention, on the other hand, it can usually only be rapidly sketched on the basis of limited information and inference. The critical elements in a useful formulation include:

a. Assessment of reality testing. Note the integrity of the person's reality testing. For the nonpsychotic patient this refers to his or her ability to grapple with reality as opposed to turning to fantasy, denial, or projection. In individuals whose tolerance for reality is weak, note what problems appear to trigger losses of reality testing.

b. **Assessment of relationships.** Note with whom the person has had his or her main relationships in the past and present. An ability to engage in and sustain meaningful relationships augurs well for the person's ability to use the clinician's help. If relationships are not so well developed, there will be clues about how the clinician can interact most acceptably with this particular person.

c. **Assessment of feelings.** Note how the person experiences feelings. Is there a broad range of feeling, as opposed to a very narrow range (constricted affect), a shallowness of feeling (blunted affect), or rapid swings among feelings (affective lability)? How does the person defend against uncomfortable feelings? Which feelings seem particularly difficult?

d. **Assessment of the reaction to the examiner.** Note the patient's attitude toward the clinician, including his or her initial attitudes as well as how the attitude changes over the course of time; hypothesize about how this might reflect the patient's patterns of interaction with other people.

e. **Hypotheses about patterns.** Given what is known about the person's history, about his or her interactions with other people, including the clinician, and about the person's current state of psychologic functioning, attempt to form hypotheses about repetitive patterns that render comprehensible the person's experience and prognosis in the current crisis.

5. **Negotiating about the nature of the problem.** Aside from establishing rapport, the most crucial step in effective crisis intervention is coming to an agreement with the patient or family about what ought to be done about it. This requires that the clinician come to an understanding of what the problem is and of the person suffering it, as described above, but it must include an opportunity for the patient or family to make clear their perspective on the problem and what it is they hope can be done. For many reasons patients are often not explicit about their fears regarding a problem or their expectations with respect to treatment. Such unstated worries or unmade requests may cause important covert conflicts between the patient and clinician about treatment. For example, in a crisis involving parents with a gravely ill child, the parent might want information about the illness, but fearing bad news, might be afraid to ask. The physician might therefore believe that the parents need an opportunity to vent their fears regarding their child's danger. In such a case the physician's emphasis on the worst outcome, while well-meaning, would be deeply hurtful. Covert conflicts of this kind can be minimized if the clinician inquires of the patient or family **how they hoped they might be helped.** Such questions should not be asked too near the beginning of the interview before the patient has become comfortable with the interviewer, but rather after a period of initial understanding. As the physician attends to the patient's perspective, he or she should be alert for unstated conflicts (see Lazare, 1979) regarding:

   a. The nature of the problem.

   b. The goals of the clinical interaction.

   c. The means to be used to solve the problem.

   d. The conditions under which the treatment is to occur.

   e. The nature of the doctor-patient relationship being sought.

6. **Negotiating solutions.** Having arrived at a sense of the nature of the problem, the first decision is whether the problem can be handled in a crisis intervention mode or whether the patient requires referral back to an already ongoing therapy, hospitalization, or some other treatment setting. Assuming that crisis intervention is indicated, the following should be considered:

a. In negotiating interventions, insofar as possible, draw on the patient's own resources and other resources that are readily at hand. The goals of the intervention should be modest, the smallest possible change that will improve the situation. Ambitious goals are rarely attainable. Elaborate solutions requiring complex orchestration are unlikely to succeed.

b. If at all possible allow the patient or family to generate solutions.

c. If possible, involve other people available to the patient in solving the acute problem. Supports provided by the patient's family and friends are more likely to be effective and sustaining than support provided by the physician alone.

d. Defend and mobilize the patient's self-esteem by acknowledging the seriousness of the difficulty, by putting the patient's reaction in as healthy a light as possible, and by treating the patient's attempts to cope with the problem positively.

e. Emphasize the short-term nature of the work, thus implying the expectation that a natural resolution of the crisis is expected. It is important to bear in mind that life is full of crises, that resolution is always partial and imperfect, and that the ordinary supports that people offer one another are usually what make troubles bearable and life worthwhile.

IV. How crisis intervention heals. Assuming that crises are inherently self-limited and tend to be integrated over time into the person's life, the goals of crisis intervention are generally to foster the healing process, to help the person make the best use of available resources, both intrapsychic and interpersonal, and to facilitate further treatment of concomitant psychiatric illness, if indicated. Some of the ways crisis intervention can be helpful are:

A. Providing support and an opportunity for ventilation. One of the most common benefits of crisis intervention is the opportunity for the patient to talk with a sympathetic, nonjudgmental listener who avoids pat answers and the meaningless reassurances of everyday life. It is often an extraordinary, even unprecedented experience for many people to share their deeper feelings with such an attentive listener. In cases like this, crisis intervention sessions provide a chance for ventilation in an atmosphere that helps the patient put his or her feelings in perspective—that is, as a response to an understandable human dilemma. For many people this sort of encouragement and empathy can bring great relief, sometimes to years of suffering.

B. Enlisting social support. In times of stress usually the best sources of support are the people who know the patient and are customarily available. Sometimes in crisis, however, the people most in need become unwittingly cut off from sources of support. For example, in situations of acute bereavement sometimes the person most bereaved must assume major responsibility for making arrangements and meeting the needs of others, to the point that the bereaved person's own needs are overlooked (see Chap. 6). In other situations the crisis itself severely strains the bonds between family or friends—for example, when an AIDS patient reveals his homosexuality for the first time. In these situations the goals of the intervention will be to foster the interpersonal network of support.

C. Creating a bridge of hope. Sometimes crises seem overwhelming because the person suffering can imagine no end to the dilemma, no time when events can be seen from another perspective. This may occur in families at times of intense discord, such as the revelation of a teenager's drug use, or in an individual facing a sudden important loss, but it may also be the result of personality disorder or depression. In instances like these one of the healing functions of the crisis intervention is to create a context (short-term treatment) in which the sufferer knows he or she will meet again with an interested person. If, however, the patient's feelings of hopelessness are strong or occur in the context of a psychiatric disorder, a full evaluation of suicide potential is needed (see Chap. 4).

D. **Getting over a developmental hurdle.** Often crises occur at times of normal developmental steps, such as a child's leaving home, final examinations in college, or first sexual experiences. The fact that such events precipitate an emergency room visit usually indicates that additional problems are complicating the apparent developmental step. Crisis intervention in these situations can often be helpful if directed at removing the immediate obstacle to developmental success. For example, interventions with the family to assist the child's leaving home, ventilation of a student's fears about failure in college, and, sometimes, avuncular encouragement about the problems and rewards of a sexual life are sufficient to let the person resume the normal course of daily living.

Selected Readings

Gordon, C. D., and Beresin, E. Emergency ward management of the borderline patient. *Gen. Hosp. Psychiatry* 3:237, 1981.

Groves, J., and Kucharski, A. Brief Psychotherapy. In T. P. Hackett and N. H. Cassem (eds.), *Handbook of General Hospital Psychiatry* (2nd ed.). Littleton, MA: PSG, 1987. Pp. 309–331.

Lazare, A. A Negotiated Approach to the Clinical Encounter II; Conflict and Negotiation. In A. Lazare (ed.), *Outpatient Psychiatry*. Baltimore: Williams & Wilkins, 1979. Pp. 157–172.

Slaby, A. E. Crisis-Oriented Therapy. In F. R. Lipton and S. M. Goldfinger (eds.), *Emergency Psychiatry at the Crossroads*. San Francisco: Jossey-Bass, 1985. Pp. 21–34.

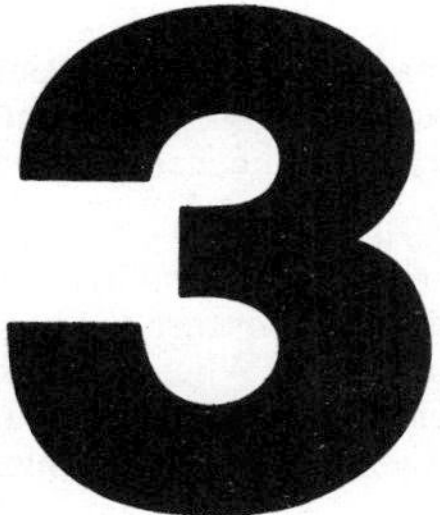

Telephone Evaluations

Steven E. Hyman

I. Many general and psychiatric hospitals provide a telephone service patients may call for medical advice. Such a telephone service is often used by patients with psychiatric difficulties and occasionally by patients who say that they are suicidal or homicidal. Calls requesting psychiatric help often represent true emergencies or honest attempts to get help and advice. However, calls may also be made by patients with personality disorders simply to relieve empty feelings or to express anger at physicians. Such calls represent attempts to engage, entangle, or even upset the physician and have no therapeutic goal. It may be difficult to sort out the motivations of the caller rapidly because the physician lacks the other tools usually available in making assessments, such as the patient's appearance and nonverbal responses to the conversation.

II. The physician's relationship to the caller depends on the caller's willingness to supply the information the physician needs to make an evaluation and recommendation. At a minimum, the caller should be asked for his or her name, age, address, and telephone number. In addition, it is helpful to obtain the name and number of the patient's physician or therapist, and the name of anyone else that the patient had been trying to reach to discuss the current problem. Patients who refuse to divulge identifying data can be asked directly why they feel it necessary to conceal their identity. If the patient is clearly psychotic, the physician should review with the patient his or her motives for calling and the need for identifying data. If a patient refuses to divulge his or her identity after a reasonable time, it is unlikely that the patient is honestly seeking help. Even if the patient claims to be suicidal, there is little that can be done if this information is not supplied. (It is rarely possible to trace calls, and even if the call could be traced, the patient who refuses to be identified is more likely to be involved in manipulative behavior than to be seriously in need of emergency intervention.) Thus, the physician should make it clear that he or she is willing to help, but unless the patient cooperates, it will be necessary to hang up.

III. Specific situations

A. The physician should obtain a brief description of the current problem and find out why the patient was unable to come to the hospital in person. The patient may live at a great distance, may be frightened, or may feel so suicidal that he or she fears that it would take too long to come to the hospital. A suicide attempt—for example, an ingestion—may already have been made. Often patients call an emergency number when they are feeling suicidal because they are isolated and cannot reach anyone else of significance. If the patient is severely suicidal or having other acute psychiatric symptoms (such as psychotic symptoms), the physician should ask the patient if there is someone who could bring him or her to the emergency department. If such a person is not available, the physician should contact the local police department.

B. Family members may call about a patient's behavior and symptoms. If more than a brief medical advice question is asked, they should also give their name and address. After hearing a brief description of the patient and the problem, the physician might suggest an appropriate means of further evaluation. If the problem sounds serious, it should be suggested that the patient be brought in. If the family member is calling because the patient refuses to be brought to the hospital, the caller should be referred to the police or to the local crisis agency if one is available.

C. **Straightforward medical advice questions** or requests for referral services should be answered directly, but if there is doubt about the nature or seriousness of the problem, the patient should be urged to come in. When questions are asked seeking **second medical opinions,** it is best to refer the patient back to his or her physician because facts are often selectively presented for manipulative reasons.

D. **Personality disordered or intoxicated patients** often use emergency telephone services. If a patient is intoxicated and can present no clear reason for calling, the physician should tell the patient that he or she is going to hang up and then do so. Personality disordered patients represent a more complex problem because they often call with a pretext that sounds reasonable at first but then becomes more confused, or they may use threats of self-destruction to involve the physician. The physician should attempt to focus the patient in order to discover whether there is any specific request for help that can be formulated. If not, the physician should not spend time dispensing a free psychiatric hour on the phone. Such hours are almost invariably frustrating to the physician and not therapeutic to the patient. If the patient is able to state what he or she needs help with, the physician must decide whether it is something that the patient should be able to do independently. It is ultimately not helpful to do for these patients what they should be able to do for themselves. For example, a physician should never call an unknown patient's therapist or spouse on the patient's behalf. In the case of nonemergency requests, patients should be referred to their own therapists, or if they have none, sources of referral should be suggested. If the patient describes a real emergency, he or she should be brought to the hospital.

E. **Requests to prescribe drugs** to unknown patients over the telephone should be denied. The patient should be told to come to the hospital if there is an emergency that requires medication.

Selected Readings

MacKinnon, R. A., and Michels, R. The role of the telephone in the psychiatric interview. *Psychiatry* 33:82, 1970.

Murphy, G. E., et al. Who calls the suicide prevention center? A study of 55 persons calling on their own behalf. *Am. J. Psychiatry* 126:314, 1969.

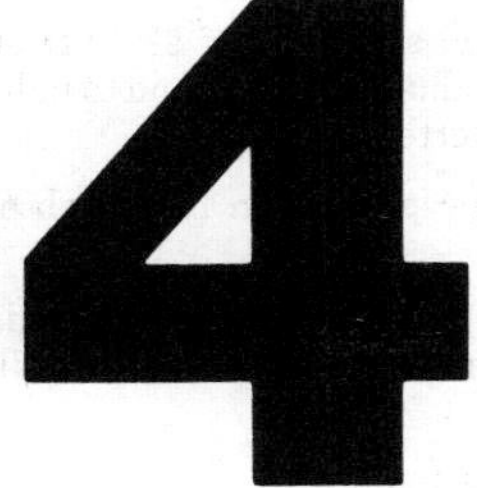

The Suicidal Patient

Steven E. Hyman

I. The scope of the problem. The suicide rate in the United States is approximately 12 per 100,000 persons per year, which breaks down to a rate of 18 per 100,000 for males and 5.4 per 100,000 for females. Overall, suicide is the eighth leading cause of death in the United States. Suicide is particularly tragic because it is one of the leading causes of death among younger age groups (indeed, the rate of suicide has increased markedly among adolescents in recent years), and because it is almost entirely preventable. Suicide also creates deep distress in surviving family and friends.

II. The problems of prediction. The assessment of suicide risk is one of the most important and difficult tasks in emergency psychiatry. Since suicide is usually preventable, the importance of good prediction and timely intervention is obvious. With proper intervention, most suicidal patients change their minds about wanting to die. Unfortunately, the task of adequate prediction is difficult even among patients who present to the physician with a complaint of suicidal ideas or intent. Although helpful in estimating the degree of the patient's danger, personal and demographic risk factors for suicide (enumerated below) are far from infallible predictors. No risk factor or combination of factors has adequate specificity or sensitivity to select those patients with suicidal thinking who will go on to attempt suicide. An adequate evaluation requires that the physician assess the degree of the patient's suicidal intent in the present and project what it is likely to be in the immediate future. In addition, the physician must judge the quality of the controls, both internal and environmental, that are available to the patient to act against the suicidal intent. In this task objective risk factors can play a part, but the physician's ability to elicit the patient's thoughts and feelings, and to make good clinical judgments, remains far more important.

III. Difficulties relating to the clinician. The task of evaluating suicidal patients is complicated by the fact that such patients often evoke strong feelings in the examining physician. Suicidal patients can provoke anxiety because of the physician's awareness that an error in management can have catastrophic consequences. In addition, some patients, such as those with histories of multiple suicide gestures, may arouse anger in the physician, making objective assessment difficult, or even resulting in punitive rather than therapeutic interventions. Perhaps most treacherous are patients who the clinician likes or identifies with. With such patients, the clinician might be tempted to deny serious risk of suicide and therefore try to reassure the patient that "everything will be all right," or to talk the patient out of his or her suicidal feelings. This makes it difficult for the patient to fully express his or her feelings and denies the patient proper evaluation and treatment. To evaluate suicidal patients, the clinician must be aware of his or her own feelings and not let them interfere with the clinical task.

IV. Patients needing evaluation for suicide

A. All patients with a major psychiatric disorder should be asked about suicidality. Depressed patients must be evaluated with particular care. Although almost all cases of suicide occur in patients with a psychiatric disorder, such as depression, alcoholism, or schizophrenia, the risk of suicide should be considered in other patients as well. **Other states potentially leading to suicide** include:

1. Deliria, such as delirium tremens, or toxic states, such as LSD or PCP (phencyclidine) intoxication, in which individuals may respond to hallucinations or delusional ideas that lead to inadvertent suicide.
2. Demoralization, terminal illness, or chronic pain, even in the absence of diagnosable depression.

B. **Patient types.** The issue of suicidality will be raised differently depending on the patient's situation. In general, the physician will be faced with the following types of suicidal patients:

1. Patients who have just survived a suicide attempt.
2. Patients who come complaining of suicidal thoughts or urges.
3. Patients who come with other complaints but who admit to suicidality during evaluation.
4. Patients who deny suicidality but who are behaving in a way that demonstrates suicide potential. These patients are often brought to the emergency room by friends or family members.

C. **General recommendations**

1. **Take all suicide threats seriously,** even if they seem manipulative.
2. Any patient who conveys a sense of hopelessness must be **questioned about suicide.** Patients who believe that there is no way out of their problems are at high risk for suicide.
3. Patients with a **history of frequent accidents** should be asked about life problems, alcohol and drug use, depression, and self-destructive feelings.
4. **Patients who have been depressed and suddenly improve** must be asked about suicide. Apparently inexplicable improvement may result from the patient having resolved all of his or her problems by deciding to commit suicide.
5. If a patient refuses to discuss suicidality at all, it is helpful to **ask friends and family** about the patient's behavior.
6. If a potentially self-destructive patient wants to leave the emergency department prior to evaluation, the patient should be **detained until the evaluation is completed.** All data and clinical reasoning should be carefully documented.

V. Interviewing the suicidal patient

A. General approach

1. Suicide is an extremely personal matter. Therefore the patient must be approached in an empathic and, at first, circumspect manner. The physician must remain calm and uncritical. Some degree of rapport must be established before the interviewer asks direct questions about suicide. It is best to proceed from more general questions to the specific. For example, the question of suicidality may be approached in the context of asking the patient how badly or how hopeless he or she feels. The patient might then be asked, "Are you feeling so badly that sometimes you would prefer not to go on living?" This can be followed with: "Have things been so bad that you have thought of hurting yourself?"
2. Although it is often useful to obtain information from family and friends, the patient may find it difficult to divulge suicidal ideas and motives unless given an opportunity to talk to the physician alone.
3. Asking patients about suicide does not put the idea into their heads. It is an error to avoid the subject for fear of doing so. Indeed, truly suicidal patients are often relieved to be asked about it.

Table 4-1. Risk factors for suicide

Major depression
Alcoholism
History of suicide attempts and threats
Male sex
Increasing age (males peak incidence at 75, females from 55–65 years)
Widowed or never married
Unemployed and unskilled
Chronic illness or chronic pain
Terminal illness
Guns in the home

4. Do not try to talk patients out of their suicidality. Premature or inappropriate reassurances may be experienced by the patient as a lack of empathy or as a lack of permission to speak. Listen and evaluate, then make a treatment decision.

B. Goals of the evaluation for suicide

1. **Evaluate the patient for:**
   a. **Suicidal thinking** (ideas, wishes, and motives).
   b. **Suicidal intent** (i.e., the degree to which the patient intends to act on his or her suicidal thoughts).
   c. **Suicidal plans**
      (1) Has the patient made a detailed plan?
      (2) Are the planned means of suicide available to the patient (e.g., pills or a gun), and does the patient know how to use them?
      (3) Are the means potentially lethal?
      (4) Has the patient made any provision for being saved?
   d. **Future orientation,** if any. If the patient has future plans, are they realistic? Has the patient recently put his or her affairs in order?
   e. **Relevant mental status.** Is the patient depressed, demoralized, hopeless, psychotic, or intoxicated?
2. **Establish sufficient rapport** with the patient so that the patient does not withhold information and will not resist the physician's eventual intervention.
3. Determine the patient's **personal and demographic risk factors for suicide.**

VI. Personal and demographic risk factors for suicide (Table 4-1)

A. Psychiatric disorder. More than 90% of patients who attempt suicide have a major psychiatric disorder.

1. **Depression** is by far the most common diagnosis associated with suicide. Fifty percent of suicides have depression as their primary diagnosis, and 15% of patients with recurrent affective disorders eventually die by suicide. If the depressed patient is also experiencing psychotic symptoms, the risk of suicide is markedly increased.
2. **Alcoholism** and drug dependence increase risk. Alcoholism is the primary diagnosis in 25% of suicides. Alcohol and drug use may be particularly

important risk factors in young people. In addition, acute use of alcohol and drugs may disinhibit depressed or chronically dysphoric patients and thereby facilitate an attempt.

3. Among females, **postpartum psychiatric disorders** are associated with some increased risk of suicide. These probably represent variants of major affective disorders.
4. **Psychoses** create risk of suicide in certain situations:
   a. If the symptoms include paranoia or command hallucinations urging self-destruction.
   b. If a **depressed patient has delusions** (such patients are at highest risk).
   c. If a patient is **schizophrenic.** Ten percent of schizophrenic patients die by suicide. Schizophrenic patients may develop secondary depression or demoralization resulting in suicide. However, schizophrenic patients who commit suicide do not fit the usual demographic profile of suicidality. They tend to be young males and often fail to communicate their suicidal intent directly (Breier and Astrachan, 1984). Therefore in evaluating schizophrenic patients, a careful clinical assessment of suicidal ideation is necessary.

B. History of attempts and threats

1. A history of suicide threats and attempts is a strong risk factor, carrying even more weight than psychiatric diagnosis. Patients with a prior history of attempting suicide have a five- to sixfold increased risk of trying again. Between one-fourth and one-half of successful suicide victims have made a prior attempt.
2. The risk of a second attempt is highest within 3 months of a first attempt, but some increased risk continues even with passage of time.
3. Even patients who make **chronic, manipulative suicide attempts** often eventually succeed in committing suicide. Because of the serious manner in which they repeatedly demand attention and medical care, such patients are easy to dislike. Nonetheless, the physician must evaluate these patients fully when they present to the emergency department. If they are already in treatment with a mental health professional, it is invaluable to confer with the clinician before making a disposition. When in doubt about these patients it is best to be conservative and admit them for at least a brief hospital stay.

C. Age

1. Suicide is uncommon (but on the increase) prior to adolescence. The suicide rate among adolescents and young adults has increased markedly in recent years.
2. Among males frequency increases with age, peaking at age 75.
3. Among females the peak for successful attempts is between 55 and 65.

D. Sex

1. Females attempt suicide 3 to 4 times more frequently than males.
2. Males are successful 2 to 3 times more frequently than females.

E. Social factors

1. Marital status affects the suicide risk as follows: Those who have never married are at greatest risk followed in descending order by those who are widowed, separated, or divorced; married without children; or married with children.

2. Patients who live alone and those who have lost a loved one or failed in a love relationship within the past year are at increased risk.

3. Urban dwellers are at higher risk than rural populations.

F. Occupational factors

1. The unemployed and unskilled are at greater risk than the employed and skilled.

2. Among professions, there is a higher rate of suicide among police, musicians, insurance agents, lawyers, dentists, and physicians (especially ophthalmologists, anesthesiologists, and psychiatrists).

3. A sense of failure in a particular role is a risk factor (e.g., someone who has been demoted or a parent who believes that he or she has failed in that role).

G. Health factors. Half of all patients who attempt suicide have a physical illness. Risk is especially increased by:

1. Chronic pain.

2. Recent surgery.

3. Chronic disease.

4. Terminal illness—for example, AIDS or cancer.

H. Family history

1. Patients with a positive family history of suicide and suicide attempts are more likely to make attempts. This increased risk is independent of psychiatric diagnosis. There may be independent genetic risks for suicide, or a family history may create a sense of permission for suicide in other family members.

2. A positive family history for affective disorders is helpful in diagnosing an underlying affective disorder in the suicidal patient.

I. Access to lethal means may be an independent risk factor for suicide. In particular the presence of firearms in the home appears to confer increased risk (Kellermann, et al., 1992).

VII. Evaluation of a suicide attempt. Some of the patients who must be evaluated for risk are patients who have just made an unsuccessful attempt. Judging their immediate risk and arriving at a disposition require an assessment of their medical stability, the seriousness of the attempt, and the circumstances under which it occurred. The psychiatric factors that must be considered are:

A. Was the method chosen a dangerous one?

B. Did the patient believe that the method would work? It is useful to ask the patient whether he or she is surprised to have survived.

C. Did the patient perform the act in a way that was likely to be discovered or not?

D. Was the patient relieved to be saved?

E. Was the patient largely attempting to get a message across, or did he or she want to die?

F. Was the attempt impulsive or planned?

G. Have the psychologic and life circumstances that led to the attempt changed?

VIII. Choice of treatment and disposition

A. The chosen disposition will depend on the physician's overall impression of the patient's risk for suicide presently and in the near future, the patient's psychiatric treatment needs, and, if an attempt has just been made, the patient's medical stability. The immediate risk of suicide and the risk of worsening suicidality in the near future will have to be judged from the evaluation. The judgment will be based on the following:

1. The degree to which the patient wants to commit suicide.
2. The strength of the patient's will to fight suicidal impulses. If the patient is psychotic, for example, or extremely impulsive by history, it must be assumed that there are no effective controls against suicide.
3. The quality of the external controls available to a patient. For example, in the mildly suicidal patient, are there family members who will watch the patient and supervise medication? If the patient is extremely suicidal or has no useful internal controls against suicidality, the physician will have to ensure that adequate external controls are provided. The strongest such controls are those provided by a locked psychiatric ward.
4. Finally, the physician must project into the immediate future and ask whether the patient's risk of suicide is likely to increase. A knowledge of the natural history of the patient's psychiatric illness and the likelihood of treatment being effective, along with a knowledge of the patient's personal and demographic risk factors for suicide, are most important here.

B. Possible dispositions in ascending order of restrictiveness are:

1. Sending the patient home, with outpatient follow-up.
2. Admission to a general hospital. This may be necessary if a patient is medically unstable following an attempt. If a patient is admitted to a medical or surgical service, ongoing psychiatric consultation will be needed.
3. Admission to an open psychiatric unit.
4. Voluntary admission to a locked psychiatric unit.
5. Involuntary hospitalization.

C. Choosing a disposition

1. Suicidality has legal implications. The physician's thinking should be well documented. If the physician is unsure of what to do after making the evaluation, it is safest to obtain psychiatric consultation, if available. Patients who are judged severely suicidal but refuse treatment will require involuntary hospitalization. In such a case, the physician will have to make application according to the local state laws.
2. Patients who are not severely suicidal and who are at low risk for immediate worsening can be sent home. It is crucial, however, that realistic provisions for follow-up be made. Patients should not be sent home if they are going to be alone. Patients who are sent home should have an emergency number to call or should be instructed to return to the emergency room if their suicidal feelings become more severe.
3. Suicidal patients should be asked to remove from the home any firearms, lethal medications, or other means of suicide the patient has considered.
4. Chronically suicidal individuals need a long-term relationship with a clinician or agency who will get to know them well. A long-term relationship will allow the clinician to judge when restrictive hospitalizations are needed and when other interventions will suffice.
5. With patients at higher risk for suicide, increasingly restrictive forms of treatment must be chosen. Hospitalization acts both to prevent suicide and to allow more aggressive treatment of the patient's psychiatric illness. It is optimal that the patient agree to hospitalization voluntarily.

a. If a suicide attempt has been made, generally at least a short hospital stay is indicated, unless the attempt was of low risk and the patient already has someone who agrees to follow him or her and agrees that discharge is reasonable. If a serious attempt has been made, inpatient treatment is necessary, preferably on a locked unit.

b. Patients who are seriously depressed should be hospitalized, especially if their illness is worsening.

c. Patients who are intoxicated must be held until they are sober and must then be reevaluated.

d. Psychotic patients who are suicidal should be hospitalized, usually on a locked unit.

e. The patients at highest risk must be kept away from anything that they can use to hurt themselves (e.g., glass, windows, sources of flame) pending transfer to a locked psychiatric unit.

Selected Readings

Breier, A., and Astrachan, B. M. Characterization of schizophrenic patients who commit suicide. *Am. J. Psychiatry* 141:206, 1984.

Fowler, C. F., Rich, C. L., and Young, D. San Diego Suicide Study II. Substance abuse on young cases. *Arch. Gen. Psychiatry* 43:962, 1986.

Kellermann, A. L., Rivara, F. P., Somes, G., et al. Suicide in the home in relation to gun ownership. *N. Engl. J. Med.* 327:467, 1992.

Marzuk, P. M., Leon, A. C., Tardiff, K., et al. The effect of access to lethal methods of injury on suicide rates. *Arch. Gen. Psychiatry* 49:451, 1992.

Murphy, G. E. On suicide prediction and prevention. *Arch. Gen. Psychiatry* 40:343, 1983.

Pokorny, A. D. Prediction of suicide in psychiatric patients. *Arch. Gen. Psychiatry* 40:249, 1983.

Robbins, D. R., and Alessik N. E. Depressive symptoms and suicidal behavior in adolescents. *Am. J. Psychiatry* 142:558, 1985.

5 The Violent Patient

Steven E. Hyman

I. The **evaluation and management** of violent and potentially violent individuals are important skills in emergency psychiatry. It should be stressed that most violent individuals in our society are not mentally ill or definable as patients.

A. **Patients.** Those violent individuals who fall within the domain of the physician are:

1. Those with a diagnosable psychiatric disorder.
2. Those who have a neurologic or organic disorder that results in violence.
3. Those who perceive their violent acts and urges as unwanted (ego-dystonic) and who request psychiatric help.
4. Those who are intoxicated or undergoing a withdrawal syndrome.

B. Those who are not mentally ill or who cannot be helped by psychiatric interventions are best handled by legal authorities.

II. **The approach to the violent patient**

A. **Overview.** The emergency evaluation of a patient who is threatening violence or who has performed a violent act is complicated by a number of factors:

1. There may be strong **pressure on the physician** from the emergency department staff or outside agencies to intervene quickly, making it difficult to perform a careful evaluation.
2. Violent patients commonly arouse strong emotions. Most commonly they evoke fear, but they may also evoke anger in the examiner. **It is important that the examiner pay attention to his or her subjective response to the patient.**
   a. The degree of subjective fear felt by the clinician may be a clue to the patient's violence potential and may therefore be useful in formulating a clinical judgment.
   b. Awareness of fear should also lead the physician to ensure that measures are available to protect his or her own physical safety (e.g., access to a door, the presence of security staff). If not, the clinician should calmly excuse himself or herself and return only when security staff are available.
   c. The clinician should ensure that subjective fear or anger do not interfere with objectivity—for example, by leading to punitive measures.
3. The evaluation of violence has **legal implications** that have profound consequences for the patient's future. It is therefore important to perform the evaluation carefully and to fully document all data and clinical reasoning.

B. **Reducing the risk to clinical personnel**

1. **Weapons.** An interview must not be conducted with weapons present.

a. If a patient is armed, the evaluation should not proceed until the weapon is surrendered. It is helpful to ask the patient why he or she feels a need to carry a weapon; the answer may help the clinician formulate a request that the weapon be given up. If a dangerous patient is unwilling to surrender a weapon, the clinician should excuse himself or herself from the room and allow hospital security or the police to deal with the person. If a patient who is armed and presumably dangerous tries to leave the emergency room prior to being evaluated, the staff should notify the police rather than chasing the patient themselves.

b. Interviewing and seclusion areas must be free of any objects that could be used as weapons (e.g., ashtrays, pens, table lamps).

2. Violent patients should not be interviewed in cramped rooms, especially if they are agitated and need to pace. The interviewing room should not be in an isolated place. It should be fitted with an alarm or "panic button" that is within easy reach of the interviewer. It should not be possible to lock the door of the interview room from the inside.

3. The patient and the examiner should be positioned in such a way that both have access to the door. A paranoid or poorly controlled patient must not be made to feel cornered.

4. Decide whether those who accompanied the patient are a stabilizing or destabilizing influence. People who appear to be provocative to the patient—for example, uniformed officers and perhaps family members—should be asked to leave. If, however, uniformed guards are the only security staff available, they should remain nearby.

5. Pay attention to the patient's speech and motor activity. Clues to **impending violence** are:

   a. Speech that is loud, threatening, and profane.

   b. Increased muscle tension, such as sitting on the edge of the chair or gripping the arms.

   c. Hyperactivity, such as pacing.

   d. Slamming doors or knocking over furniture.

6. The staff should be drilled in emergency procedures, including **restraint.** Clinicians should attempt to calm patients verbally, but when patients are too agitated to be calmed by talking, restraints should be used (Table 5-1).

C. Interview technique

1. **Show concern.** The patient should not be humiliated or made to feel rejected. The patient's requests should be treated in a forthright manner. The patient should be allowed to make some choices, such as where he or she would like to sit. An offer of food may help calm an agitated patient.

2. **Develop some rapport** with the patient before asking specific questions about violence. When asking about violence, questions should be direct and honest.

3. **Assure the patient** that you will do what you can to help him or her stay in control of violent impulses. Set limits firmly but do not threaten or display anger. Limit-setting can involve talk, sedatives, or, if necessary, physical restraint.

4. **With paranoid patients** who are threatening violence, the interview is best conducted as though interviewer and patient are facing the problem together. Do not be confrontational—that is, this is not the time to tell the patient that he or she is deluded. Be aware of whether the patient has begun to incorporate you into his or her delusional system; if that occurs

Table 5-1. The method of physical restraint

1. Restraint must be performed by a large number of persons, ideally at least five. A show of force may gain cooperation by itself.
2. There should be a specific plan, e.g., each person taking a limb and one protecting the head.
3. The approach is preferably made with the patient's attention distracted.
4. Parenteral sedatives should be readily available (see sec. **V**) and administered as soon as possible after restraint is complete if the patient continues to struggle.
5. Leather restraints are safest. They should be checked at frequent intervals by the staff for comfort and security. It is important that limbs are not contorted in a way that could cause a nerve traction or compression injury.
6. The reason for the restraints should be calmly explained to the patient.
7. Restraints must never be removed without adequate staff present.
8. Intoxicated patients should be restrained in the left lateral decubitus position and closely observed to guard against aspiration.

there is increased risk of being assaulted because you may have become part of what the patient perceives as threatening. Give the patient adequate physical space. Paranoid patients may feel threatened at normal interpersonal distances.

III. The evaluation

A. The patient's mental status and psychiatric diagnosis

1. An attempt should be made to diagnose any **major psychiatric disorder** because this will have important implications for long-term treatment. Major psychiatric and neurologic disorders that may underlie violent behaviors include mania, depression, schizophrenia, substance abuse, personality disorders, posttraumatic stress disorder, attention deficit disorder, mental retardation, brain injuries, delirium, dementia, and partial complex seizure disorders.

2. For the short-term risk of violence, certain **mental states** may have more import than the underlying psychiatric illness. These include:

    a. **Paranoid states** regardless of etiology, including geriatric patients (whose potential for violence is often overlooked).

    b. Patients with **command hallucinations** ordering violence.

    c. Patients who are **intoxicated** with alcohol or drugs, especially cocaine or other stimulants, phencyclidine (PCP), and central nervous system (CNS) depressants, and patients who are undergoing withdrawal syndromes, especially from alcohol or other CNS depressants.

    d. Patients with delirium, especially if they are agitated.

    e. **Manic patients,** especially if they are paranoid or irritable rather than elated.

3. Physicians often mistakenly fail to consider the possibility of violence in **depressed patients.**

    a. Depressed patients may be irritable and agitated.

    b. Some extremely depressed patients commit homicide and then suicide, either because of delusional ideas or to spare others what they believe to be some worse fate.

c. Women with severe postpartum depression may attempt to kill their children.

B. **The patient's past history of violence** is probably the most reliable predictor of current violence potential. This is not true, of course, if the patient has never exhibited the present mental state before (e.g., the lack of a history of prior violence is noncontributory if the patient is currently paranoid for the first time).

1. Under what circumstances has the patient been violent in the past?

2. What is the frequency of violence? If episodic, what is the duration and how does the patient behave between episodes?

3. What is the intensity of the violence? It may be useful to ask the patient what is the most violent thing he or she has ever done. What means has the patient used to perpetrate violence?

4. Obtain a past history of arrests (juvenile and adult).

5. Ask for a history of automobile misuse (such as a history of getting into fights with other drivers or a history of multiple moving violations).

C. **The mode of referral** is an important source of information.

1. Note who brought the patient to the emergency department.

a. Self? Family or friends? Police?

b. Obtain whatever information is available from third parties who have accompanied the patient. (This is often most safely done out of the patient's presence.)

2. What brought the patient to psychiatric attention?

a. Does the patient fear violence?

b. Does the patient plan violence?

c. Is the patient currently violent?

d. Has violence already occurred?

D. **Who are the intended victims, if any?**

1. Violence may be directed at specific individuals or groups, or it may be diffuse and poorly directed.

2. If well directed, are the intended victims easily accessible? (See Chap. 10, sec **II. B** on the duty to warn potential victims.)

E. **What means does the patient have to commit violence?**

1. Has the patient made a plan?

2. Does the patient possess weapons that he or she knows how to use? Has the patient recently obtained lethal equipment? Is the patient trained in martial arts?

F. What **environmental stresses** have predisposed the patient to violence? What has the patient done in similar situations in the past?

G. The quality of the patient's **self-control** should be noted.

1. Does the patient want to control himself or herself, and if so, is he or she able to do so?

2. Is the patient overcontrolled with brittle defenses? It is important not to ignore threats of violence made by such patients.

H. In addition to assessing the nature and quality of the patient's self-control, the physician should assess the **external constraints on the patient's behavior** (e.g., if the patient is a child, are the parents able to control the violent behavior?).

I. The patient's **demographic characteristics** give the physician an idea of the base rate of violence in the patient's peer group. Of course these statistical data do not allow the physician to make predictions about the individual patient. Characteristics of groups with increased risk for violent behavior are:

1. Male sex.
2. Age group 15 to 24 years.
3. Poverty.
4. Low educational level; few employment skills.
5. Nonwhite.
6. Absent roots (low employment stability, many moves, no family ties).

J. A history of childhood abuse and neglect is a risk factor for violence.

K. **Physical examination** should be done if possible but should not be forced on an extremely agitated or paranoid patient until control has been established.

1. If violence has already occurred, the patient should be examined for fresh injuries.
2. Examine for scars from fights and from bullet and knife wounds.
3. Examine the hands and face for evidence of old fractures.
4. Perform a neurologic examination. Rule out head injury or any acute neurologic illness.

IV. Acute management of violent patients

A. **The agitated, threatening individual; violence imminent.** The violent patient who is acutely agitated requires interventions that will restore his or her self-control.

1. Talk and an offer of sedatives will be helpful.
   a. Staff members of the opposite sex may be calming, especially if the patient has homosexual concerns.
   b. If the patient reports fear of going out of control, it should be acknowledged that this is an unpleasant state.
   c. If the patient is unaware of how threatening and angry he is, the clinician should help the patient recognize what is happening in a nonconfrontational way.
2. Limits must be set firmly but without anger. Patients who fear losing control respond well to limit-setting, but if the staff does not set limits calmly, the patient may see it as a confirmation that he or she is already dangerously out of control.
3. Patients who refuse to talk and begin to escalate must be placed in physical restraints (see Table 5-1).

B. **The combative, actively violent patient**

1. At this stage verbal interventions are not effective and only make the patient angrier.
2. Physical restraint is necessary.

3. Once restraint has been accomplished, parenteral sedation should be administered as soon as possible.

V. Acute pharmacologic interventions

A. If the patient is only moderately agitated, oral sedatives can be offered. In cases of extreme agitation or actual violence, oral preparations are too slow-acting and IM or IV medication should be used.

B. For mild to moderate agitation, PO benzodiazepines are usually effective. Lorazepam (Ativan), 1–2 mg, or diazepam (Valium), 5–10 mg, can be given. Diazepam has the advantage of having the fastest onset of oral benzodiazepine drugs.

1. Rarely, benzodiazepines can paradoxically disinhibit a patient, potentially resulting in violence. To minimize the risks of such reactions, it is prudent to withhold benzodiazepines in patients with a history of CNS depressant abuse or a prior history of benzodiazepine-induced disinhibition. For such patients a neuroleptic drug, such as haloperidol (Haldol), 5 mg, given as the liquid concentrate for rapid absorption, is preferable.

2. For patients who become disinhibited after benzodiazepines are given, haloperidol, 5 mg IM repeated every 20–30 minutes as necessary, should be calming.

C. For **seriously agitated or violent** individuals, medication should be administered IM or IV.

1. The first choice for rapid reliable sedation with minimal side effects is a parenterally administered benzodiazepine. Of the benzodiazepines, lorazepam is probably the best absorbed IM; diazepam may be absorbed if given in the well-perfused deltoid muscle. Chlordiazepoxide is absorbed erratically, if at all, IM and should not be given by that route. For **extremely agitated patients** many clinicians administer lorazepam, 1–2 mg slowly IV. When benzodiazepines are given IV they should be administered slowly to minimize the risks of respiratory depression.

2. Alternatively, haloperidol, 5 mg, can be given IM or IV (IV use does not have Food and Drug Administration approval). This agent is not as reliably sedating as a benzodiazepine but is effective in many patients. The dose can be repeated after 20–30 minutes. If a patient has not responded to two doses, it is worth adding lorazepam. The combination is usually extremely effective and may have fewer side effects than high doses of either agent alone. If given carefully, the greatest risk is oversedation.

3. **For psychotic patients** a neuroleptic or neuroleptic plus benzodiazepine is the treatment of choice (see Chap. 19).

D. The success during the acute situation of any of the drugs described in this section **is not an indication for prescribing them over the long term.**

VI. From the data obtained in the examination, it is often possible to recognize **patterns of violence.**

A. If violence is due to a **major psychiatric disorder,** such as mania, long-term treatment will be determined by the specific diagnosis, but short-term management, of the sort described above, may be needed in the interim.

B. In the absence of a major psychiatric disorder it is useful to think about violent patients in terms of chronic or episodic violence, undercontrolled or overcontrolled personalities, and those exhibiting well-directed or poorly directed violence (i.e., directing violence at a specific victim or randomly lashing out).

1. **Chronically violent and undercontrolled individuals.** In the absence of a major psychiatric disorder, these patients are often males with an aggressive "macho" style, sometimes with clear antisocial features, and often with histories of drug and alcohol abuse. There is usually a history of problems

Table 5-2. DSM-IV draft criteria for intermittent explosive disorder

A. Several discrete episodes of loss of control of aggressive impulses resulting in serious assaultive acts or destruction of property.
B. The degree of aggressiveness expressed during the episodes is grossly out of proportion to any precipitating psychosocial stressors.
C. The episodes of loss of control are not better accounted for by antisocial personality disorder, borderline personality disorder, a psychotic disorder, a manic episode, conduct disorder, or attention deficit hyperactivity disorder; and are not due to the direct effects of a substance or a general medical condition.

Source: Reprinted with permission from the *Diagnostic and Statistical Manual of Mental Disorders, Fourth Edition, Draft Criteria:* 3/1/93. Copyright 1993 American Psychiatric Association.

beginning in youth, with truancy, delinquency, and school failure. Often there is a history of cognitive impairment and of soft neurologic signs. Many of these individuals have been abused or have witnessed abuse during childhood. There are often histories of adult crime and almost always of frequent fighting. It is crucial to approach such patients with the understanding that violence may seem culturally appropriate to them. If this is the case psychiatric intervention is extremely difficult. Successful psychiatric treatment requires that the patient begin to experience violence as ego-dystonic because it has a negative impact on his or her life.

2. Episodic violence

a. Individuals who appear overcontrolled. When there is a single extremely violent outburst, the clinician must examine the patient carefully for paranoid ideation. In the absence of paranoia, these patients are often inadequate, overcontrolled personalities under stress. Their outburst usually comes as a surprise. Management requires that stresses leading to pent-up frustration and rage be explored so that the patient can avoid further outbursts. It is important that referral for treatment be made at the time of the event.

b. Intermittent violent outbursts in the form of **well-directed brief explosive rages** with little provocation.

(1) There is often a history of normal behavior between episodes, occasionally loss of contact with reality during outbursts, postictal-like states after episodes, and a history of extreme disinhibition with alcohol. Many such individuals have histories of childhood abuse or neglect and social maladjustment. Some have a history of prior neurologic illness.

(2) In the absence of a diagnosable major psychiatric disorder, the *Diagnostic and Statistical Manual of Mental Disorders, Fourth Edition, Draft Criteria* (DSM-IV) would call this intermittent explosive disorder (Table 5-2); other authorities would call this the *episodic dyscontrol syndrome.* These are descriptive terms that do not represent validated diagnoses. As suggested by DSM-IV, this is a diagnosis of exclusion; a concerted search must be made for a major psychiatric disorder, especially antisocial or borderline personality disorder, substance abuse disorders, mania, organic mental disorders, or posttraumatic stress disorder.

(3) If a specific neuropsychiatric disorder is diagnosed, specific treatment may effectively terminate the violence, especially in the case of affective disorders, where treatment is often extremely effective.

If a seizure disorder is diagnosed, anticonvulsant therapy is indicated but may not improve violence if it is due to the interictal personality disorder of partial complex epilepsy. Psychotherapy and symptomatic pharmacotherapy will still be necessary.

(4) If intermittent explosive disorder is diagnosed, or if there is residual episodic violence after treatment of another psychiatric disorder, both psychologic and pharmacologic management may be helpful.

(a) For intermittently violent patients, it is critical that physician contact be available at times of stress. These patients may make excellent use of the emergency department for help in regaining control of their impulses.

(b) Especially if there is a history of disinhibition with alcohol or other CNS depressants, these patients should not receive prescriptions for benzodiazepines because of the risks of disinhibition or abuse.

(c) Rare prn use of sedating neuroleptics, such as chlorpromazine (Thorazine), 25–50 mg, or thioridazine (Mellaril), 25–50 mg, can be helpful when the patient feels that the risk of violence is great. The major immediate risks are postural hypotension or dystonias. Patients should not be given supplies large enough to make parkinsonism or tardive dyskinesia likely.

c. If violence is **episodic but poorly directed,** consider mental retardation, dementia, brain injuries, or intoxication. The ictus of partial complex seizures may cause patients to lash out, but this is rare and when it occurs, is most likely in the context of an attempt to restrain the patient's freedom of movement.

(1) When cognitive impairment or brain injury is present, management of episodic violence is a difficult empirical process. Often a combination of pharmacologic agents and behavioral maneuvers must be used.

(2) In using pharmacologic agents, the physician often must walk a tightrope between worsening violence and further clouding of the patient's sensorium. (Patients with organic mental disorders are often exquisitely sensitive to the CNS side effects of psychotropic agents.)

(a) The use of **propranolol** has been described for episodic violence in patients with organic brain syndromes. These have generally been uncontrolled patient series; in most cases patients have continued to receive other drugs, including neuroleptics, in addition to propranolol. The effective doses of propranolol have been high, ranging from 40–520 mg/day usually divided into two daily doses. It is the best practice to increase dosages slowly as needed; the major side effects are hypotension and bradycardia. Beta-adrenergic blockers should be avoided in patients with asthma; even $beta_1$-selective agents may cause problems at high doses. Propranolol is not effective in emergency situations.

(b) **Lithium** (at levels of 0.8–1.0 mEq/liter) and **carbamazepine** (Tegretol) have both been reported to be useful in such patients. Orderly empirical trials are indicated for patients whose violence is otherwise uncontrollable. Like propranolol, neither of these agents is useful in an emergency.

VII. Making a **disposition** involves the physician's assessment of the risk that violence will continue or recur. The degree of the patient's dangerousness will determine how restrictive a disposition is necessary. This sort of assessment is extremely difficult, requiring the integration of all of the information obtained in the examination, including the physician's subjective response to the patient.

A. If violent behaviors appear unlikely to subside in the emergency department or appear likely to recur in short order and are judged by the physician to be amenable to psychiatric intervention, hospitalization on a locked unit will be necessary. If the violence is unrelated to a psychiatric disorder, the civil authorities should be called.

B. If the cause of acute violence is believed likely to be short-lived (such as alcohol intoxication), the patient can be kept in the emergency department as long as he or she can be safely contained.

C. More complex is the case of the patient who has already been violent or has violent urges but is not currently violent. Determination of the risk of future violence requires that the physician judge the severity of the patient's violent impulses in relation to his or her internal and external controls. It is important to recall how the patient acted before in similar circumstances.

1. Patients who present with violent urges and who calm down may be sent home as long as they are not at high risk for worsening.

   a. If the circumstances that precipitated their violence have not changed, patients should not be returned to that environment without treatment.

   b. **Follow-up** is the key element in prevention of violence in patients thought well enough to send home. The patient should be encouraged to return to the emergency department if violent impulses return. In addition, a referral should be made for further treatment. Chances of compliance are enhanced if a clear plan is presented to the patient, preferably with a follow-up appointment time; it may be useful to contact the patient after discharge from the emergency department to make sure that the referral has been acted on.

2. If the patient is unable to gain control of violent impulses, is psychotic, or otherwise appears to be at high risk for continued or recurrent violence, hospitalization on a locked unit is necessary. It is much preferred if the admission is voluntary. It should be made clear to the patient that the decision to hospitalize is not meant punitively.

Selected Readings

GENERAL

American Psychiatric Association Task Force on DSM-IV. *Diagnostic and Statistical Manual of Mental Disorders, Fourth Edition, Draft Criteria:* 3/1/93. Washington, D.C.: American Psychiatric Association.

Bach-Y-Rita, G., et al. Episodic dyscontrol: A study of 130 violent patients. *Am. J. Psychiatry* 127:1473, 1971.

Lewis, D. O., and Pincus, J. H. Epilepsy and violence: Evidence for a neuropsychotic-aggressive syndrome. *J Neuropsychiatry* 4:413, 1989.

Lion, J. R., Bach-Y-Rita, G., and Ervin, F. R. Violent patients in the emergency room. *Am. J. Psychiatry* 125:1706, 1969.

Monahan, J. The prediction of violent behavior. Toward a second generation of theory and policy. *Am. J. Psychiatry* 141:10, 1984.

Rosenbaum, M., and Bennett, B. Homicide and depression. *Am. J. Psychiatry* 143:367, 1986.

Widom, C. S. The Cycle of Violence. *Science* 244:160, 1989.

PROPRANOLOL

Arana, G. W., and Hyman, S. E. *Handbook of Psychiatric Drug Therapy*. Boston: Little, Brown, 1991.

Greendyke, R. M., Schuster, D. B., and Wooton, J. A. Propranolol in the treatment of assaultive patients with organic brain disease. *J. Clin. Psychopharmacol.* 4:282, 1984.

Ratey, J. J., et al. Beta-blockers in the severely and profoundly mentally retarded. *J. Clin. Psychopharmacol.* 6:103, 1986.

Yudofsky, S., Williams, D., and Gorman, J. Propranolol in the treatment of rage and violent behavior in patients with chronic brain syndromes. *Am. J. Psychiatry* 138:218, 1981.

Acute Grief and Disaster Victims

Anthony J. Rothschild
Adele C. Viguera

I. Acute grief reactions

A. Definition. Grief, mourning, and bereavement are terms used synonymously to describe a syndrome precipitated by a significant loss, such as loss of a loved one, a body part, or a valued job. An uncomplicated grief reaction is a normal response to loss and generally runs a benign course. Its course is affected by the abruptness of the loss; the extent, if any, of preparation for the loss, the significance of the lost person or object to the survivor and the manner of death (i.e., natural vs. unnatural). Extensive investigations of bereaved persons have demonstrated that most recover well and seldom seek psychiatric help. However, when the normal grieving process does not occur, the bereaved is at high risk for the development of secondary psychiatric and physical problems.

B. Overview. Recognition and management of acute grief reactions are important skills in the emergency department. The physician will be faced with three general groups of patients who may need help with grief and bereavement.

1. **Family and friends** of patients who are dying in the emergency department. The psychologic consequences of sudden death or serious trauma for patients and families are an often neglected aspect of care in a busy emergency department. The physician can play a critical role in facilitating a normal grief reaction when there is unexpected death due to accident, trauma, cardiac arrest, stillbirth, sudden infant death, murder, suicide, or other causes. The physician should be able to help the grieving process progress and to identify those who may need further consultation.

2. **Patients** who come to the emergency department with somatic or psyschologic complaints that may be due to a recent bereavement. It is not uncommon for bereaved persons to develop diverse somatic and psychologic symptoms. Since these symptoms will respond to treatments aimed at facilitating the grieving process, the physician must be alert to the possibility of grief as the cause of a variety of symptoms.

3. **Survivors of a disaster.** The psychologic care of survivors of disasters such as fires, plane crashes, or natural disasters is a crucial component of their overall care.

II. Clinical features of grief reactions.

A person's reaction to loss will vary depending on character, style, cultural background, and the way in which losses were experienced in the past. A depressive syndrome consisting of feelings of sadness, insomnia, poor appetite, and loss of interests is frequently seen. Guilt, if present, is usually in regard to things that could have been done for the deceased. Thoughts of dying are common, but these are usually limited to thinking that it would have been better to have died with the deceased than to go on living. Prolonged functional impairment, marked psychomotor retardation, or a morbid preoccupation with feelings of worthlessness are not usually seen and suggest that the grief reaction is complicated by a major depression (see Chap. 17). Normal grief is generally a phasic process with somewhat indistinct transitions from one phase to the next. The usual phases are:

A. The first hours to days. This initial phase consists of shock and disbelief. Often the bereaved denies the loss in his or her mind in order to be protected from the painful reality. People in this phase will often refer to themselves as numb.

B. The first several weeks up to 6 months. After the phase of numbness, the bereaved enters a phase in which the reality of the loss enters full awareness. The bereaved person feels yearning for the deceased and is often preoccupied with the loss. In addition, the bereaved often expresses anger and resentment over the loss. This second phase is marked by sadness, guilt, shame, and feelings of helplessness, hopelessness, and emptiness. Crying, sleep disturbance, poor appetite, loss of interest in usual pursuits, impairment of work performance, and somatic complaints are often present. The bereaved often finds social interaction with others difficult, yet finds solitude intolerable. Feelings that life is not worth living are also common during this second phase.

C. Six months to a year. This final phase of grief is one of reorganization in which normal functioning and behavior are restored. During this phase the bereaved fully accepts the reality of the loss and its impact on life. Although the symptoms of the second phase of grieving should have ended during the first 6 months, these symptoms may be prolonged if the relationship with the deceased has been extremely important. Cultural practices may also affect the time course of the phases of grieving. Indeed, reappearance of aspects of the first two phases are not uncommon during the final phase, particularly when the bereaved is caught off guard by reminders of the loss. Normal feelings during this final phase include anger at the deceased as well as anxiety about being left behind.

III. Management of uncomplicated grief reactions

A. Patients may come to the physician or the emergency department during the first two phases of grief with a variety of psychologic complaints (especially depression and anxiety) or somatic complaints. The somatic complaints often include lethargy, insomnia, or bodily pains, but they may be modeled on the symptoms of the terminal illness of the deceased. Most people go through the grieving process accepting their feelings and reactions as appropriate and seldom seek professional help. Therefore, those who do come to the physician or emergency department deserve an evaluation since they are at risk for developing other psychiatric difficulties.

B. Evaluation of the bereaved

1. The evaluation must include an assessment of the degree of depression; the presence or absence of psychosis, alcoholism, or drug abuse; and suicide potential. Particular attention should be paid to those individuals bereaved as a result of a suicide, because data suggest that this group of people are themselves at increased risk of suicide. If, in addition to normal grief, a second psychiatric condition is discovered, it should be treated appropriately. It can be particularly difficult to tell grief from major depression. Severe vegetative signs or suicidality suggest that the grieving process has been complicated by major depression.

2. In evaluating the patient whose period of grieving is extremely protracted, the physician should entertain the possibility of an underlying psychiatric disorder or the possibility that the patient has been unable to proceed normally with the grieving process (what has been called the syndrome of unresolved grief). The failure to grieve normally can result from social factors (such as isolation of the bereaved, or his or her having taken on the role of the strong one) and psychologic factors (such as guilt or feeling overwhelmed by the loss).

C. Management of the grieving patient. Whether or not grief has proceeded normally, management consists of treatment of any superimposed disorders and facilitation of the mourning process. If there is no superimposed disorder requiring immediate attention or hospitalization, treatment can begin in the emergency department. This can be accomplished as follows:

1. Arrange an appropriate setting. A private room with seating should be available.
2. The patient should be encouraged to talk about his or her feelings concerning the deceased. The physician's questions should be asked in such a way that the patient is encouraged to review the relationship with the deceased and to express affects of grief, such as sadness, anger, and despair.
3. It is important that the physician be able to tolerate the patient's sadness and allow it expression. The physician should avoid nullifying the patient's feelings with clichés ("It's God's will"), simplistic reassurances ("At least you still have children"), or commands to stop grieving ("Life must go on").
4. The patient should be reassured that symptoms such as insomnia, somatic distress, social withdrawal, and preoccupation with the image of the deceased are normal reactions to loss and gradually pass with time and expression of feelings.
5. The patient should be reassured, if necessary, that he or she is not becoming insane or losing his or her mind.
6. Do not discourage the expression of angry or hostile feelings should the patient bring them up. Angry feelings toward the deceased are common. Anger toward the physician or hospital are also common and should not be taken personally.
7. Special attention should be given to those individuals bereaved as a result of a suicide. Studies suggest that bereavement due to suicide is different from bereavement due to other types of death. Affected individuals tend to have a complicated bereavement course and seldom fully resolve their feelings of guilt and anger and sense of failure to save the deceased. They also tend to be preoccupied, searching for some meaning to the tragedy. One should encourage these patients to become involved at an early phase of their grief work in "suicide survivor" peer groups to prevent the social isolation to which they are vulnerable.
8. Medications should be used sparingly.
   a. Attempts to block mourning with heavy sedation are ill-advised. This will only result in postponing the work of mourning or, worse, cause the bereaved to feel guilty later for not having been fully alert during parts of the mourning process.
   b. At times mild sedation is indicated to treat severe anxiety or insomnia resulting from grieving. Moderate doses of benzodiazepines may be given, such as lorazepam (Ativan), 1 mg tid or 1–2 mg hs, or diazepam (Valium), 5 mg tid or 5–10 mg hs. Barbiturates should be avoided because of their toxicity in combination with alcohol and because of their danger if taken in overdose.
   c. The use of antidepressants is not indicated for the sadness of mourning; they are used only if a major depression develops as a complication.
   d. Neuroleptic drugs have no use in the management of bereavement.
9. Assess the patient's social supports. Are family members, coworkers, or friends available to help the bereaved? People with established relationships to the bereaved are likely to provide considerable support. With the patient's permission, family and friends should be notified that the patient has come to the emergency department. They should be encouraged to talk about the deceased in the presence of the bereaved once the evaluation is complete. Besides emotional support, some patients may require help with

basic needs and personal care such as obtaining food and medications as well as making funeral arrangements. Attempts should be made to enlist the help of friends and family for these tasks.

10. Do not assume that quiet patients who refrain from emotional outbursts are handling the situation. These patients may simply be numb or for a variety of social and psychologic reasons find it difficult to grieve. If they were not in distress, they would not have come for help.

11. The patient should be encouraged to return to past activities such as work or school. Most bereaved persons benefit from returning to work within 3–6 weeks after the death of a loved one. The therapeutic effects of work on self-esteem and the effects of contact with concerned coworkers can be an essential part of the recovery process.

12. When sent home, the patient should be accompanied by family or friends. Patients should be made aware of the availability of further outpatient and emergency services (such as self-help groups, when they exist) and should be encouraged to use these services if they need them.

13. If a patient is found to have a superimposed psychiatric or physical disorder, an appropriate follow-up referral should be made (see below).

IV. Abnormal grief reactions

A. A psychiatric referral and the beginnings of treatment in the emergency department are indicated when a severe or abnormal grief reaction is present or when there is an underlying psychiatric disorder.

B. Psychiatric treatment is indicated for any of the following conditions:

1. In the case of **unresolved grief,** the patient will often come to the emergency department with apparently unrelated complaints, such as somatic complaints or depression. Such patients may strenuously deny the importance of the loss. Treatment can begin in the emergency department by facilitating the grieving process—for example, by helping the patient to remember the deceased and the nature of their relationship. A referral for a brief course of supportive psychotherapy is usually indicated. It is important that the physician not miss the diagnosis of a major depressive disorder just because the patient's state of depression was preceded by a loss.

2. If the patient has severe signs of **major depression** or if the patient has remained nonfunctional for an extended period of time, further specific treatment is indicated (see Chap. 17).

3. If the patient appears to be **suicidal,** a full evaluation will be necessary (see Chap. 4).

4. **Psychotic** patients will require treatment after diagnostic evaluation is made.

5. Patients who are **abusing drugs or alcohol** in excess of previous use will require intervention.

6. Patients who begin to visit the emergency department or physician's office **frequently** with physical complaints may be suffering from unresolved grief, depression, or social isolation. Appropriate evaluation and referral should be made.

V. The management of family and friends of patients who are critically ill in the emergency department

A. If the patient is still alive

1. If possible the family should be seated in a private waiting area. If relatives come alone, other family members or friends should be called in.

2. The availability of a staff person to answer questions at frequent intervals is helpful to the family.

3. If possible, the family should be allowed to see the patient. This will not be feasible or helpful if full-scale resuscitative efforts are being made.

4. In the case of observing Catholics a priest should be called in order to administer last rites.

5. It is helpful if the physician speaks with the family and asks about their well-being. Often the presence of an emergency staff member may comfort the family. Attention should be paid to the family's physical needs. Providing a quiet, comfortable room in which to meet, coffee, and a box of tissues is often the best means of communicating with a distraught family.

B. **Viewing the body.** For some survivors, reviewing the last hours of the deceased may be helpful. The emergency department physician should also offer the family a chance to view the body if the patient dies. The family's fantasies, imagination, and fears of the unknown are often far more horrible than reality. In order to be able to grieve, many people need a chance to say good-bye. It is recommended that before the family sees the body, the deceased's eyes be closed, visible blood be wiped off, and any equipment used in the attempted resuscitation be removed from the room. The body should be covered, with only face and hands exposed. If the body is mutilated, the family should be warned of the disfigurement. A staff person should be present with the family to answer questions and to help if a family member becomes overwrought. The bereaved family members will often touch the body and say the things they want the deceased to know. Most families will stay with the deceased for less than 15 minutes.

VI. Victims of disasters

A. **Introduction.** The emergency department physician may rarely but unexpectedly be faced with victims of a disaster. Therefore, he or she should be aware of the psychologic distress caused by traumatic events that are outside the range of such common human experience as bereavement, chronic illness, or job loss. A disaster can be of natural causes (flood or earthquake), man-made (plane crash or fire), involve a relatively small number of people (a car accident), or a whole community (a flood). Data from a number of studies suggest that the severity of psychopathology is greater if there are many casualties and if the cause of the disaster is natural as opposed to human in origin. Psychologically, the victims are more apt to tolerate the negative consequences of a human disaster than a natural disaster (which is seen as an "act of God" or out of one's control) because there may be easier assignment of blame. In general, a disaster will produce four classes of victims:

1. **Severely physically injured.** These patients will, of course, need immediate attention to their physical injuries. However, if the victims are conscious, an attempt should also be made to relieve any psychologic distress. Since disasters occur without warning, the victims will often have many questions about what happened and whether friends or family were injured. If the facts are known, the victims should be told them, unless it appears that the information would be too overwhelming. If that is the case, or if the facts are not yet known, the victims should be told that an attempt will be made to find out what took place.

2. **Uninjured survivors.** There is considerable psychologic morbidity for those persons who were not actually physically injured in the disaster. Survivors often have painful guilt feelings about having escaped injury when others did not and about what they had to do in order to survive. The survivors will often come to the emergency department with feelings of helplessness at their inability to have prevented or reduced injuries during the disaster. As in the case of the physically injured, the survivors will have many ques-

tions about what happened that the clinician should address empathically but honestly.

3. **Relatives of victims.** The members of the victims' families may appear in the emergency department having heard sketchy reports about the disaster. An attempt should be made to inform the family about the victim's condition and the extent of the disaster. Feelings of guilt and helplessness are commonly seen in this group.

4. **Disaster workers.** The people who provided aid to the disaster victims should be considered to have experienced a severe psychologic trauma themselves. In addition to possible physical injury, disaster workers experience frustration, anger, guilt, and helplessness, which may need to be addressed.

B. **Management.** The long-term psychologic morbidity of all four classes of disaster victims can be reduced by giving attention to their fears and their feelings as soon as the emergency department staff has time to do so. For all four groups:

1. A sympathetic, flexible attitude toward the variety of victims' reactions should be adopted.

2. Places to sit or rest and hot drinks can be provided to those who are not undergoing emergency treatment.

3. Victims should not be left alone. It is often useful to group several victims in a room together during treatment. The exception to this are extremely disturbed or disturbing patients, who should be separated from the others.

4. Allow the victims to express their feelings about the experience.

5. Provide accurate and responsible information to the survivors and their relatives. Quash all unfounded rumors.

6. Use psychotropic medication sparingly and only when definitely indicated. Moderate doses of benzodiazepines may be needed for extremely agitated patients.

7. Victims who show clear emotional disturbances beyond the expected sadness and numbness should be referred for further psychiatric assessment. All victims should be told of the availability of individual counseling if they desire it.

8. Several reports suggest that group therapy is particularly useful in providing longer-term support for disaster victims. The uninjured survivors, relatives, and disaster workers should also be invited to participate.

9. Disaster workers should be encouraged to participate in "debriefing sessions," which give them the opportunity in a private, quiet setting to express their feelings of helplessness, fear, and sadness regarding the rescue effort and to contemplate the impact of the disaster on themselves and others.

Selected Readings

Bartone, P. T., Ursano, R. J., Wright, K. M., Ingraham, L. H. The impact of a military air disaster on the health of assistance workers: A prospective study. *J. Nerv. Ment. Dis.* 177:317, 1989.

Clayton, P., Desmarais, L., and Winokur, G. A study of normal bereavement. *Am. J. Psychiatry* 125:64, 1968.

Edwards, J. G. Psychiatric aspects of civilian disasters. *Br. Med. J.* 1:944, 1976.

Engel, G. Is grief a disease? *Psychosom. Med* 23:18, 1961.

Gonda, T. A. Death, Dying, and Bereavement. In H. I. Kaplan and B. J. Sadock (eds.), *Comprehensive Textbook of Psychiatry*. Baltimore: Williams & Wilkins, 1989.

McHorney, C., and Sherwood, S. Secondary morbidity among the recently bereaved. *Am. J. Psychiatry* 143:158, 1986.

Ness, D. E., and Pfeffer, C. R. Sequelae of bereavement resulting from suicide. *Am. J. Psychiatry* 147:279, 1990.

Rubonis, A. V., Bickman, L. Psychological impairment in the wake of disaster: The disaster-psychopathology relationship. *Psychol. Bull.* 109:384, 1991.

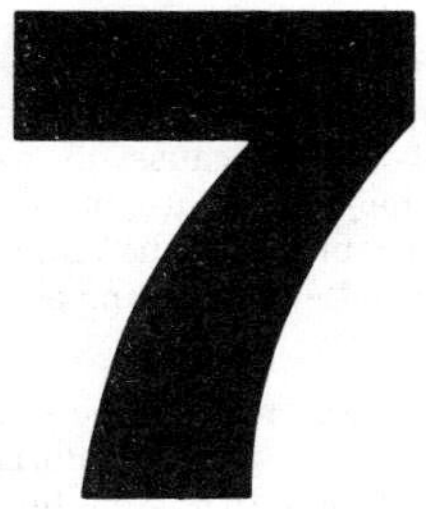

Treating the Family in the Emergency Department

Anne Fishel
Christopher Gordon

I. Although families occasionally come to an emergency department explicitly complaining of a family problem, they most often identify a single member (the designated patient) as the person in need of help. However, when an individual is accompanied to the emergency department by family members, it is common that the patient's problems reflect those of the family. Even when the problem is largely that of an individual, family members can provide an invaluable resource to the clinician in an emergency situation, particularly when the patient is a poor historian. Also, when the family is a participant in the suffering of the individual brought to the emergency department, a family interview can provide an opportunity for members to express their points of view, register concern, and ask questions. This process itself may decrease the stress in the family and activate members to help resolve the crisis. In addition, family members are often a crucial aspect of the solution. For example, a family might offer a round-the-clock vigil for a suicidal patient or agree to ongoing family therapy for a troubled child. In any case, involving the family in an emergency situation can increase the family's ability to deal with future crises, alleviate scapegoating of the patient, and often avoid unnecessary hospitalization.

II. **Indications for interviewing the family.** The most obvious clue about when to include family members in the interview is their presence. In a study of cases presenting to a psychiatric emergency department (Rubenstein, 1972) it was found that 50% of all patients were accompanied by family members. Of these cases 80% were judged by clinicians to have problems related to intrafamily stresses.

A. **Indications for involving the family in the treatment of an individual.** Whenever a patient in an emergency situation is a member of a family, that family will be affected by the crisis and should be a consideration in the patient's care. A family's involvement may run the gamut from shaking hands with the treating clinician to being actively solicited for participation in ongoing treatment. The following instances provide some guidelines for determining when family participation is warranted.

1. The clinician may be able to solicit support from the family when the patient is resistant to treatment recommendations. For example, a wife may offer to accompany her alcoholic husband to his first Alcoholics Anonymous meeting when he is afraid to go on his own.

2. The family can provide support and observation to avoid hospitalizing a patient. In a family meeting, arrangements can be made to watch a suicidal patient. The family can construct a schedule for taking turns with a plan to enlist other relatives as well.

3. The family can be enlisted to participate in the solution to a crisis. For example, a brother can help find his sibling employment.

4. The family can make modifications in family life that will benefit the patient. For example, a mother may agree to stop talking to relatives about an adolescent's problems, or parents may agree to move their 5-year-old out of their room and into his own room.

5. When, in the individual's description of his or her problem, there is mention of family disagreement regarding the problem, family involvement is usually warranted. Statements such as, "I'm only here because my parents think I should be," or, "I think my problem is the job pressure, but my wife thinks I should lay off the booze," offer an opportunity for the clinician to involve those family members mentioned by the patient as having pertinent information about the problem.

6. When there are allegations of child or spouse abuse or when the clinician suspects abuse, family involvement is indicated to gather information quickly, to assess the safety of individual members, and to make alternative living arrangements for endangered individuals, if needed. Of course it is best to ask the victim about the abuse in private (see sec. **VI.B.** and Chaps. 11 and 12).

B. Indications for treating the family

1. When the family is very much involved with the identified patient's problem, as with an adolescent who has an eating disorder, any strategy that does not take the family into account is likely to be counterproductive.

2. Family treatment may be helpful when the identified patient is actively resistant to treatment while the family is more agreeable, or alternatively, if the family is standing in the way of the identified patient's treatment—for example, because of its belief system or because the identified patient's illness takes the pressure off other family members.

3. When a patient has a long history of unsuccessful individual therapy it is useful to consider whether family therapy focused on changing the individual's context in the family rather than individual therapy focused on the individual's symptoms might have a greater chance of success.

4. When there is an irreconcilable disagreement, as with a stalemate about whether to divorce, family treatment should be considered.

5. Family treatment is recommended when the family is having difficulty negotiating a life transition—for example, when a grown child develops serious psychologic symptoms when preparing to leave home for the first time.

6. If a whole family has suffered a tragedy or trauma, such as the sudden death of a family member, there is often no identified patient and treatment of the whole family makes sense.

7. Although the emergency department is not usually well equipped to function as the site of ongoing treatment, the clinician should consider whether this setting would suffice to see the family for a few crisis meetings or whether to refer the family elsewhere for treatment.

III. Interviewing families. Families cope with medical or psychiatric emergencies in the same fashion that they deal with other problems of life. It is necessary to understand the style, coping strategies, and characteristic defenses that they have used both in the past and during the present crisis.

A. The clinician should try to understand the present crisis from the **family's perspective.**

1. Why is the present situation a crisis in the family's eyes? The clinician should not assume that he or she understands why the stated problem is a problem. It is important to ascertain all the different perspectives on the problem in the family, emphasizing how the problem affects each individual member. For example, an adolescent's anorexia may present a crisis to her mother because "my husband and I have started fighting about it" or "my mother is on my back about it," whereas her father may feel that, "I'm afraid she's going to die," or, "I'm afraid her younger sister is going to stop eating." Even the youngest family member's view is of great importance.

2. Have there been similar crises before? If so, what was done about it? Was it helpful? What was harmful? How was the crisis resolved? How long did it take?

3. What shifts in family structure have occurred? These shifts may be due to developmental changes (such as making room for the birth of a child, increasing flexibility needed for adolescence, renegotiation of the marital relationship as older children leave home) or to unusual losses or additions (remarriage, miscarriages, deaths in the family, a relative coming to live with the family). Families typically experience more stress at times of family restructuring, even when these changes are expected, wanted, and positive. At transition points families' characteristic coping strategies are taxed and an additional, even minor stressor may be the last straw precipitating a crisis. Also, a family whose coping patterns are narrow and rigid will have difficulty making the adjustments required to get through transition points and may experience a new developmental stage as a crisis. For example, parents who react to an adolescent's first attempts at autonomy and risk-taking by re-emphasizing the rules that worked during childhood may invite worsening of the very behaviors that they seek to curtail.

4. How does the family feel about coming to the emergency department? Often such a visit is the last resort after seeking help from relatives, teachers, clergy, pediatricians, and mental health professionals. The family may feel angry, distressed, and hopeless. It is important to ask about the family's history of seeking help and to find out what experiences and beliefs are helping to shape the current encounter. The clinician should listen for attitudes of defiance or compliance, pessimism or hope, as the history of prior attempts to get help is elicited. Do outsiders know that they have come to the emergency department? Did anyone suggest it? Are there demands from outside agencies such as school or court insisting that the family change? Is the family trying to change or is it digging in its heels?

B. Understanding the family's resources

1. **Family cohesiveness**—that is, bonds of affection and economic interdependence. What activities do family members participate in together? What is mealtime like at the house? Who is apt to notice first when the designated patient is upset, and how do they respond?

2. **Extended family.** Who can help to provide support, relief, material resources? Who else in the family knows about the present crisis? How have they been helpful with this crisis or with troubles in the past?

3. **Ability to use outside resources.** Have any clinicians or agencies been helpful in the past? If so, in what ways? If not, why not?

4. **Adaptability**—that is, the family's capacity to meet obstacles and shift its course of action. Such information can be inferred from the family's description of previous crises but can be inquired about directly by asking questions such as, "Could someone tell me about a time when a change was necessary in the family and how it was accomplished?"

C. Understanding the family's style. It is important to be able to enter the family's world, to appreciate the way they perceive and structure their world. The clinician who can interview a family without violating their beliefs will increase the family's willingness to share information and will strengthen their interest in attending subsequent meetings.

1. **Language.** Does the family use metaphor, concrete examples, hyperbole, or erudite philosophizing to explain their current difficulties? Do they describe the identified patient as a "bad seed," crazy, naughty, or immature? In recommending interventions the clinician should use the family's own language for the greatest impact.

2. **Power hierarchy.** Is decision making shared by the parents, or does one member make all of the decisions? Does one parent have nominal power while the other makes actual decisions? In an egalitarian marriage, for example, where decisions about finances and child rearing are shared, the couple will feel misunderstood if certain questions are directed only to one of them.

3. **Cultural matrix.** Developmental changes, expression of affect, mental illness, and encounters with mental health professionals all have different meanings according to the family's cultural background.

4. **Expression of affect.** Is open expression of feelings encouraged to promote closeness and support, or discouraged because feelings are seen as a sign of weakness? Interventions that are too discrepant with the amount of expression tolerated in a given family will be rejected.

D. **Understanding the family's defense mechanisms**

1. **Level of involvement among family members.** Are individuals overly involved so that they have no room to function independently, or so oblivious to one another that even dangerous behaviors can be engaged in by an individual without someone else reacting?

2. **Scapegoating versus self-blaming.** Are family members quick to point the finger at one individual as being the source of all problems, or do they all try to blame themselves for the difficulties? In the interview the clinician must avoid being drawn into either of these styles.

3. **Tolerance for difficulties.** Is the family in a constant state of chaos, going from one crisis to another? Or is there something unique about this set of conditions that has prompted a crisis in a family that otherwise has negotiated changes and developmental shifts without seeking help?

IV. **The crisis interview.** Throughout the meeting the clinician should look for opportunities to accomplish the following tasks, which help lower the level of stress: developing a trusting relationship, offering realistic hope, empathizing with expressed emotion, and showing an understanding of the family's way of perceiving the world. The interview may be conducted in several stages, and the clinician should allow about 1½ hours for it.

A. **The opening phase**

1. At the outset the clinician must often offer **a rationale** for a family interview if the family was expecting that only an individual family member would be seen. The critical element is to involve the family without making all members feel that they are to blame or that there are many patients instead of one. The clinician can emphasize that he or she needs all of the family members to share information, and that everyone will be needed to solve the crisis. For example, it could be stated that, "All members of the family must have their unique way of understanding X's problem and I could benefit from hearing everyone's observations," or, "This problem affects everyone in the family and I thought we could meet to gather information and to decide whether further family meetings might be helpful."

2. **A brief period of introduction.** If the introductory phase is too long, the family will feel that the crisis is not being appreciated. For example, one might introduce oneself, ask for the names and ages of adults and children, and ascertain how family members occupy themselves, focusing on any recent changes in daily routine that may have disrupted family life. For example, if a parent has switched from working days to the night shift, the clinician will be interested in understanding why this occurred and how other family members have adjusted. The goal of this introductory phase is to differentiate family members and to present oneself as a friendly, interested, and neutral professional.

B. Ask about the problem

1. **What is the family's definition of the problem?** Ask each member what has brought him or her to the emergency department. Find out whose idea it was to come. Find out what the precipitating event was and why the family decided to come today and not yesterday or tomorrow.

2. **Expand the family's definition of the problem.** One goal of the family interview is to convey to the family that they are mutually affected by one another and that problematic behaviors may be part of family patterns of interaction. Certain types of questions (Penn, 1982, 1985) aid in shifting the focus from the individual's problem to the concept of family members' interconnectedness:

   a. Ask questions that help focus on the current situation: Who in the family knows about the problem? Who worries most? Who least? Who is the most, who the least affected by the problem? What does X do when Y acts that way? What do other members do? What explanation does each member have as to the nature of the problem and what is needed for it to improve? What have family members already tried to do to remedy this problem? What came of these efforts?

   b. Place the problem in a time perspective. When were things different in this family? When did things start to change? In the future, if things were to change, who would notice first? Who would be most affected? If you were not worried about X, who would you be most worried about? Has anything like this ever happened to this family before? What would have to change now to return the family to its previous state? What else was different then?

C. Taking a break. A 10-minute recess provides an opportunity for both the clinician and the family to gain perspective on the problem. While the clinician steps out of the room, the family is asked to review the session, discussing among themselves whether there were important questions unasked by the clinician and what might be helpful given the definition of the problem. Meanwhile the clinician can review and think about:

1. The acute crisis of the individual.

2. Whatever larger problems the family may be facing.

3. A way to formulate the problem for the family that confers dignity on the individual patient and elicits cooperation from the rest of the family in dealing with the current difficulty.

D. Feedback to the family

1. Comment on the family's strengths and coping abilities. In the beginning it is important to convey to the family an appreciation of their positive qualities, whatever they may be. Doing so diminishes defensiveness and elicits cooperation. Moreover, by emphasizing what is positive about the family as a whole, one begins to shift attention from the identified patient to family relationships in a way that is palatable to family members. For example, a family whose members have been loud, angry, and interruptive may be described as "lively" or "passionate."

2. Show an appreciation for the intensity of the family's concern or distress about its difficulties.

3. "**Normalize**" the family's problems whenever possible by identifying stressors and situational factors, placing the problem in developmental perspective (e.g., "Many families have difficulty figuring out how much responsibility and freedom to afford an adolescent"), and noting that the family's responses are common and understandable given their present situation. In

normalizing the crisis situation one hopes to interrupt the typical cycle of blame, anger, and guilt that is rarely constructive in problem solving.

4. **Use the family's own language** to redefine the problem in a way that points to a new direction that will be constructive. Often the family's conceptualization of the problem has led to well-intentioned solutions that have only exacerbated the problem.

E. Problem solving

1. Assuming that it is reasonable to involve the family in dealing with the present problem, negotiate changes that individual members can make. What small change would indicate that something positive has begun to happen? How much improvement would be needed to minimally satisfy each member? Ask each member what small change needs to be made for the situation to be "tolerable" or "safe." The focus should be on setting up reasonable, achievable goals that will help the family see the problem as solvable.
2. Negotiate decisions regarding hospitalizations, individual or family therapy, and medication. Whenever possible, while not abdicating responsibility for critical medical decisions, it is useful to involve members in decision making to foster their active participation in the solution.

F. Ending the interview. Set up the next appointments, suggesting the approximate number of further meetings you want to schedule, who should attend, and the interval between meetings. In general it is optimal for everyone who was at the initial meeting, and for any other significant members you have learned about, to attend subsequent meetings. The interval between the initial and second meeting should be no longer than 1 week.

V. Special problems in interviewing families

A. The silent patient. Sometimes a child, often an adolescent, refuses to talk in order to register protest about being "dragged" to the emergency department. Other times, a child is mute from fear of the surroundings or afraid that he or she will be punished afterward for speaking the truth. Try to ascertain whether the individual is silent out of anger or fear. With the oppositional adolescent, paradoxical techniques that do not confront the patient's resistance head-on will be most helpful (see below). With the fearful child, it will be more useful to reassure the child that this is a safe place and that he or she is free to speak without fear of reprisal. If child abuse is suspected, however, special interventions will be needed (see Chap. 12).

1. **Paradoxical strategy with oppositional patients.** Side with the patient's resistance by commenting positively on it—for example, "I see that you know the importance of privacy. Please do not be too hasty to join in." Or, "I want you to really size up the situation and make sure that it is safe to talk here; after all, you don't know me yet at all." This approach of positively framing the adolescent's recalcitrance as helpful is aimed at loosening his or her commitment to this position (since it is difficult to be defiant when one is asked to do so) and to make the parents feel less embarrassed by their child's behavior.
2. **Other techniques for silent patients.** Ask questions that require only "yes" or "no" or other one-word answers, but that yield useful information—for example, after asking, "Who in the family knows most about why you are here?" the silent member can be asked if there is someone in the family he or she would designate to answer this question. Suggest that the mute individual indicate whether or not the answer is on target by raising his or her finger.

B. Active, restless, young children

1. Make the room comfortable for them by providing a snack and toys, such as markers, blocks, and puppets.

2. Obtain a pictorial description of the family by asking the child to place family members in characteristic positions showing relationships to one another as if posing for a family picture.

3. Ask the family to remember a recent time when the problem occurred and then invite them to act out what happened. Parents and children alike can be encouraged to coach one another to play their parts realistically. Ask the family to show what happens before and after the problem occurs.

C. **Angry, hostile parents.** The combination of worry about a child's illness, anxiety about possible hospitalization, and a long wait often make parents angry and ready to lash out at staff. Kahn (1979) offers some guidelines (modified here) for handling enraged parents.

1. Allow, even encourage, the parents to ventilate their angry feelings in the privacy of an office, not in the waiting room.

2. Find out from the parents what they want and what they think would remedy the problem. Usually parents want to express their anger and to feel that they have been heard.

3. The clinician should outline a specific plan of action and assure the parents that they will be kept abreast of the progress of the plan.

D. **The absent family member.** A family rarely presents with all relevant family members at the first family meeting. Often, even when the clinician asks that additional members attend subsequent sessions, certain members continue to be absent, either because of their own reluctance to participate or because of the family's wish to exclude or protect them from the meetings. Sometimes a letter written to the missing member, and mentioned in passing to the family, can bring him or her in. The letter should include statements that will pique curiosity by indicating that the absent member is being discussed and that rules and interventions affecting him or her will be decided on. The letter should also state that the missing individual is an important member whose perspective on the family situation is valuable.

VI. **Contraindications, dilemmas, and pitfalls**

A. **The violent patient.** If, in the initial description of the problem, it becomes clear that family members can provoke violence in the patient, family meetings may be dangerous and should be avoided.

B. **In instances where sexual abuse or incest is suspected,** the victim should be interviewed separately prior to any family meeting. (This topic is discussed in detail in Chap. 12). A victim will disclose details of abuse more freely in the safety and privacy of an individual interview, without involved family members denying, threatening, disqualifying, or otherwise inhibiting such disclosures.

C. **Family meetings should not be a substitute for other treatments.** Obviously, even when it has been determined that a psychotic or depressed patient's symptoms have been worsened by a dramatic change in the family, which family meetings can address, the patient's psychosis must still be thoroughly evaluated medically and treated comprehensively. Similarly, individual therapy, hospitalization, referral to a social worker, or other interventions should not be ruled out because family meetings are scheduled.

Selected Readings

Fraser, J. S. The crisis interview: Strategic rapid intervention. *J. Strategic Systemic Ther.* 5:71, 1986.

Kahn, A. V. *Psychiatric Emergencies in Pediatrics.* Chicago: Year Book, 1979.

Langsley, D., et al. Family crisis therapy—results and implications. *Fam. Process* 7:145, 1968.

Murphy, G. E., et al. Who calls the suicide prevention center? *Am. J. Psychiatry* 126:314, 1969.

Penn, P. Circular questioning. *Family Process* 21:267, 1982.

Penn, P. Feed-forward: Future questions, future maps. *Family Process* 24:299, 1985.

Perlmutter, R. Family involvement in psychiatric emergencies. *Hosp. Community Psychiatry* 34:255, 1983.

Rubenstein, D. Rehospitalization versus family crisis intervention. *Am. J. Psychiatry* 129:715, 1972.

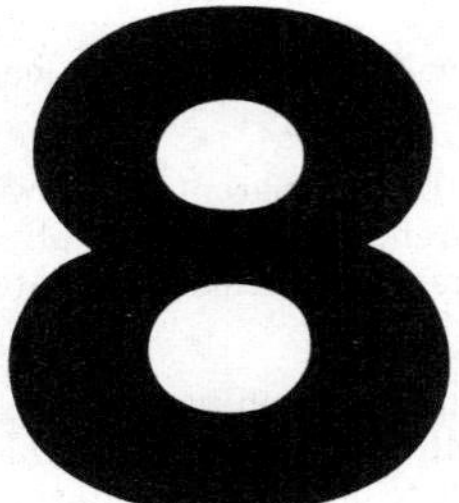

Child Psychiatric Emergencies

Paula K. Rauch
Nancy Rappaport

I. The psychiatric assessment of children as well as adults requires consideration of both medical and psychiatric etiologies. Children's behaviors should be evaluated in the context of developmental norms and within the framework of the supports and capacities of the family or agency who protects and cares for the child. Emergency department presentation may be the result of a significant change in the child or a change in the family's tolerance for disturbed behavior.

The majority of pediatric psychiatric emergencies occur in adolescents. Half of the cases involve suicidal gestures or ideation and the remainder involve morbidity associated with axis I psychiatric diagnoses, unmanageable behavior, psychosomatic illness, psychologic trauma, and substance abuse.

II. General approach

A. Safety. Whenever possible, the child should be evaluated in a safe place.

B. Restraints. In general, it is best to avoid the use of mechanical restraints on children. However, failure to restrain a severely agitated child because of the clinician's discomfort with restraining or because of a wish to be gentle may have dire consequences for both the patient and the staff. A combative or violent adolescent requires some form of mechanical restraint until he or she exhibits the ability to maintain self-control. Younger children whose behavior is out of control may also require holding or restraints for protection and safety.

C. Supervision. The suicidal or hyperactive child requires vigilant supervision. The emergency department with its potentially hazardous equipment and medications poses particular danger for self-destructive and agitated patients. Parents, even those who appear to be supportive, should not supervise suicidal or behaviorally disordered children. The child's presentation to an emergency department should be regarded as presumptive evidence of the parents' or caretaker's inability to protect the child. Emergency department staff must fulfill the supervisory function until safety has been assessed and is assured.

D. The interview room. Ideally, evaluation of the child should take place in a setting that is both emotionally and physically safe. For older children, a quiet room removed from the bustle and intrusions of the emergency department may be adequate. A space with toys and art materials is recommended for younger children. When such accommodations are not available, it may be helpful to pull a curtain to screen out distractions, and for younger children, to provide toys (e.g., puppets, a family of dolls, crayons and paper) for play and for use during the evaluation.

E. Parents. Parents can have either a calming or a provocative effect on the child. Those parents who are judged to be provocative should be kept separate from the child.

III. The interview has the same format as that used for adults, including review of the chief complaint, the history of present illness, and the mental status examination. Adolescents may be able to tell most of their own story, much as an adult would, but in younger children history taking relies heavily on information provided by the parent or guardian.

A. Alliance formation. Establishing an alliance with a teenager can be time-consuming and requires patience.

1. It is best to address the adolescent first and then the parents; otherwise the adolescent may view the interviewer as a parental figure and an ally of the parents. Important information from the parents can be obtained later during the interview.

2. A healthy alliance is also fostered by a nonthreatening style of interviewing. It is best to begin the interview with inquiry about neutral topics (e.g., age, school, interests) before progressing to more challenging or upsetting material (e.g., chief complaint, symptoms, family problems).

B. History. Adherence to the following principles should facilitate the gathering of history:

1. Integrate history provided by both the child and the parent(s). Reliance on information provided by only one party is insufficient and potentially misleading.

2. Begin with open-ended questions and proceed to more specific ones.

3. When interviewing the latency-aged child (i.e., ages seven to twelve), question the child as long as he or she can tolerate it. Further information gathering can be facilitated by the use of other vehicles of expression (e.g., playing with dolls, drawing).

4. The "interview" of the preschooler (ages two to six) relies almost exclusively on observation of the child's play.

IV. The mental status examination is performed using the adult format. It is important to interpret one's observations of a child in the context of expected developmental milestones.

A. Appearance

1. Observe for evidence of **abuse** (e.g., bruises or other signs of injury) or **neglect** (e.g., poor hygiene, inappropriate clothing for the weather) (see Chap. 12).

2. Determine if the child looks his or her chronologic age.

B. Behavior

1. Note the **level of activity** and **impulsivity.** Overactivity may signify fear of the emergency department setting. In general, however, intimidating circumstances foster inhibition of activity and calming of the hyperactive child.

2. Parents should be asked to provide pertinent observations of the child's behavior. The parents are better historians of the behavior of all age groups than is the child.

C. Speech and language

1. The child's speech and language skills should be assessed in the context of expected developmental milestones.

   a. Two-year-olds have the ability to speak in at least two-word sentences.

   b. Most of a three-year-old's words should be intelligible to a non-family member.

   c. Essentially all of a five-year-old's words should be intelligible.

2. The language content of a three- to five-year-old does not always make sense unless the listener is familiar with the child's world.

D. **Mood and affect**

1. Adolescents can describe their own mood and often report more sadness than has been recognized by their parents.

2. Children under thirteen can describe the mood state of the moment but cannot reliably report on their mood over time.

3. Children under ten are generally unable to provide an accurate report of their mood, so parental input is required.

E. **Thought**

1. **The normal adolescent's thought process has fully matured.** Therefore, thought disorder in an adolescent (e.g., flight of ideas, loosening of associations, delusions) is evidence of psychopathology.

2. **Logical, generally concrete thinking is typical of a seven- to twelve-year-old.** The presence of an isolated hallucination or delusion in this age group is of questionable diagnostic significance. Delusions should be considered an indication of psychosis only if they occur in the context of bizarre thinking (e.g., the child believes that hidden monsters or wild animals are in constant pursuit of him or her) and abnormal behavior (e.g., urinating into cups and placing them in patterns throughout the house). Latency-age delusions are also clinically significant if they occur in the context of deteriorating daily function, social skills, or school performance.

3. **Fantasy (or magical thinking) is typical of the preschooler.** For example, it is normal for the child under seven to have one or more imaginary friends. The correct identification of thought disorder in the preschool-aged child generally requires special training. Inferring a child's real life situation from observations of the child's fantasy play should be reserved for the trained child psychiatrist. The clinician should strongly suspect significant psychopathology when there is a history of certain unusual or abnormal behaviors: grossly bizarre behavior (e.g., headbanging, automatisms, or unprovoked wailing); impulsivity; destructive play (e.g., ripping off the head of a doll or purposefully breaking toys); and lack of relatedness to parents or others.

V. **Categories of childhood psychiatric illness**

A. **Childhood psychosis** occurs in all age groups but presents most commonly during adolescence.

1. Hallucinations and delusions in a teenager strongly suggest a psychotic disorder such as schizophrenia or bipolar disorder, which often have their onset in this age group.

2. Primary psychotic illness is uncommon in preschool and latency-age children. When it occurs the child typically exhibits bizarre behavior and thinking that parents report as significantly different from previous behavior. As in other age groups, a marked change in behavior due to psychosis is also often associated with a significant decline in social functioning and self care.

3. New-onset psychosis requires a comprehensive inpatient assessment. The **differential diagnosis** includes organic etiologies (e.g., ingestions, intoxications, delirium, seizure activity), trauma (e.g., physical and/or sexual abuse), obsessive-compulsive disorder (which can initially mimic psychosis), mania, and a primary psychotic disorder (e.g., schizophrenia).

B. The recognition of childhood **depression** may be difficult.

1. Some children manifest an adult pattern of depressive illness with neurovegetative disturbances (e.g., impaired sleep, energy, appetite, and concen-

tration), sad, constricted affect, and self reports of dysphoria similar to adults.

2. The majority of depressed younger children, however, are unable to describe depressed mood and often present a picture of irritability rather than sadness. The depressed child may also exhibit social withdrawal, poor school performance, erratic or inappropriate conduct, anxiety, and somatic complaints.
3. The adolescent is able to give an accurate description of his or her current affect as well as the predominant mood. However, because adolescents frequently do not talk about their mood, parents and others are likely to be unaware of their sadness or sense of hopelessness.
4. **Suicidal ideation** is common in adolescents and there is a high risk of attempted and completed suicide in this age group. In general, evidence of either a suicide gesture or a suicide attempt warrants mandatory inpatient evaluation. The assessment may occur either on a pediatric ward with consultation by a child psychiatrist or in an inpatient psychiatric facility.
5. Depression without suicidal ideation can in most instances be assessed and treated on an outpatient basis.

C. Children who present repeatedly with nonspecific or atypical physical complaints may be suffering from a **psychosomatic illness.**

1. Depression, trauma, and family dysfunction are important and common causes of psychosomatic symptoms.
2. The psychiatrist can play an important protective role by advocating for a comprehensive psychiatric assessment prior to any further invasive tests.
3. It is best to begin the assessment by accepting the patient's point of view—namely, that the symptom is the source of distress. The clinician can then gradually interject questions about other types of stresses on the child and the family. To suggest too soon that the symptom is psychologic may be heard as "It's all in your head" and is likely to alienate the patient and family.

D. **Anxiety disorders** commonly manifest as school refusal (separation anxiety), phobic behavior, and, in the adolescent, panic attacks.

1. Anxiety symptoms may either be new or represent a disabling exacerbation of a chronic condition. The child may be afraid to go to school, to sleep, or to separate from parents, afraid that a catastrophe might befall either them or the child.
2. Ritualized behaviors may occur.
3. Parents may bring the child to the emergency department because they are overwhelmed by the child's anxiety or because they fear that some unknown trauma is responsible for the change.
4. The **differential diagnosis** of anxiety includes the following. **Separation anxiety disorder** is characterized by fear of being away from the primary caretaker. **Avoidant disorder** is characterized by fears about social situations. **Overanxious disorder** is characterized by generalized fears in all settings. **Obsessive-compulsive disorder** and **panic disorder** present as they would in adults. Physical and sexual abuse may present with any combination of anxiety features (see Chap. 12).
5. Outpatient psychiatric assessment is appropriate except when the anxious behavior is incapacitating, when outpatient treatment has failed, or when trauma is suspected.

E. **Violent and impulsive behaviors and disorders of conduct**

1. The degree of emergency is determined by the level of risk attributable to

the behavior and the capacity of the caretakers to manage the child. Some behaviors (e.g., fire-setting, threats of assault with dangerous objects or weapons) may be beyond the control of the family. Behaviors that are generally managed in an outpatient setting (e.g., hyperactivity, oppositional behavior, petty theft) can also occasionally overwhelm an overstressed family and necessitate an emergency department visit.

2. Problematic behaviors (e.g., stealing, fire-setting, truancy) may present alone or in combination.

3. An acute onset of violent or impulsive behaviors raises the possibility of depression, mania, substance abuse, or family crisis.

4. A history of chronic conduct difficulties can be associated with either attention deficit with hyperactivity disorder, oppositional disorder, a chaotic family setting, or a conduct disorder. Sometimes, particularly in an adolescent, conduct disturbance can be the heralding sign of an incipient thought disorder.

5. **The decision to hospitalize** a child depends principally on the child's safety and the safety of others. Discharge from the emergency department can be considered if:

   a. It is determined that the child can be managed safely at home;

   b. The clinician is assured that the family will seek outpatient treatment; and

   c. If the clinician is satisfied that the circumstances of the disturbed behavior have changed or that the emergency department visit has been therapeutic. Discharge of the patient to the same circumstances and stressors that precipitated the emergency department visit is likely to result in relapse and return.

6. Legal intervention should be considered for the conduct-disordered adolescent who displays a pattern of chronic disregard for the rights of others and has failed previous psychiatric treatments.

F. Pathological **fire-setting** is characterized by unsupervised play with matches or lighters, repeated intentional fire-setting, and an inappropriate fascination with fire.

1. A child that sets a number of small fires or one large fire presents a significant threat to both his own safety and that of others.

2. Due to the enormous risk of this type of behavior, **inpatient psychiatric assessment is indicated.**

VI. **Trauma** is any event that overwhelms the child's coping skills. The trauma may be either physical or pyschological.

A. Being witness to a traumatic event (e.g., fighting between parents), being the victim of trauma (e.g., sexual or physical abuse), or living through a natural disaster are examples of traumatic experience.

B. When a victim of trauma presents to the emergency department, the clinician may be asked to help the victim make sense of the extraordinary events.

1. It is important for the clinician to recognize that a child may also be traumatized by events generally regarded as less dramatic (e.g., birth of a new sibling, move to another city, illness in the family, illness in the child). If the traumatic nature of the event is not appreciated, an associated change in the child's behavior may also be misunderstood.

2. Assuming that the trauma and its consequences have been appreciated, the traumatized child needs an emotionally safe setting in which to tell or play out the traumatic experience.

3. The child should be encouraged to recount the experience in words, with drawings, or with toys.
4. The child should be encouraged to ask questions to clarify possible confusion or distortion of the experience.
5. Special attention should be devoted to the victim's common inclination to feel guilty and responsible.
6. Though some children may be able to verbalize some of their feelings or describe the events, many will not be ready to do so in the emergency setting.

C. The need for outpatient psychiatric follow-up depends on the gravity of the event and on the family's capacity to tolerate, if not facilitate, the child's retelling of the trauma. If outpatient follow-up is not scheduled, the parents should be advised to return or to seek care elsewhere if symptoms of distress (e.g., anxiety, nightmares, easy crying) or regression (e.g., helplessness, baby talk, enuresis) last longer than two weeks.

VII. **Substance abuse** may manifest either as acute intoxication and/or as the behavioral sequelae of intoxication (e.g., injury, suicidal behavior, assaultiveness).

A. The substance most commonly abused by children and adolescents is alcohol.

B. Substance abuse is more likely when the parents are substance abusers or when they are tolerant of the child's use.

C. **An emergency department visit prompted by any form of substance use is clinically significant.**

1. A thorough and complete history of substance use should be obtained. It should include answers to questions about patterns of use and the consequences of use on academic performance and social functioning.
2. The emergency evaluation of substance abuse should include screening toxicology for alcohol as well as other substances.
3. Some form of follow-up, either inpatient or outpatient, is mandatory.
4. It is important that substance use is identified as a problem. If the patient and/or the family minimize the problem, as commonly occurs, the clinician has the opportunity to confront and educate them about the dangerousness of continued substance abuse.

D. **Inpatient psychiatric assessment** should be considered in the following circumstances:

1. When the child is younger than 14.
2. If outpatient treatment has failed.
3. Life-threatening behavior has occurred either during or around the period of intoxication.
4. When the clinician doubts the child's or family's stated intention to pursue outpatient treatment.

E. It is useful to keep a list of inpatient and outpatient referral sources as well as a schedule of Alcoholics Anonymous meetings for teens.

F. It should be remembered that substance abuse treatment often involves many interventions and treatment failures along the road to recovery.

VIII. **Psychiatric presentation of medical illness.** Children and adults who present with psychiatric symptoms must be fully assessed for underlying medical illness. Consideration must be given to infectious, metabolic, and toxic etiologies. Children should receive the same physical examination, laboratory, and diagnostic assessment afforded adults (see Chaps. 1 and 5).

IX. Disposition

A. Guiding principles

1. Err on the side of safety.
2. Consider symptoms and behaviors in the context of the family or guardian's capacity to protect the child and respond to the child's needs.
3. Outpatient assessment and treatment is appropriate when there is no immediate danger and when the family is assessed to be motivated to get treatment.
4. Inpatient assessment is indicated when the presenting behavior(s) are dangerous to the child or others (such as suicide gestures, fire-setting, or suspected abuse), or outpatient treatment has been unsuccessful. All suicide gestures are significant in children.
5. In the emergency department lists for referral, assessment and treatment resources for children with information about 24-hour accessibility should be available.

Selected Readings

Jellinek, M. S., and Herzog, D. B. (eds.). *Massachusetts General Hospital Psychiatric Aspects of General Hospital Pediatrics.* Chicago: Year Book, 1990.

Tomb, D. A. Child Psychiatric Emergencies. In M. Lewis (ed.), *Child and Adolescent Psychiatry: A Comprehensive Textbook.* Baltimore: Williams & Wilkins, 1991.

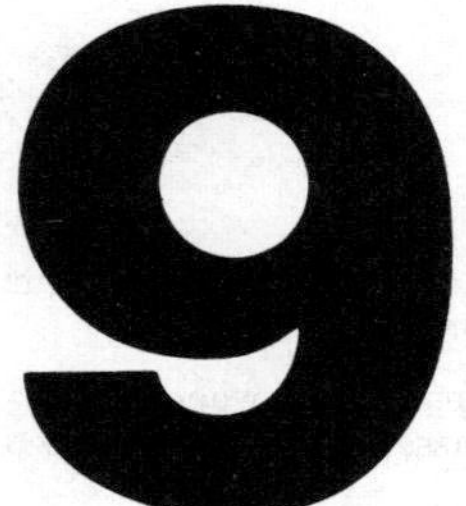

Geriatric Emergencies

Michael A. Jenike
M. Cornelia Cremens

I. Since Americans are living to older ages, the prevalence of psychiatric illnesses i the elderly is increasing. Persons over the age of 65 years constitute the fastes growing segment of the United States population, with an eightfold increase fror 1900 to 1980; the number of people over age 65 is expected to more than double from 26 million in 1980 to 67 million by the middle of the next century.

A. Overview

1. It is particularly challenging to evaluate and treat elderly patients wit psychiatric symptoms because they often suffer concomitant medical il nesses that may mimic or exacerbate psychiatric disorders. The majority o the medically ill elderly present with an acute confusional state or cloudin of consciousness that can be confused with a psychiatric disorder. In addi tion, they are likely to be taking a number of drugs that may themselve cause mental symptoms and have potential interactions with psychotropi agents. Fewer than 5% of those over the age of 65 use no medications.

2. Psychiatric problems frequently encountered in the elderly include demen tia, delirium, depression, psychosis, rage, violence, anxiety, and insomnia

B. General approach to the elderly patient in an emergency situation. Elderl patients are likely to be embarrassed by any signs of dementia or mental illness Older patients are less likely to accept help for psychiatric problems and are more likely to deny symptoms. It is safest to take a straightforward, medica approach in questioning an elderly patient. The elderly overwhelmingly resen being addressed by their first name, especially by younger physicians and staff The presence of cognitive difficulties among demented or depressed patients requires that the history must also be obtained from a friend or family member

C. Mental status examination. As a general rule, one should routinely assess three main areas in all elderly patients: cognition, presence of affective symptoms, and presence of psychotic symptoms.

1. **Cognition.** Often elderly patients are disoriented or have extremely poor memory but are socially adroit enough that the casual observer will not pick up difficulties unless direct questions are asked. It is best to tell the patient that these are questions you ask everyone as part of your routine examination. A full mental status examination is presented in Chap. 1; cognition can be grossly evaluated by means of the Mini-Mental State Examination (see Fig. 1-1).

2. It is important to ask about symptoms that would suggest an **affective illness.** Although some elderly depressed individuals present atypically, most can be diagnosed according to standard criteria (see Chap. 17 for symptoms of depression). However, depressed elderly individuals may initially complain primarily of multiple somatic problems in several body systems. When a patient's complaints do not fit a recognizable pattern or when chronic pain is a component, the possibility of depression should be considered. Finally, depressed elderly patients may have symptoms of cognitive

decline that are entirely secondary to depression (pseudodementia) or that represent a concomitant dementing process.

3. The elderly patient should also be evaluated for **psychosis.** Routinely, the elderly should be asked about auditory and visual hallucinations, thought insertion, thought broadcasting, ideas of reference, and paranoia. It is useful to corroborate the patient's answers by talking to the family. As with dementia, some elderly patients may be quietly psychotic and deny any symptoms.

II. Common syndromes affecting the elderly

A. Dementia

1. The current prevalence of severe dementia in the United States has been estimated at about 1.3 million cases, of which 50–60% are of the Alzheimer's type. Over age 65, 5–7% of the population suffers from Alzheimer's disease; over age 80 the figure rises to 20%. About half of all patients living in nursing homes in the United States suffer from dementing illnesses. Frequently these patients present to emergency departments with acute clinical deteriorations, without previously having been correctly evaluated or diagnosed. Any superimposed medical illness, such as a urinary tract infection or pneumonia, may produce a global decompensation in functioning or an acute confusional state.

2. When cognitive deficits are present, it is important to determine whether they are acute. If the deficits are long-standing, the physician must see that a medical workup has been performed. If the patient has severe cognitive deficits but was functioning normally the week before, the likelihood is a delirium (acute confusional state) rather than a dementing illness. The *Diagnostic and Statistical Manual of Mental Disorders, Fourth Edition, Draft Criteria* (DSM-IV) for dementia of the Alzheimer's type and for vascular dementia are listed in Tables 9-1 and 9-2. A suggested medical workup for the demented patient is listed in Table 9-3. Reversible causes of dementia are outlined in Table 9-4.

3. Dementing patients may concomitantly suffer from reversible psychiatric conditions such as depression, psychoses, agitation, delirium (see sec. **II.G**), and severe insomnia (see sec. **II.F** for treatment).

4. Almost all communities have access to a local chapter of the Alzheimer's Disease and Related Disorders Association (ADRDA), an organization that offers information, a monthly newsletter, family support (including groups), and advice about local resources. The national organization can be reached by writing to: ADRDA, 919 North Michigan Street, Chicago, IL 60611. The national organization will give addresses of local groups and will put families on the mailing list for the newsletter.

5. **Troublesome behaviors.** The most frequent difficult behaviors in the dementing patient include physical violence and hitting, catastrophic reactions (massive emotional overresponse), suspiciousness and accusatory behavior, waking at night, and incontinence.

   a. **Catastrophic reactions** can be minimized by teaching caregivers to avoid or remove the precipitating task or stress, to remain quiet and calm, and to gently change the focus of attention. Neuroleptics are sometimes helpful but only as an adjunct to these techniques. Hitting and violent resistance to care are extreme catastrophic reactions and often can be eliminated or made less frequent or less severe by the same interventions.

   b. **Night awakening and wandering** by the dementing patient can cause caregivers to suffer chronic fatigue. Useful interventions include placing locks on doors to prevent wandering out of the house at night, or keeping the patient physically active during the day and preventing daytime

Table 9-1. DSM-IV draft criteria for dementia of the Alzheimer's type

A. The development of multiple cognitive deficits manifested by both:
   1. Memory impairment (inability to learn new information and to recall previously learned information)
   2. At least one of the following cognitive disturbances:
      a. Aphasia (language disturbance)
      b. Apraxia (inability to carry out motor activities despite intact motor function)
      c. Agnosia (failure to recognize or identify objects despite intact sensory function)
      d. Disturbance in executive functioning (i.e., planning, organizing, sequencing, abstracting)

B. The course is characterized by gradual onset and continuing cognitive decline.

C. The cognitive deficits cause significant impairment in social or occupational functioning and represent a significant decline from a previous level of functioning.

D. The cognitive deficits in A are *not* due to any of the following:
   1. Central nervous system conditions that cause progressive deficits in memory and cognition (e.g., cerebrovascular disease, Parkinson's disease, Huntington's disease, subdural hematoma, normal pressure hydrocephalus)
   2. Systemic conditions known to cause dementia (e.g., hypothyroidism, vitamin B_{12} or folic acid deficiency, niacin deficiency, hypercalcemia, neurosyphilis, HIV infection)
   3. Substance-induced conditions

E. The deficits do not occur exclusively during the course of delirium.

F. Not better accounted for by another axis I disorder (e.g., major depressive disorder, schizophrenia).

Source: Reprinted with permission from the *Diagnostic and Statistical Manual of Mental Disorders, Fourth Edition, Draft Criteria:* 3/1/93. Copyright 1993 American Psychiatric Association.

Table 9-2. DSM-IV draft criteria for vascular dementia

For **vascular dementia,** criteria B and D in dementia of the Alzheimer's type are replaced by:

B. Focal neurologic signs and symptoms (e.g., exaggeration of deep tendon reflexes, extensor plantar response, pseudobulbar palsy, gait abnormalities, weakness of an extremity) or laboratory evidence indicative of cerebral vascular disease (e.g., multiple infarctions involving cortex and underlying white matter) that are judged to be etiologically related to the disturbance.

D. The cognitive deficits do *not* occur exclusively during the course of delirium.

Source: Reprinted with permission from the *Diagnostic and Statistical Manual of Mental Disorders, Fourth Edition, Draft Criteria*: 3/1/93. Copyright 1993 American Psychiatric Association.

Table 9-3. Medical workup for a dementing patient

1. History from patient and relative or friend
2. Mental status examination
3. Physical examination with vital signs
4. Neurologic examination
5. Computed tomography (CT) scan, electroencephalogram
6. Thyroid function tests, serum vitamin B_{12}, serum folate
7. Chest x-ray, electrocardiogram
8. Complete blood count, urinalysis, VDRL, glucose, blood urea nitrogen (BUN), calcium, albumin, electrolytes, alkaline phosphatase, erythrocyte sedimentation rate

Other tests as indicated:

1. Drug levels
2. Toxic screen
3. Brain scan
4. Lumbar puncture

Source: M. A. Jenike. *Handbook of Geriatric Psychopharmacology*. Littleton, MA: PSG, 1985.

Table 9-4. Potentially treatable causes of dementia

Drugs and alcohol
- Propranolol and other beta-blockers, methyldopa, clonidine, neuroleptics, phenytoin, phenobarbital, long-acting benzodiazepines, cimetidine, steroids, procainamide, disopyramide, anticholinergics, bromides, alcohol

Tumors
- Direct central nervous system invasion; remote effects (mostly from adenocarcinomas)

Nutritional
- Vitamin B_{12} deficiency (dementia may precede anemia); pellagra, Wernicke-Korsakoff syndrome, folate deficiency

Infection
- Syphilis, encephalitis, abscess, AIDS

Metabolic
- Electrolyte abnormalities, hepatic failure, renal failure, hypoxia

Inflammatory
- Lupus

Endocrine
- Hypo- or hyperthyroidism, Cushing's syndrome, Addison's disease, hyperparathyroidism

Neurologic
- Subdural hematoma, normal pressure hydrocephalus

Psychiatric
- Depression (empirical trial of antidepressant may be needed)

Source: Adapted from M. A. Jenike. *Handbook of Geriatric Psychopharmacology*. Littleton, MA: PSG, 1985.

napping. Sedative-hypnotics at night, such as short-acting benzodiazepines (e.g., lorazepam [Ativan], 0.5–1.0 mg, or chloral hydrate) may be helpful. Low doses of a neuroleptic may occasionally be needed. Trazodone in low doses has been reported to cause sedation and to decrease agitation.

c. **Suspiciousness and accusations** may result from the dementing or brain-injured person's efforts to explain misplaced possessions or misinterpreted events. If the family understands this, frustration, hurt, and anger may be reduced. Making a special effort to keep the home in orderly condition, or even a simple procedure such as placing a sign pointing to where an object is kept, may help. Again, neuroleptics may be used as a last resort.

d. **Incontinence** in the elderly demented patient often prompts the family to seek medical attention. Although incontinence has been considered a late manifestation of dementia, studies of nursing home populations do not confirm this impression. A careful search for an underlying etiology within the nervous system (e.g., normal pressure hydrocephalus, spinal stenosis) or outside it (e.g., urinary tract infection) is warranted.

e. **Inappropriate sexual behavior** is very uncommon and in the rare instances when it occurs, self-stimulation is the usual form. Dementing patients are not child molesters.

f. **Driving.** Patients may want to continue driving when it is clearly no longer safe to do so. If possible, avoid confrontation. Simple techniques such as hiding keys, disconnecting distributor wires, or providing a nonfunctional set of keys have often been successful in discouraging a patient from driving. Family members can be encouraged to assume responsibility for driving by coordinating their schedules around the transportation needs of the patient. Sometimes the patient will follow instructions in letter form from a physician when he or she ignores requests from family members.

g. **Smoking and cooking** become potentially dangerous activities. Environmental modifications, such as removing stove knobs, having a stove cutoff switch placed in an inconspicuous place, locking rooms or closets, and locking away matches improve safety.

h. **Lack of time for themselves and sleep disturbance in patients** are the least tolerable aspects of home care for primary caregivers. Family support is the major variable in keeping the dementing elderly person at home. Families do best when relatives and friends visit frequently and when provisions are made for the primary caregiver to have regularly scheduled breaks in responsibilities. Visiting nurses or day care centers can be invaluable, until the need for placement in a nursing home becomes necessary.

B. Depression

1. In some studies of community-dwelling elderly, the prevalence of depression has been reported as high as 13%, and as many as 20–35% of elderly with concurrent medical illness are depressed. Those over age 65 account for about 11% of the United States population but commit 25% of all suicides. Untreated major depression lowers life expectancy and is associated with increased risk of cardiac disease. Depressed elderly patients are often malnourished and agitated for months or even years.

2. **Differential diagnosis**

a. **Psychiatric disorders** that may produce an episode of major depression include major depressive disorder (unipolar), bipolar disorder, and major depression with psychotic features. It is important to differentiate among these because the treatments differ. Bipolar patients will benefit from lithium in addition to antidepressants; depressed patients with psychosis are unlikely to respond to therapy with an antidepressant alone but require either a combined regimen with a neuroleptic or, alternatively, electroconvulsive therapy (see Chap. 17, sec. **IV.B.4**). Psychiatric disorders that can mimic a primary depression include schizophrenia, alcoholism with secondary depression, and unresolved grief. Grieving patients may appear depressed (see Chap. 6). Uncomplicated grief may last for 6 months or more, and in one study, 17% of bereaved persons were clinically depressed 1 year after the death of a spouse or close family member.

b. Physical illnesses. Many physical conditions may be associated with depression. They are listed in Table 17-3.

(1) All severely depressed elderly patients require a thorough medical history, physical examination, mental status examination, and basic laboratory tests.

(2) One important organic cause of depression that is frequently overlooked and undertreated is depression after **stroke.** The incidence of poststroke depression is higher than what would be expected for the degree of disability alone (compared with other neurologic disorders). More important, the condition responds well to tricyclic antidepressants.

3. Suicide assessment is fully discussed in Chap. 4. It is particularly important to ask about suicide in elderly depressed or alcoholic patients. The suicide rate for men increases with age and for women peaks between ages 55 and 65 years, but remains high in older age groups.

4. Drug treatment of depression

a. Tricyclic and other cyclic antidepressants. Drug treatment of depression may be difficult in the elderly because they are prone to side effects.

(1) Choice of agent. Since the tricyclic antidepressants are generally considered to be equally effective, the choice of drug should be based on side effects. In general the most anticholinergic drugs, such as amitriptyline (Elavil) or protriptyline (Vivactil) should be avoided in the elderly (see Appendix II). If a patient has had a prior positive response or if he or she has a relative who had a good outcome from a particular drug, it may be best to begin treatment with that drug. If postural hypotension is a problem, nortriptyline (Pamelor) might be tried because of its reputation as the tricyclic antidepressant least likely to cause this side effect. Otherwise the choice of antidepressant can be based on the clinical picture. For example, if the patient is sleeping more than usual, the nonsedating, relatively nonanticholinergic agent desipramine (Norpramin) would be worth trying. If, on the other hand, the patient is unable to sleep, a more sedating agent like doxepin (Sinequan) or the atypical agent trazodone (Desyrel) should be started, with most of the dose given at bedtime.

(2) Prior to starting any antidepressant medication in the elderly, an electrocardiogram (ECG) should be performed.

(3) In the elderly **treatment should begin** with a very low dose, a maximum of 25 mg for most patients (10 mg for nortriptyline, which is twice as potent as the others, and 50 mg for trazodone). The dosage can be raised slowly every few days. Subjective response and heart rate must be monitored, and the clinician must be alert for anticholinergic, cardiovascular, and central nervous system (CNS) side effects. Elderly patients often need lower final doses than younger individuals. Blood levels can be used to guide therapy in the case of nortriptyline, imipramine, and desipramine.

b. Monoamine oxidase inhibitors (MAOIs)

(1) MAOIs can be safely used in the elderly when certain precautions are taken. Many patients who do not respond to tricyclics or atypical antidepressants will improve with MAOIs. Also, MAOIs may have a special advantage in treating depression related to dementia.

(2) It is essential that all patients on MAOIs receive dietary and drug precautions (see Table 24-4).

(3) The side effects of MAOIs that cause the most problems for the elderly are postural hypotension and insomnia. Insomnia can be minimized by giving the last daily dose no later than 4 P.M. Some patients, however, feel drowsy on these agents, particularly phenelzine (Nardil), and can be given the drug at bedtime. Orthostatic hypotension, which may peak in severity between 3 and 4 weeks after MAOIs are begun, is the more dangerous side effect for geriatric patients because they tolerate falls poorly.

(4) The most serious adverse effect associated with MAOIs is the uncommon but frightening occurrence of a hypertensive crisis caused by a toxic interaction with certain drugs or tyramine-containing foods. The elderly patient, who may have underlying vascular disease, is at risk for a stroke or myocardial infarction during the crisis. Intravenous phentolamine, an alpha-adrenergic blocker, is the treatment of choice for severe hypertensive reactions (see Chap. 24, sec. **V.C**).

c. Newer antidepressants

(1) Fluoxetine (Prozac), a selective serotonin reuptake inhibitor (SSRI), has been used in the elderly with promising results. In studies of geriatric patients treated with either fluoxetine or standard cyclic antidepressants, fluoxetine appeared to be as effective and to produce fewer anticholinergic, cardiovascular, and sedating side effects. Fluoxetine and other SSRIs appear to have no impact on atrioventricular conduction time, although they may produce bradycardia, particularly in susceptible individuals. Although these characteristics recommend its use in the elderly depressed patient, prospective studies of its use in medically ill geriatric patients (e.g., those with cardiac disease) have not been completed. Older patients can tolerate 20 mg daily but may need to initiate treatment at lower doses (e.g., 5–10 mg daily, or 20 mg every second or third day). Fluoxetine, which is highly protein bound, may displace other protein-bound drugs (e.g., warfarin), requiring careful monitoring of their dosage and serum levels. Also, fluoxetine, an inhibitor of hepatic microsomal enzyme activity, may raise the levels of concurrently used drugs (e.g., cyclic antidepressants, digoxin, anticonvulsants, certain antiarrhythmic agents).

(2) Bupropion (Wellbutrin) is an antidepressant that generally exerts a stimulant rather than sedative effect. Older patients should be started on 100–200 mg daily with the dosage increased weekly as tolerated up to a maximum of 450 mg per day.

(3) Sertraline (Zoloft) is an SSRI with a profile of therapeutic and adverse effects similar to that of fluoxetine. In contrast to fluoxetine, it has a shorter half-life (i.e., approximately 24 hours) and does not appear to interfere with the hepatic metabolism of drugs.

(4) Paroxetine (Paxil), recently marketed in the United States, is the most selective of the available SSRIs. It should offer similar benefits to other drugs of this class.

d. Psychostimulants

(1) Studies advocate the use of stimulants such as methylphenidate (Ritalin) or dextroamphetamine in medically ill depressed patients and for adjustment reactions in patients recovering from chronic illnesses or surgical procedures. At least one double-blind study of endogenously depressed patients demonstrated superiority of amphetamine over placebo in improving mood and psychomotor activity. At least two studies have shown the effectiveness of methylphenidate in treating depressive symptoms in patients with concurrent dementia.

(2) Dextroamphetamine is roughly twice as potent as methylphenidate. Therapeutic effects are usually achieved with daily doses of 10–20 mg of dextroamphetamine given PO in two divided daily doses, preferably 30 minutes before meals, or with 20–40 mg of methylphenidate divided into three or four daily doses. The last daily dose should be administered by 4 P.M. to avoid insomnia. If there is no therapeutic response in 48–72 hours, the medication should be increased or discontinued.

e. Electroconvulsive therapy (ECT)

(1) ECT may be the best treatment for the elderly depressed patient whose illness is accompanied by catatonia or self-destructive behavior, such as suicide attempts or refusal to eat. In these cases, a drug trial lasting 4–6 weeks may be associated with significant risk. ECT, which characteristically begins to exert a significant beneficial effect within the first week, may be lifesaving.

(2) Many depressed elderly patients, especially those with psychotic symptoms, do not respond to drugs but do respond to ECT. In one study, remission occurred in 80–85% of patients who had not responded to medication.

(3) Not only is ECT more effective than pharmacologic agents, it may be safer for the patients with serious illness, particularly for patients with cardiac conduction disturbances. Relative contraindications to ECT include recent myocardial infarction or stroke or severe hypertension. The only absolute contraindication is increased intracranial pressure.

C. Mania

1. It is unusual for mania to occur for the first time after the age of 65, although such cases do occur. Most elderly patients with mania have a prior history. It is critical that organic causes of mania be considered (see Table 20-2) when it occurs for the first time late in life.
2. As in younger patients, the agent of choice for treatment and prophylaxis is **lithium.**
3. **Special precautions in the elderly when using lithium.** Glomerular filtration rate (GFR) decreases with advancing age, and since lithium is almost exclusively renally excreted, dosages of lithium that produce therapeutic serum levels will be smaller than in younger patients. It may be prudent to start therapy with 300 mg bid or less in some cases. In addition, there is some risk of lithium producing a confusional state in the elderly, especially if the patient has a dementing process.
4. **Drug interactions.** In the elderly, thiazide diuretics are frequently taken for hypertension or congestive heart failure. These agents cause decreased

renal clearance of lithium and raise serum lithium levels. Whenever a thiazide is added to ongoing lithium therapy, the lithium dosage should be halved and then reestablished using blood levels. Conversely, to avoid subtherapeutic levels, the dosage may have to be increased when a thiazide is discontinued. Nonsteroidal anti-inflammatory agents (NSAIDs), such as indomethacin and ibuprofen (available over-the-counter), have been reported to reduce lithium clearance and raise serum lithium levels by 25–60%.

D. Psychosis and violence

1. Violent, psychotic, or aggressive elderly patients are among the most difficult to manage. The majority of such patients suffer from moderate to severe dementia while a smaller percentage may have a lifelong psychotic process. Such disturbances of behavior may also be present in elderly patients who are delirious or manic, or who have an agitated depression.

2. **Neuroleptics are the mainstay of treatment** but have many potentially severe side effects.

   a. These drugs should be used at the lowest possible dose to minimize unwanted effects. Haloperidol (Haldol) in doses of 0.5 mg once or twice daily or thiothixene (Navane), 1 mg twice daily, are reasonable starting doses in the elderly. In the very frail elderly, doses as low as 0.25 mg of haloperidol at bedtime may have a therapeutic effect.

   b. Low-potency agents such as chlorpromazine (Thorazine) or thioridazine (Mellaril) have more associated sedation, orthostatic hypotension, and anticholinergic effects than the high-potency agents, but the latter cause more extrapyramidal effects (see Appendix I). For this reason low-potency agents are preferred in patients with preexisting Parkinson's disease (PD). High-potency agents at low dose are preferred in patients with cardiovascular disorders. Neuroleptic side effects are fully discussed in Chap. 24, sec. **II.**

3. **Clozapine** (Clozaril) is an atypical antipsychotic drug that produces significantly less inhibition of nigrostriatal dopamine activity than conventional neuroleptic agents and therefore has been advocated for the treatment of psychosis and agitation in PD patients. In addition to sialorrhea, orthostatic hypotension, tachycardia, and constipation, clozapine can produce life-threatening agranulocytosis and seizures. The risk of agranulocytosis necessitates weekly monitoring of white blood cell and granulocyte counts as long as clozapine treatment continues.

4. **Propranolol**

   a. **Severe belligerence and violence** of some previously unmanageable patients with organic brain disease have been controlled by high doses of propranolol (see Chap. 5, sec. **VI.B.2.c.(2).(a)**). In most of the cases reported thus far, a therapeutic response was noted between 10 and 21 days after beginning treatment, with doses ranging from 60–550 mg/day divided into two to three daily doses. There was no improvement in cognition, confusion, or memory. Many of the patients were still on substantial doses of neuroleptics. Side effects of propranolol include bradycardia, precipitation of heart failure, and bronchoconstriction.

5. **Trazodone** (Desyrel), prescribed for agitation at doses of 50–100 mg daily, can produce rapid calming.

6. **Buspirone** (Buspar) has been reported to control agitation at doses ranging from 5–60 mg daily. The effect may not be immediate, taking as long as 2–12 weeks to achieve a full therapeutic response. One of the reported side effects of buspirone, restlessness, can paradoxically exacerbate preexistent agitation.

E. Anxiety

1. Anxiety is a universal human experience and generally is not an indication for medication. It can, however, reach disabling proportions and can also be associated with phobias and panic attacks. Numerous factors, such as loss of friends and loved ones, failing health, intellectual decline, feelings of helplessness and worthlessness, and loss of control over the immediate environment, make the elderly particularly susceptible to anxiety states.

2. It is important to rule out medical causes of anxiety (see Table 18-3). Panic disorder should be treated as described in Chap. 18, but onset of panic symptoms late in life deserves a thorough medical workup.

3. Although older sedative-hypnotics are still on the market, in the elderly (as in younger patients) benzodiazepines are the agents of choice for generalized anxiety. Benzodiazepines are less addicting than the older agents, have a greater margin between anxiolysis and sedation, and are safer in overdose.

4. All of the benzodiazepines are effective. Thus the choice of agents should be based on the potential for side effects. Lorazepam (Ativan) and oxazepam (Serax) are especially attractive choices for use in the elderly because they have a short half-life and no active metabolites, and their metabolism is affected only slightly, if at all, by the physiologic changes that accompany aging. Initial dosage in the elderly should be oxazepam 10 mg or lorazepam 0.5 mg two or three times daily. Lorazepam is the only benzodiazepine that is reliably absorbed IM and may therefore be particularly useful when oral dosing is impossible. The longer-acting agents, such as diazepam (Valium), chlordiazepoxide (Librium), and flurazepam (Dalmane), have long half-lives and active metabolites, and their metabolism is profoundly affected by aging. Thus they are best avoided in the elderly. They can easily accumulate to high levels, producing deleterious clinical effects including a long-lasting delirium.

5. **Antihistamines,** such as diphenhydramine (Benadryl) or hydroxyzine (Atarax), are sometimes prescribed for anxiety or insomnia and are common ingredients in over-the-counter medications. Although they may be effective, these agents have many potential side effects, including disturbed coordination, weakness, inability to concentrate, urinary frequency, palpitations, and confusion. Their anticholinergic properties make them poor choices for patients taking other anticholinergic drugs, such as tricyclic antidepressants, low-potency neuroleptics, antispasmodics, and antiparkinsonian agents. Polypharmacy with anticholinergics may produce an anticholinergic syndrome with delirium (see Chap. 24).

F. Insomnia

1. Difficulties with sleep are among the most common complaints of elderly patients, and emergency physicians will encounter these problems frequently. Physicians should use medication for insomnia only as a last resort.

2. With aging there are natural changes in sleep architecture that cannot readily be altered by medication. With increasing age the lengthy deep sleep of younger years evolves into lighter, shorter, and interrupted sleep. Sleep latency (the time it takes to get to sleep) lengthens, and sleep is normally interrupted by an increased number of awakenings. It is important that clinicians be aware of these *normal* changes with aging so that unnecessary treatment can be avoided.

3. **Sleep problems should be carefully worked up and diagnosed.** Sleep logs may be helpful. A careful medical and drug history may illuminate potential causes of insomnia. Caffeine, nicotine, and alcohol should be stopped temporarily. Depression and anxiety commonly produce sleep disturbance

and should be ruled out. If depression is causing insomnia, a sedating antidepressant, such as doxepin, may be useful.

4. Advising the patient that normal elderly patients require less sleep an that their sleep is typically lighter with more awakenings is often therapeutic by itself.

5. **Avoid hypnotic medications initially** and try to get the patient to avoi daytime naps and to get regular exercise when possible.

6. Advise patients to set regular times for going to bed and awakening.

7. If **nocturia** is a problem, rule out urinary system pathology and have th patient avoid drinking fluids in the evening.

8. If nonpharmacologic approaches fail, a brief trial of medication should b considered. Chloral hydrate is safe and effective with minimal side effects short-acting benzodiazepines, such as lorazepam and oxazepam, are helpfu for short-term treatment.

G. Acute confusional states

1. The diagnosis and treatment of agitation and delirium are covered in Chap 23. Acute confusional states are usually reversible. Patients who are dementing may develop confusional states secondary to medications and systemic medical illnesses (such as pneumonia or a urinary tract infection and will improve dramatically with treatment of the precipitating problem

2. **Sundowning** refers to deterioration of an elderly person's mental status a the evening progresses. This is presumably secondary to sensory deprivation and is most likely to occur when delirious or demented patients ar moved to a new environment (such as a hospital). The key to managin these patients is to increase sensory input and feedback. Use of good lighting, television, radio, calendars, and clocks, as well as the presence o friends or family members, is often helpful. Occasionally low doses of high potency neuroleptics (e.g., 0.5 mg of haloperidol) given early in the evenin may be effective.

H. Alcoholism

1. In the elderly, alcoholism can easily be mistaken for other medical conditions, necessitating a high index of suspicion for its presence.

2. The **clinical presentation** of alcohol abuse in the elderly is often characterized by one or more of the following: poor hygiene, self-neglect, falls an injuries, uncontrolled hypertension, depression, insomnia, lability of affect malnutrition, bloating, incontinence (of urine, feces, or both), diarrhea, unusual behaviors, and, occasionally, confusion.

3. The consequences of chronic alcohol abuse (i.e., delirium tremens, alcoholi hallucinosis, the alcohol withdrawal syndrome [including seizures], an Wernicke's encephalopathy) are more likely to occur in the elderly than i younger patients.

4. The **treatment** of choice for alcohol withdrawal in the elderly is a benzodiazepine. Either lorazepam or oxazepam is the preferred drug in elderly patients, particularly in those with hepatic dysfunction. Both drugs have shor half-lives and do not accumulate in patients with abnormal liver function Hospitalization is indicated if alcohol withdrawal is severe and does no respond to oral medication.

5. All intoxicated patients who present to the emergency department shoul receive **thiamine,** 100 mg IM and 50 mg PO each day for one week. Olde alcoholic patients, particularly those who are poorly nourished, are at hig risk for developing the Wernicke-Korsakoff syndrome.

I. Obsessive-compulsive disorder

1. The onset of obsessive-compulsive disorder (OCD) is rare after the age of 50. However, the percentage of elderly who suffer from OCD is significant. The lifetime prevalence in the general population has been reported as high as 2–3%.

2. The **diagnosis** of OCD requires that either obsessions or compulsions are a significant source of distress or interfere with social and occupational functioning (see also Chap. 18).

   a. **Obsessions** are defined in the *Diagnostic and Statistical Manual of Mental Disorders, Fourth Edition, Draft Criteria* (DSM-IV) as recurrent and persistent ideas, thoughts, impulses, or images that are experienced as intrusive and inappropriate, and cause marked anxiety or distress.

   b. **Compulsions** are described in DSM-IV as repetitive behaviors (e.g., handwashing, ordering, checking) or mental acts (e.g., praying, counting, repeating words silently) that the person feels driven to perform in response to an obsession or according to rules that must be applied rigidly.

3. **Medical evaluation** is indicated but results are usually normal. Late onset of illness is associated with a greater likelihood of associated medical or neurologic illness.

4. **Treatment** principles are the same for the elderly as for younger patients, although the greater risk of adverse effects of pharmacologic treatment in the elderly requires careful titration of dosage and monitoring of medication response.

   a. The recommended treatment should be based on a comprehensive behavioral, psychodynamic, and family evaluation.

   b. The pharmacologic treatments of choice are either fluoxetine or clomipramine (Anafranil). If these are ineffective, then therapeutic trials of a MAOI (e.g., phenelzine, tranylcypromine) and/or a benzodiazepine (e.g., clonazepam) may prove fruitful.

   c. Medication should be started at a low dose and increased gradually to minimize the risk of treatment-emergent adverse effects. Clomipramine, which has potent anticholinergic and hypotensive properties, should be used cautiously if at all in the elderly.

5. The Obsessive Compulsive Disorders Foundation can help patients and their families with information and a monthly newsletter. For more information, write to OCD Foundation, P.O. Box 9573, New Haven, CT 06535.

J. The documented prevalence of **elder abuse** likely underestimates its true prevalence since approximately 40% of abused elders decline investigation. Abuse is generally not relegated to isolated incidents but often is part of a pattern of violence in which the older person is harmed repeatedly. Physicians need to maintain a high index of suspicion for elder abuse and entertain it as a cause of unexplained injury or signs of neglect.

1. Elder abuse is defined by the Congressional Select Committee on Aging as "the infliction of physical pain, injury, or debilitating mental anguish, unreasonable confinement, or willful deprivation by a caretaker of services which are necessary to maintain mental and physical health of an elderly person."

2. **Types** of elder abuse include physical abuse, psychological abuse, material abuse, and neglect.

3. The presence of one or more of the following **risk factors** places the older patient at an increased risk for abuse:

a. Psychopathology in a family member (e.g., major mental illness, dementia, mental retardation, or substance abuse).

b. Being dependent on a family member for financial, emotional, or functional support and housing.

c. Being isolated with no opportunity for interaction with others or for pursuit of interests and enjoyable activities.

d. A family history of violence particularly if it has been multigenerational.

e. Stressful life events within the family (e.g., death of a spouse, relocation, or loss of job).

4. All 50 states require that alleged incidents of elder abuse be **reported** to a protective service agency. There is no federal law protecting elders against abuse. Unlike children, adults have the right to privacy and self-determination. Correspondingly, elders have the right to refuse medical assistance unless refusal poses a danger to the patient or others or the patient has been judged mentally incompetent.

5. **Treatment** is best initiated by a team composed of a protective service worker, a social worker, an attorney, a psychiatrist, and a psychiatric caseworker. The protective service worker's primary task is to coordinate the activities of the team members.

Selected Readings

American Psychiatric Association Task Force on DSM-IV. *Diagnostic and Statistical Manual of Mental Disorders, Fourth Edition, Draft Criteria:* 3/1/93. Washington, D.C.: American Psychiatric Association.

Jenike, M. A. *Handbook of Geriatric Psychopharmacology*. Littleton, MA: PSG, 1985.

Jenike, M. A. Alzheimer's Disease. In E. Rubenstein and D. D. Federman (eds.), *Scientific American Medicine*. New York: Scientific American, 1987.

Salzman, C. (ed.). *Clinical Geriatric Psychopharmacology*. (2nd ed.). Baltimore: Williams & Wilkins, 1992.

Special Problems and Patient Populations

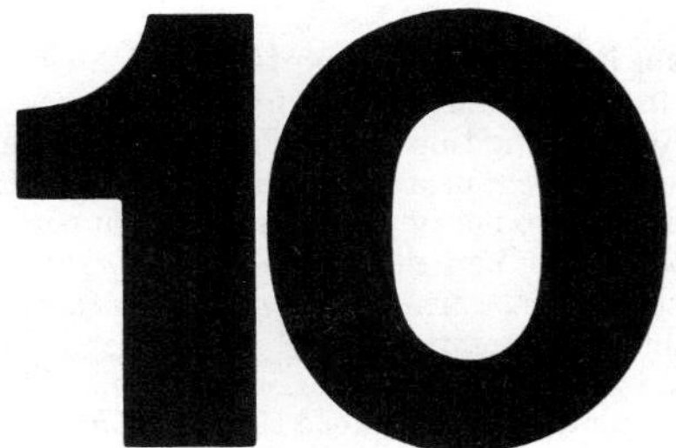

Legal Issues

Ronald Schouten
Steven K. Hoge

I. Psychiatrists face unique medicolegal challenges in emergency assessments. Patients frequently present with scanty history and often lack the ability to provide urgently needed information. Typically no prior relationship exists between patient and physician, and patients may not be compliant with treatment recommendations despite the fact that the crisis at hand may require an immediate response. In such stressful conditions it is common for clinicians to feel caught between clinical and legal responsibilities. An understanding of the basic legal principles that govern the practice of emergency psychiatry will enable the psychiatrist to perform his or her duties more efficiently and with less anxiety. When these guidelines prove insufficient and time does not allow consultation with an attorney, the best course is to focus on clinical issues and to act in what appears to be the patient's best interests.

II. Confidentiality. Physicians have a duty to maintain confidentiality concerning matters disclosed during the course of treatment. The patient's right to privacy of communication with his or her psychiatrist is supported by professional ethics and in many jurisdictions by laws and regulations. In addition to general requirements concerning confidentiality, many jurisdictions have special laws or regulations concerning specific matters such as HIV infection. Society's interests are served by the promise of confidentiality: Patients are more likely to seek treatment and to discuss their private problems candidly if they are assured that their privacy will be protected. But the right to confidentiality is not absolute. Countervailing interests—for example, the safety of the patient and third parties—must be considered. When in doubt about the technicalities of breaching confidentiality, consultation with a knowledgeable attorney or colleague is advisable. In the absence of these resources, decisions made in good faith and based on clinical common sense are usually more consistent with the principles of confidentiality than decisions based on legalistic concerns about malpractice.

A. The emergency exception. Psychiatrists evaluating potentially suicidal or dangerous patients usually need information from family, friends, and other caregivers. When the patient is unwilling or unable to give permission to seek necessary information, the psychiatrist is justified in overriding the patient's wishes. In breaching confidentiality, the clinician should divulge only that information necessary to obtain the cooperation of the third party. Therapists receiving such calls from colleagues should comply with requests for information relevant to the emergency assessment. When a patient is transferred to another facility or committed, the emergency exception allows the transferring psychiatrist to follow good medical practice and forward information pertinent to the initiation of treatment. In transfer situations, the psychiatrist should be aware of special requirements concerning disclosure of HIV status that may apply in his or her jurisdiction. Psychiatrists often receive requests for information about patients from family members, lawyers, and police officers. Confidentiality generally requires that such information not be disclosed without the patient's permission, except to the extent that disclosure is necessary for emergency management of the patient.

B. **Responsibilities to third parties.** In recent years, courts have defined a new responsibility for psychiatrists: to protect third parties from harm perpetrated by patients. The requirements for fulfilling this responsibility vary among the different jurisdictions. Fulfillment may require a breach of confidentiality in the form of warning the intended victim or notifying law enforcement personnel. It is often best, if possible, to obtain the patient's permission to warn the intended victim or to enlist the patient in the warning personally. The responsibility may be fulfilled by arranging for voluntary or involuntary hospitalization or by increasing the intensity of treatment. Not all jurisdictions have adopted the duty to protect, but most commentators recommend that clinicians act as if the obligation exists. A number of states have passed laws that limit the duty to protect or specify how the duty can be fulfilled. This duty is analogous to other responsibilities to prevent **future harm** to third parties that fall on the medical profession, such as the duty to report suspected child abuse or neglect. However, when a patient reports that a crime has been committed in the **past,** the psychiatrist is under no obligation to report this to the authorities, although he or she may not actively conceal the crime.

III. **Civil commitment laws** vary from state to state in the procedures required for emergency detention; physicians should familiarize themselves with their local laws. The substantive criteria in nearly every state are based on dangerousness; the patient must be dangerous to himself or herself or others, or so gravely disabled as to endanger life, by reason of mental illness. Some states require a recent act as proof of dangerousness; others require only threats. Dangerousness standards are based on the police power of the state and replaced the older "in need of treatment" standard during the 1970s. Many psychiatrists have protested that the newer criteria place the clinician in the role of an agent of social control and undermine the doctor-patient relationship. These standards have also been criticized as being too restrictive, allowing many seriously ill patients to go untreated. More recently there has been a movement to ease the barriers to commitment and to return to a paternalistic basis for involuntary hospitalization. A few states have already broadened the standards for commitment.

IV. **Competency to consent to treatment** is a frequent assessment in emergency psychiatry. Medical and surgical colleagues call on psychiatrists when their patients seem unable to make reasoned decisions or do not seem to be acting in their own best interests. It is important to note that competency is a **legal** concept and ultimately a matter for judicial decision. All patients are presumptively competent until a court decides otherwise.

A. **Assessment.** Competency, information, and voluntariness make up the requisite components of informed consent, which is required to permit any medical intervention. The information that must be transmitted to the patient must include the risks, benefits, alternatives to the recommended treatment, and the likely outcome of treatment. The legal definitions of competency are circular and vague, at best, and clinicians have proposed an array of standards to meet them. It is generally acknowledged that the patient must:

1. Recognize the presence of an illness
2. Understand the risks, benefits, and alternatives to treatment
3. Be able to reason about this information to some extent

B. **Documentation.** The psychiatrist should document the patient's mental status and capacity to understand and manipulate the relevant information, using the patient's own language. Optimally, psychiatrists should refer to the patient's "capacity to make informed decisions" and avoid the legal term *competent.*

C. **Emergency exception.** In an emergency, when delay may result in harm to the patient, there is an exception to the requirement to obtain informed consent; clinicians should act in what appears to be the best interests of the patient. If time permits, the hospital attorney should be consulted. Generally a substitute decision maker is needed to give informed consent when the patient cannot. In some jurisdictions the patient's family may be able to fill this role; in others more formal mechanisms may be necessary. In the latter case a guardian may be appointed or the court itself may make decisions. The emergency exception should not be relied on to authorize a prolonged course of treatment in the absence of informed consent from the patient or a substitute decision maker.

V. **Documentation.** As in all medical settings, documentation of the data, clinical reasoning, and recommendations are crucial. In the event of a lawsuit the record will become the most important piece of evidence. Areas commonly neglected by psychiatrists in emergency department documentation include the following:

   A. **Disposition.** Clinicians are usually careful to note the data supporting the emergency commitment of a patient but frequently fail to note adequately why a patient was felt to be safe to release. In the event of a bad outcome, suicide, or assault, a poorly documented, even if clinically appropriate, decision not to hospitalize a patient may seem retrospectively to have been negligent. Documentation should outline the reasoning process regardless of the final disposition.

   B. **Seclusion, restraint, and forced medication** are frequently used in emergencies and frequently not adequately documented. The symptoms and behaviors that justified these measures should be recorded somewhere in the medical chart. Periodic assessments of the need for continuing prolonged seclusions or restraints should be performed and documented with the times noted. Many states and institutions require that seclusion and the use of mechanical or chemical restraints be documented with special forms, which must then be available for review by regulatory authorities.

Selected Readings

Appelbaum, P. S., and Gutheil, T. G. *Clinical Handbook of Psychiatry and the Law* (2nd ed.). Baltimore: Williams & Wilkins, 1991.

Beck, J. C. (ed.). *The Potentially Violent Patient and the Tarasoff Decision in Psychiatric Practice.* Washington, D.C.: American Psychiatric Association, 1985.

Hoge, S. K., Appelbaum, P. S., and Geller, J. L. Involuntary Treatment. In A. Frances and R. Hales (eds.), *American Psychiatric Association Annual Review* Vol. 8. Washington, D.C.: American Psychiatric Press, 1989.

Tardiff, K. (ed.). *The Psychiatric Uses of Seclusion and Restraint.* Washington, D.C.: American Psychiatric Association, 1987.

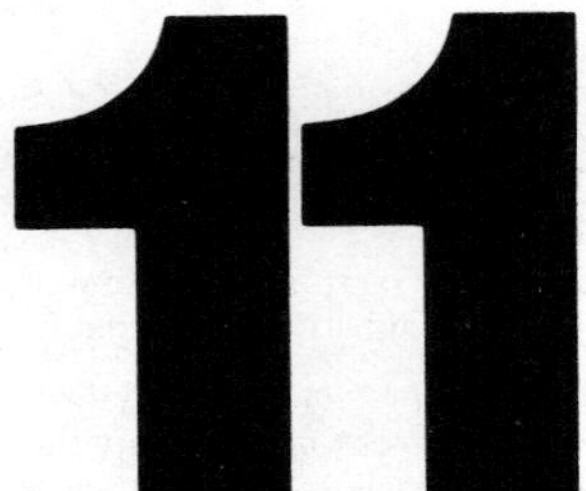

Domestic Violence

Julia M. Reade

I. Domestic violence is not a new or trivial problem in the United States. Up to half of U.S. marriages involve physical violence at some point, nearly one-fifth of the nation's homicides occur within the family, and half of these are due to a spouse killing a spouse.

A. Women are far more frequently injured or killed by domestic violence than men. Up to 25% of adult women are physically abused by their male partners, and as many as 40% of female homicide victims are killed by their husbands. More succinctly put, a woman is battered by her husband every 7.4 seconds in this country.

B. Little has been documented regarding violence between same-sex couples or regarding battered husbands. It is believed that the prevalence of the latter is very low.

II. Presentation

A. Domestic violence produces enormous morbidity and accounts for significant numbers of hospitalizations and emergency department visits. Among women presenting for medical care, battering is estimated to account for more injury episodes than motor vehicle accidents, muggings, and rapes combined.

B. About one-third of women who present to an emergency department, regardless of the chief complaint, are being battered. Most women, however, do not present with injuries but with general medical, behavioral, or psychiatric problems. They are more likely to complain of depression, anxiety, and family, marital, or sexual problems. Of those who present with physical trauma, about 40% are being battered, and the vast majority of these women will continue to be abused further. Indeed, the abuse usually increases in severity and frequency over time. The injuries are more likely to be axial (i.e., involving the face, breasts, chest, and abdomen).

III. Detection

A. Detection is poor in the absence of a specific interview protocol or of systematic questioning of all patients about family violence.

B. Most women will acknowledge the battering if asked, but few will volunteer the information spontaneously. They are often quite ashamed of the violence and feel responsible for its occurrence and humiliated for staying in the relationship. Some women may see the violence as an inevitable consequence of a relationship with a man or may fail to associate the violence with their presenting symptoms. Other women may avoid discussion of the violence so as not to experience homicidal rage or suicidal despair. Still others may have tried in the past to discuss the violence with others but found their disclosures unhelpful, since they were blamed or exhorted "to forgive and forget."

IV. Characteristics of battered women

A. Battered women comprise a heterogeneous group, drawn from all ages, social classes, income levels, ethnic groups, and types of marital status.

B. Only **widowhood** decreases the risk of battering. There are no predictors of being battered that are victim-specific.

C. Many, but by no means all, women in violent relationships grew up in violent or abusive homes and were either witness to or subject to physical or sexual abuse, often by fathers or father-surrogates. A history of childhood abuse may be a more significant factor in a woman's ability or inability to leave her abusive partner.

V. Characteristics of batterers

A. Batterers are a demographically heterogeneous group.

B. They are often needy, fragile men terrified by their dependency needs and enraged at their spouses for any sign of autonomy. They frequently have poor self-esteem, intense jealousy of their partners, and a need to dominate or control their wives.

C. Many are alcohol or substance abusers and may blame their violence on disinhibition, but many also abuse their partners when sober.

D. Many battering men were abused as children, but, as with the women they beat, many were not. The most powerful predictor is a history of having as children watched their fathers abuse their mothers.

VI. Characteristics of the violent relationship

A. Early phase and development. In most cases, the violence does not begin right away. It may emerge after the marriage, during a pregnancy, or following the birth of a child. It is frequently rationalized by both partners as due to some external stressor and thought unlikely to recur. In most cases, however, the violence does recur and becomes cyclical. Following a tension-building phase comes a violent outburst and then a period of reconciliation.

B. Types of violent acts. The threats and violence are often terrifying and life-threatening and may involve a variety of weapons, including fists, feet, clubs, knives, and guns. Some women are also sexually assaulted and any or all of the violence may take place in front of the couple's children.

C. Dynamics of the batterer-victim relationship. The woman is often accused by her partner of having extramarital sexual liaisons (although the man commits adultery far more frequently). The woman is progressively restricted from any relationships or activities seen as a threat to the man. Frequently she becomes progressively more isolated from friends and family, is often unable or not allowed to drive, has no control over the family's finances, may not have access to a phone, and may not be allowed to work. The woman is often terrified to leave the relationship or tell an outsider about the violence. She is frequently threatened by the batterer with death, loss of her children, or the suicide of the batterer if she makes any move toward leaving. During periods of reconciliation, the batterer is often intensely remorseful toward his partner, who may, in turn feel sorry for him. At this juncture, feeling hopeful about the future, the woman may find it particularly difficult to leave the relationship.

D. Why women stay in violent relationships

1. The battered woman may be trapped economically and have no other options for housing, food, or child support.
2. Many women blame themselves for the violence and may stay in the relationship convinced that they can remedy the problem by working harder to meet their partner's needs.
3. For other women, the violence may be a commonplace—that is, something she expects as the price of a relationship with a man.
4. She may be too frightened to leave. Many women have made efforts to leave,

only to find inadequate legal, medical, or social supports. Often, leaving the relationship does not stop the violence but may escalate it.

VII. Consequences of battering. As a result of chronic battering, most women, regardless of their prebattering psychological make-up, come to see themselves as worthless, incompetent, and unlovable. Many live in a state of chronic stress akin to that experienced by soldiers in combat and show symptoms of **posttraumatic stress disorder,** evincing periods of autonomic hyperarousal intermingled with episodes of psychic numbness, withdrawal, and apathy. The incidence of **depression** is high, as are **suicide attempts,** which occur in up to 50% of battered women. Many **abuse alcohol or other substances,** a response that is believed to be largely secondary to the battering. A minority may appear to be **psychotic.**

VIII. Assessment

A. General considerations. All patients should be asked about domestic violence as a matter of course in history taking, but the index of suspicion should rise for women presenting with unusual injuries or repeated trauma and unlikely explanations for their injuries. These patients will often seem guarded or evasive when questioned about the partner.

Presentation to an emergency department by a battered woman may signal an increased risk of injury from her partner, towards her children or against herself. Attention should be paid to the patient's subjective experience, not just to the severity of her injuries or physical symptoms.

B. The interview. The physician needs time, a willingness to listen, and tactfulness. The woman should be interviewed alone, and family members should be asked diplomatically to leave the room.

C. Emergency evaluation. An emergency evaluation should include the following:

1. A thorough **physical examination** with careful documentation of findings. This should include **photographs,** if possible, since the medical record may be needed in court. The physician should detail the patient's history without editorializing or ruling on its veracity.

2. A careful **psychiatric evaluation,** with particular attention to evidence of posttraumatic stress disorder, depression, suicidality, alcohol or drug abuse, and homicidal ideation.

3. Evaluation of the **woman's coping ability.** How has she dealt with violence in the past? Has she ever told anyone? What was the outcome? Has she sought legal recourse? Has she made plans to leave? Is she able to function at home or work? Have there been recent changes in behavior or mental status?

4. Assessment of **social supports.** Does she have friends, access to a car, use of a phone, mobility? Whom can she trust or confide in? Is there evidence of isolation or social withdrawal?

5. Assessment of **current danger.** Is the batterer pathologically jealous? Has there been an escalation in the violence or threats to kill the patient? Is there a weapon in the house? Is the batterer a drug or alcohol abuser?

6. Assessment of **risk to children.** Are there children in the house? There is a 50% chance that if the spouse is being abused, the children are also being victimized.

IX. Treatment

A. Primary psychiatric disorders should be treated. As described below some changes to the usual approach (i.e., to these disorders) are required.

1. The physician may need to **hospitalize** a battered woman earlier than he or she might otherwise with a nonbattered, depressed, or suicidal patient.

One cannot use the family as a resource in monitoring symptoms, supervising medications, and containing self-destructive behavior. This holds for substance-abusing patients as well.

2. The physician must exercise caution with **prescriptions,** weighing the risks of abuse, overdose, and dulling of the patient's vigilance.
3. Ideally, **close follow-up** should be arranged, but the patient may not be able to follow through. She may be too frightened, too entrapped, or not ready to address the abuse.
4. **The clinician should not attempt any form of couples therapy in an emergency setting.** This may put the woman at further risk of injury once the couple leaves.

B. Every effort should be made to **understand the patient's behavior in context.** She may be suspicious of the clinician, secretive or protective of her assailant, and, despite the clinician's recommendation, not ready to leave her partner. She may be reluctant to accept the physician's offer of help at the time, but if the encounter was a positive one in which she felt understood and treated respectfully, she is more likely to return at a later date or avail herself of other resources.

C. The physician should become familiar with **hospital and community resources for battered women** and inform the patient of her options. These should include referrals to:

1. Battered women's shelters.
2. Safe houses.
3. 24-hour hot lines.
4. A battered woman's advocate.
5. The National Coalition Against Domestic Violence can provide referrals to state and local programs and other useful information (1-800-333-SAFE).

D. The clinician should **plan and anticipate** with the patient how she will get help when the violence erupts again. The patient should be asked if she would like to press criminal charges against her batterer or get a restraining order, and then be referred to the appropriate legal authority. Most shelters know of legal advocates who can help advise or represent the patient.

E. The clinician may also need to notify the appropriate state social services agency and the hospital's child protection team if there is reason to suspect **child abuse.**

X. Clinician resistances

A. Many physicians are reluctant to ask about abuse or histories of violence for diverse reasons, including:

1. Fear of offending the patient.
2. Dismissal of the battered woman as masochistic.
3. Assumption that a high socioeconomic status precludes battering.
4. Assumption that poverty diminishes the likelihood of following through with treatment.

B. Some of these resistances derive from ignorance of the prevalence of domestic violence across all social strata and the heterogeneity of the victims of violence. Other resistances derive from the clinician's often unconscious responses to victims. These include a sense of helplessness, fear of contamination, or anxiety about the rage that violence often engenders. Efforts to distance oneself from the victim may result in harm to the patient. Her complaints may be belittled or taken out of context, she may be blamed and punished with inappropriate medication, or she may have inadequate follow-up or safety planning (see also Chap. 12, sec. **II.B**).

Selected Readings

Carmen, E., and Rieker, P. P. A psychosocial model of the victim-to-patient process: Implications for treatment. *Psychiatr. Clin. North Am.* 12:431, 1989.

Dickstein, L. J., and Nadelson, C. C. *Family Violence: Emerging Issues of a National Crisis.* Washington, D.C.: American Psychiatric Association Press, 1989.

Hilberman, E. The "wife-beater's wife" reconsidered. *Am. J. Psychiatry* 137:1336, 1980.

McLeer, S. V., and Anwar, R. A. H. The role of the emergency physician in the prevention of domestic violence. *Ann. Emerg. Med.* 16:1155, 1987.

McLeer, S. V., et al. Education is not enough: A system's failure in protecting battered women. *Ann. Emerg. Med.* 18:651, 1989.

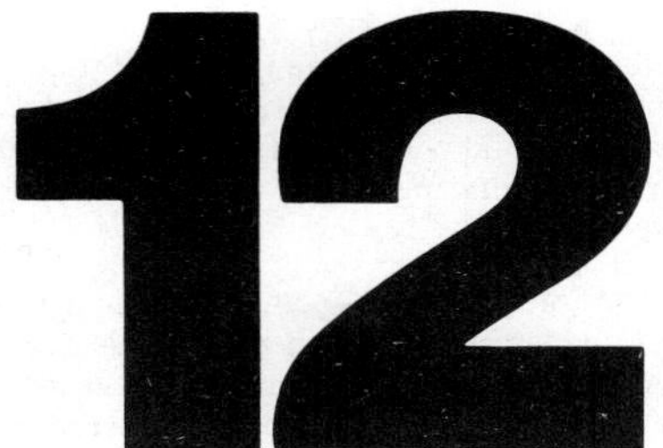

Child Abuse

Abigail R. Ostow

I. Descriptions of **physical abuse, neglect, and sexual molestation** can be found in the Bible and in the literature of virtually every culture since. Only in the past 150 years or so has society been willing to assume responsibility for the protection of children and the censure of those who mistreat them. Only within the past 30 years have physicians recognized child abuse as a clinical entity for which medical and social intervention is indicated.

II. The physician's role

A. Despite increasing public attention to the problem of domestic violence, physicians frequently ignore the possibility of abuse, especially in well-to-do patients. The result is **underreporting** of child abuse and, far more disastrous, failure to initiate treatment. Given the serious ambivalence of most families about seeking help for domestic violence, hesitation on the part of the clinician can be seen as "permission" to avoid airing their difficulties. Increasingly, evidence confirms that perpetrators of abuse of every type are far more likely than others to have either been victims of or witness to abuse in childhood. Furthermore, spouse abuse, child abuse, and sexual abuse tend to occur concomitantly within families. Thus, **identification and intervention may prevent other domestic violence.**

B. Physicians must become aware of their own feelings about violence and abuse so that they will be comfortable in looking for it and diagnosing it. Although the last 20 years have seen increasing attention paid in medical research and training to social problems, many physicians remain personally uncomfortable with cases of abuse. Disbelief or fear of being unfairly judgmental leads many physicians to avoid confronting suspicious situations. Lack of experience and anxiety about becoming involved in a legal battle may lead others to ignore their own observations.

C. The emergency physician has a limited but important role in the management of child abuse. He or she must provide acute care and facilitate further interventions.

1. First, he or she must evaluate the child's **safety.** If there is any risk of further abuse, the physician must make provisions to remove the child from the home. If the child's behavior is overly impulsive, self-destructive, or suicidal, hospitalization may be required for containment and support.

2. The physician is mandated by **law** to refer all cases of suspected abuse or neglect to the local child protection agency. Further investigation and treatment requires the coordinated services of law enforcement and courts, social service, and mental health personnel.

3. Acute **medical complaints** must be investigated. In suspicious cases, it is important to document any physical evidence that would not be available later.

4. It is very important to **support the family member who brought the child in.** The child's presence in the emergency department is an indication that

at least one of his or her caretakers is afraid and wants help. If that motivation can be encouraged and hope for change generated, it is more likely that the family will cooperate with follow-up efforts. On the other hand, if a family feels that the visit was humiliating or punitive, its members may actively resist further interventions.

5. **The initial emergency department encounter** is an opportunity to screen for acute problems and engage the family in treatment, not the occasion for a definitive diagnostic assessment. In most situations, it cannot be known at the time of presentation whether or not abuse actually occurred. Further evaluation is almost always indicated. Optimally, a member of a centralized child abuse or sexual abuse team will be on-call and available to assist in emergency management and initiate follow-up services.

III. Physical abuse and neglect

A. Definition. The federal government and all states have laws that define child abuse and require professionals to report suspected cases. Definitions vary, but generally abuse is said to involve the intentional infliction by a caretaker of physical injury that places the child at risk of death or serious impairment. Close confinement, such as tying a child to a chair, habitual verbal assault, and other overtly exploitative or punitive behavior has been defined as emotional abuse. In some states, neglect (acts of omission such as failure to provide health care, shelter, supervision, or education) is included as a form of abuse.

B. Incidence. The true incidence is unknown. Child abuse, like all forms of domestic violence, is vastly underreported. There are over 1000 reported cases of death from child abuse each year in the United States. The most serious injuries are found in children under the age of 3 years. If left untreated, a significant number of abusive situations end in the death of the child.

C. Etiology. Studies on causes of child abuse are confounded by coincidental factors. Abuse occurs in association with chaotic interpersonal relationships, drug and alcohol problems, violence between spouses, and environmental stress. Child abuse involves the interaction of a violence-prone parent or marital pair, a child who is seen as different, and a stressful situation.

1. **The abuser.** In addition to parents, caretakers such as baby-sitters and friends can abuse children. They demonstrate a wide range of psychopathology. A few are psychotic. More commonly they have personality disorders with emotional lability; many meet criteria for borderline or antisocial personality disorder. Many have drug and alcohol problems. A significant number were themselves abused as children. Many are immature and have unfulfilled dependency needs. Abusive parents tend to be isolated in their communities and distrustful of outside sources of support. They often have underlying feelings of rage and poor self-esteem. In stressful situations they may look to their children for comfort, interpreting the child's inability to satisfy them as willful. They often feel indignant when frustrated and self-righteous in their punishments. This does not preclude later remorse. Some abusers are explosive or impulsive and regain perspective once the aggression has stopped; others remain consistently rigid and punitive. In general, abuse recurs repeatedly.

2. **Spouses of abusers** often appear depressed on evaluation and can be unable to support either the child or the abusing parent emotionally.

3. **The abused child.** In some families many children are abused, but more commonly a single child is victimized. The abused child is distinctive in some way. Some are seen as fussy, hyperactive, poor sleepers, or unresponsive to affection. Others were born prematurely or have been seriously ill over a protracted period. A large number have neurologic or other physical

abnormalities that seem to have antedated the onset of abuse. They may be more or less intelligent than their siblings.

4. **The environment.** Parental history of having been abused, social isolation, and familial stress are all risk factors for child abuse. Abuse commonly increases when the family equilibrium is disturbed in some way (e.g., financial setback, loss of a caretaker, birth of a new child). It is important to be aware of environmental factors and to assess their impact so that previous levels of functioning can be restored.

D. Presentation. Parents may bring the abused child to the emergency department with an acute injury. They may delay seeking medical attention longer than would be expected or make repeated visits to the pediatrician with a variety of vague complaints. The physician should be alerted to the possibility of abuse if the story does not seem to make sense or if the family's guardedness appears out of proportion to the situation. If abuse is suspected, alternative explanations for the injuries should be considered. The psychiatrist may be enlisted as consultant to the pediatrician. The psychiatrist is asked to assist in assessment of the child's and the family's emotional state and to determine the child's immediate needs for containment or protection. Alternately, evidence of abuse might be noted during the psychiatric evaluation of a child brought in with acute behavioral problems or a suicide attempt.

E. Behavioral manifestations of abuse have been seen as resulting from the child's attempt to deal with a hostile environment, from the experience of neglect or rejection by the mother, and from the attempt to manage his or her own aggressive response. Abused children may withdraw from the external world and appear constricted, or they may be anxious, hypervigilant, or paranoid. They commonly are unable to describe what has happened or how they feel. They may deny their experience or, in severe cases, dissociate themselves so that they truly cannot recall the abuse. They may behave in a manner that seems overly mature or be excessively cooperative with or fearful of the parent. Indiscriminate or overly compliant attachment to strangers in preference to parents may also be seen. Abused childen may exhibit poor impulse control and increased food intake. They may behave in a provocative manner. They may be prone to attacks of rage and can be destructive or abusive of themselves or peers. Developmental delays are common, especially in the area of expressive language. No one behavior is pathognomonic and in some circumstances, abused children can appear fairly normal.

F. Guidelines for interviewing

1. **Parents and perpetrators of abuse are generally ambivalent about asking for help.** They feel frightened by the situation and guilty about their role in it. They are emotionally isolated and often feel overwhelmed. They tend not to trust external sources of support and view authority figures such as hospital staff as critical of them and potentially punitive. Typically, parents do not openly admit to concerns about abuse, even when they are not themselves the abusers. The initial interview is an important opportunity to support the parent's motivation to take responsibility for the child's well-being and to assuage guilt that might otherwise lead to denial or avoidance.

2. Interviews should be conducted in a dignified, unhurried manner in a location that ensures privacy and freedom from interruption. **The physician should avoid making accusations,** encouraging the patient to describe his or her experience. A mother can be asked, for example, how she copes with the stresses of parenthood, rather than whether she strikes out when her child cries. If a history of violence of any type is elicited, the physician should ask tactfully about family problems, including child abuse or spouse battering, about drug and alcohol dependence, and about legal difficulties. In addition, obtaining psychiatric history concerning those most directly

involved is important so that underlying problems can be delineated and treated.

3. **If several family members are present,** they should be seen separately, so that each has an opportunity to tell his or her story. Whenever domestic violence is investigated, the equilibrium of the entire family must be considered. All members have some awareness of the problem and have some role, possibly unconscious, in allowing it to continue. Furthermore, change will affect everyone to some degree. If this is not taken into account, resistance to treatment can come from unanticipated sources.

4. Given the guilt, discomfort, and fear this problem generates, inconsistencies and dissembling in the history should be expected. The physician must interpret the data cautiously and err on the side of protecting the child. Thus, if there appears to be any risk of severe injury or death within the family, the physician must intervene decisively to remove either the endangered individual or the source of violence from the home. Thereafter, investigation can proceed at a more leisurely pace. Despite initial resistance, many families will react to the physician's willingness to assume control with relief and may ultimately respond with trust.

G. Evaluation and emergency management

1. The child should be examined carefully for **evidence of trauma** and lesions that appear to be of different ages. Burns, welts, and ecchymoses may be found in unusual places.

2. **Neurologic evaluation** should be made to look for evidence of brain injury.

3. **Photographs** should be made to document all findings.

4. **Radiologic studies** may demontrate evidence of old fractures and periosteal reaction to chronic torsion of the extremities.

5. **Interviews.** On questioning, most children will deny that they have been abused; they feel guilty and fear further punishment. All available family members should be carefully questioned. Abuse of the spouse and other children should also be looked for. Rarely, a child will complain of abuse directly; this should be taken seriously, since children almost never make up such allegations.

6. If there is any doubt about the **safety** of the home, the child should be hospitalized or placed in foster care until the situation can be clarified.

7. **The physician must report suspicion** to the local child protection agency, which is then responsible for follow-up evaluation and further intervention.

8. Many hospitals have **child abuse teams** comprised of physicians, social workers, and administrators. Optimally, a specialist is on call to aid in assessment and to coordinate management of cases.

H. Treatment. Ideally, all victims and perpetrators of child abuse should have access to intensive evaluation, crisis-oriented support, and long-term treatment. Unfortunately, many state programs are understaffed and ill equipped. For most families follow-up is provided by a single caseworker, and no psychiatric evaluation is made. Immediate treatment should provide crisis-oriented support. Long-term individual or group psychotherapy is indicated for both the abusive parent and the child to provide a more adaptive coping style, resolve conflicts, treat associated psychiatric problems, and improve self-esteem. The family should also be seen together to identify sources of stress, modify dysfunctional interactions, and improve communication. Hotlines and similar services help impulsive parents by providing support for them when they fear they might abuse their children. Support groups for abusive parents, based on the model of Alcoholics Anonymous, have also proved useful.

IV. Sexual abuse of children

A. Definition. The term *sexual abuse* refers to any form of sexual contact between a child and another, usually significantly, older person. *Incest* traditionally refers to sexual contact between biologically related individuals but currently is often used in a broader sense to include relations between children and parental figures such as stepparents or other parental mates.

B. Incidence. As with other forms of abuse, true estimates are impossible to obtain. There has been a steady increase in reported incidence over the last several years, but this is probably due to greater public awareness and likelihood of reporting the problem. Investigators have estimated the prevalence of father-daughter incest alone at 1% of the population.

C. Types of abuse. The term *sexual abuse* covers a wide range of phenomena. Perpetrators may be unknown to the victim or may be people placed in a position of trust (such as teachers, caretakers, or baby-sitters) or members of the child's family. Incest is by far the most common form of sexual abuse. In one study, only 3% of perpetrators of sexual abuse were complete strangers to the victim. The type of contact can range from exhibitionism to fondling to anal, oral, or vaginal penetration with ejaculation accompanied by other physical violence or even murder. Molestation may occur only once or regularly over a period of years. Children can be physically forced or enticed into cooperation with various rewards. Contact can be painful and frightening or a gentle source of pleasure and comfort to the child. Thus, the effects of abuse will be extremely variable and interventions must be tailored to the specific situation.

D. Offenders

1. In general, child sex offenders are people with poor impulse control and poor capacity to delay personal gratification. Sexual activity can be used to meet less specific needs, such as for personal contact or the release of aggression, or the need to feel loved. Abusers are most commonly male, and most repeat their offenses. The offender may be an individual whose sole form of sexual gratification comes from contact with children, or someone who has at another time experienced satisfying sexual relations with adults.

2. Incest can occur in chaotic families; it can also occur in situations where the family maintains a stable but unhealthy equilibrium. For example, a mother may consciously or unconsciously permit her daughter to act as a sexual substitute. Incest offenders will sometimes assault several children serially.

3. Though it is less frequently reported, sexual activity among siblings has been estimated to be the most common form of incest. It can range from "experimentation" to a more chronic and pathological pattern.

E. Abused children. Children of all ages can be targets of sexual abuse. Girls are molested about twice as frequently as boys.

F. Clinical manifestations

1. **The impact of abuse on a child will vary widely** depending on the nature of the abuse, the relationship of the child to the abuser, the duration of the abuse, and the age or developmental capacities of the child at the time of the abuse. Thus, no one behavior or set of behaviors is indicative of abuse, nor does normal psychological functioning indicate that abuse has not taken place.

2. **Children usually do not report abuse.** They may be fearful because of threats made against them by offenders. They may suspect that parents are unable or unwilling to believe and protect them. They may feel too guilty,

especially if the contact is enjoyable to them, or they may feel loyal toward the offender.

3. **Acutely traumatized children** may display all the symptoms of a posttraumatic stress reaction, including panic attacks, painful affects, and morbid fears. Anxiety-related symptoms such as sleep disturbance, nightmares, and somatic complaints can be seen, as well as regressive behaviors such as clinginess, thumb-sucking, and enuresis. In older children, overt depression and suicide attempts can occur. Adolescents frequently run away from home.

4. **Chronically abused children** can exhibit poor self-esteem, shame, and guilt. Often sworn to secrecy, they may feel isolated from parents. Preoccupation with the experience can lead to depression, impaired peer relationships, poor concentration in school, acting out, and general social withdrawal. Abused children are often aggressive toward their parents or themselves. Active repetition of the experience through hypersexual behavior (sexual talk and play, excessive masturbation, attempts to seduce other children and adults) can place the child at risk for further sexual abuse. On the other end of the spectrum, victims can be phobic and avoidant, either of all males or of sexual situations. They may manifest hysterical and dissociative symptoms. In extreme cases, multiple personality disorder may develop. In general, victims of chronic sexual abuse have difficulties with trust and impaired development of adult sexual function. Borderline personality disorder, drug abuse, and alcohol abuse are common findings among adult incest survivors.

G. Presentation

1. Many children are brought to the emergency department because some adult already suspects that abuse has taken place. Police or family may bring children immediately following an event such as rape. Family or child care workers may ask that a child be checked for suspected abuse.

2. Infrequently, a child may claim to have been molested. Such allegations are rarely false.

3. **False allegations** of sexual abuse are being made with increasing frequency by parents during litigation involving custody or visitation. On occasion, a child will corroborate the false accusation out of loyalty toward the accusing parent or out of real confusion. A child who makes a false allegation may tend to discuss the incident with less hesitation than do true victims. During the interview, he or she may look to the accompanying parent for approval. He or she may use adult terminology in describing body parts. Affect may be bland or inappropriate rather than anxious, secretive, or depressed, as would be expected in a child reporting a real experience. False stories tend to vary less with repetition.

4. In some cases, sexualized behavior, such as excessive masturbation or using overt sexual themes in social interaction and play, can result from overly permissive or unconsciously seductive parenting, rather than from molestation. It may take several interviews and a great deal of observation of the child with his or her parent before this distinction can be made with certainty. This is one reason why careful evaluation by experienced clinicians is so important.

5. Physicians should suspect abuse in children who present with genital injuries, irritations, discharges, foreign bodies in the vagina or rectum, sexual promiscuity, excessive masturbation, or pregnancy. Venereal diseases such as gonorrhea, syphilis, condylomata, and genital herpes are almost certain signs of abuse when seen in young children. Behavioral problems and abrupt behavioral changes are less specific signs of childhood distress but can also be caused by molestation.

H. Management

1. Interviewing adults

a. Accompanying adults should be interviewed alone so that they can give any relevant history. Other forms of domestic violence and sexual deviation should be looked for. It is important to inquire about the safety of other children in the home.

b. Parents feel frightened and extremely guilty, even in cases of accidental molestation by a stranger. They need to be reassured about the child's physical and emotional condition. They should be told that a straightforward and supportive approach to the child will minimize further emotional trauma. They can be enlisted to help the child verbalize his or her feelings and "work through" the event.

c. Confrontation of an alleged or suspected abuser should not be undertaken until arrangements have been made to remove either the child or perpetrator from the home. There is a high risk of retribution and possibly death to the victim. **It is imperative that the child's safety be the primary consideration.**

d. If a parent confronted with suspected abuse denies it, it is best to honestly explain that the law requires reporting of the suspicion and to discuss the process of investigation.

2. Interviewing children

a. It is preferable to have all interviews with the child done by a member of a specialized child sexual abuse team. The experienced clinician knows how to help a child feel most comfortable with the disclosure. Familiarity with principles of child development enables the specialist to ask the child questions in a way he or she can understand, which increases the chances that the child will be able to respond accurately. Finally, knowledge and experience will minimize the chance of technical errors, such as leading questions that might invalidate a legal case. In some instances, arrangements can be made to videotape the interview. This may spare the child further interrogation.

b. Most children will initially deny that molestation has taken place. It often takes several interviews before a child can trust that speaking of the event will be helpful to him or her. Children may be overwhelmed or fearful of punishment. The child's defenses should be respected in any case and confrontation should be avoided, even when abuse is known to have occurred.

c. Children may become anxious after revealing that abuse has occurred. They may have questions about whether they will be damaged by the event. They often fear recurrence or retribution by the perpetrator. Support and reassurance about these and any other expressed worries is the best way to minimize emotional trauma.

3. Physical examination should be thorough, careful, and respectful of the child's privacy. The child should be told what will be done and reassured that it will not hurt. Unless trauma has occurred within 72 hours before the examination or pregnancy is a possibility, the examination need not be done immediately but can wait until the child is feeling more comfortable and appropriate examination facilities are available. Examination should be made by an experienced clinician to ensure adequate documentation of evidence and minimize further trauma.

a. Physical injuries and condition of the genitals should be carefully documented. In girls, the size of the vaginal ring and condition of the hymenal opening should be noted.

b. If there is evidence of vaginal trauma, girls may need hospitalization and internal examination under anesthesia.

c. Most hospitals have a **rape protocol** that dictates collection of specimens and physical evidence such as torn or soiled clothing. This should be carefully followed. Evidence is labeled and turned over to the appropriate law enforcement agency.

d. Cultures of the oral, anal, and vaginal orifices should be made to test for gonorrhea. Serologic tests for syphilis must be repeated at one-month intervals for three determinations.

e. Girls should be questioned about menstrual periods. If there is risk of pregnancy, a "morning after" pill for contraception can be considered.

4. Referral to the local child protection agency is mandatory in all states.

I. **Further evaluation and treatment.** In many communities centralized programs are being developed to deal with reports of child sexual abuse. Services provided include extended evaluations of children and their families to document abuse and to delineate its impact on child and family, diagnostic assessments of involved individuals, medical examinations, and referral to counseling services. As this area is only recently being researched, little is known about what therapeutic approaches will prove most valuable.

Selected Readings

Finkelhor, D. *Child Sexual Abuse.* New York: Free Press, 1984.

Kashani, J. H., et al. Family violence: Impact on children. *J. Am. Acad. Child Adolesc. Psychiatry* 31:2, 1992.

Lewis, Dorothy O. From Abuse to Violence: Psychophysiological Consequences of Maltreatment. *J. Am. Acad. Child Adolesc. Psychiatry* 31:3, 1992.

Newberger, E. H. (ed.). *Child Abuse.* Boston: Little, Brown, 1982.

Oates, Kim (ed). *Child Abuse: A Community Concern.* New York: Brunner/Mazel, 1982.

Schetky, D. H., and Green, A. H. *Child Sexual Abuse: A Handbook for Health Care and Legal Professionals.* New York: Brunner/Mazel, 1988.

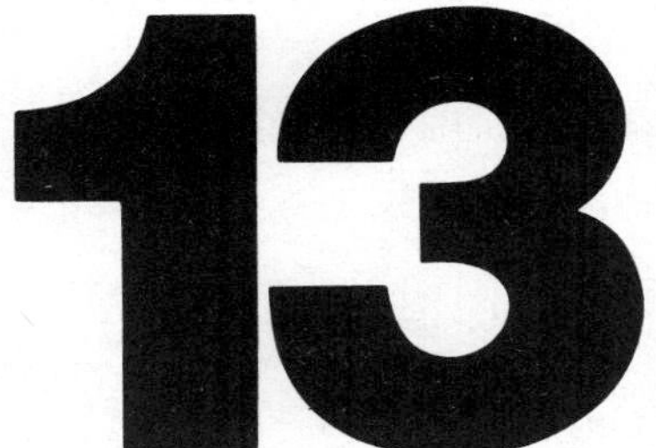

The Rape Victim

Patricia Mian
Paul Summergrad

I. **Social and epidemiologic issues.** Rape is a violent crime with medical, psychological, legal, and social implications.

A. **Definition.** More than a sexual act, rape is an aggressive assault with a sexual expression. It initiates complex emotional reactions on the part of the victim, often more significant than the physical damage.

Rape is a legal term rather than a medical diagnosis. In most states, the legal criteria for the definition of rape include lack of consent, use of force or threat of force, and penetration by a body part or object.

B. **Incidence.** Rape is one of the fastest growing violent crimes. Only about 50% of all rapes are reported. It has been estimated that nearly half of all women in the United States experience a rape or attempted rape in their lifetime.

C. During the past decade, the social and psychological views of rape have evolved significantly. **Rape has come to be perceived as a crime of violence** that may or may not include sexual arousal for the assailant. In most cases the motivation of the rapist appears to be the degradation and domination of the victim rather than the achievement of sexual relations not otherwise available. These findings help explain the victim's experience of the assault and the psychological sequelae that may occur.

D. **Male sexual assault victims** have generally not sought medical or legal help, and the incidence of male rape is not known. These men seem to be victims of pejorative stereotyping and myths, so it may be even more difficult for them to come to the emergency department. The care of men who have been sexually assaulted should follow the guidelines for women victims except for the reference to gynecologic care. Although limited, the work that has been done with male victims has demonstrated that their psychological reactions to the trauma are strikingly similar to those of female victims.

II. **Psychological issues.** The constellation of psychological reactions to a rape or attempted rape constitutes the **rape trauma syndrome.** This syndrome includes both the acute phase of the reaction and the long-term reorganization process.

A. **The phase of acute disorganization** begins at the time of the rape and may last for several weeks. It is during this time, just after the assault, that the victim is most likely to come to an emergency department for care. Rape is an experience that often overwhelms the normal expectations and the characteristic psychological coping mechanisms of the victim. Some victims come to the emergency department in an affectively labile state that may include tearfulness and expressions of anger, fear, shock, and disbelief. Other victims may appear composed, well controlled, and emotionally distant. It should not be assumed that the latter group are coping well; their surface control may mask feelings that are as equally painful and confused as those of the emotionally labile patients. During the period immediately following the assault, patients may report a wide variety of symptoms, such as fatigue and headaches. There may also be pain due to the physical trauma to the victim during the assault.

Sleep disturbance is common, including awakening from sleep at the hour the assault occurred. Psychological responses in the early period include:

1. Self-blame.
2. Fear of being killed.
3. Feelings of degradation and loss of self-esteem.
4. Feelings of depersonalization or derealization.
5. Recurrent intrusive thoughts.
6. Anxiety.
7. Depression.

B. The long-term reorganization process begins when the victim starts reorganizing her lifestyle. This process usually starts 2–3 weeks after the assault, although the time course varies among individuals. Life changes such as moving, changing one's telephone number, and turning to family members not normally seen for support are common. Many of the reactions rape victims experience reflect the events of the rape itself and mirror its violent nature. These include:

1. Fear of walking or being alone.
2. Fear of people behind them and crowds.
3. Fear of the indoors or outdoors (depending on where the rape occurred).
4. Sexual fears.
5. Repetitive nightmares recapitulating the assault.

III. Emergency department care. Because of the complex implications of rape, the victim will require medical care, collection of materials for use as legal evidence, and psychological support. The skills of various clinicians, carefully coordinated, can provide sensitive and comprehensive care for these patients. Generally, the physical examination and collection of evidence is performed by either a gynecologist or emergency department attending physician. Psychological support can be provided by a skilled nurse, clinical nurse specialist, or psychiatrist. The degree of psychological intervention is determined by the patient's needs.

A. The clinician's approach. One of the significant factors that seems to influence how the victim copes is the way she is treated by the individuals she has contact with immediately following the rape. The physician should introduce himself or herself and explain to the patient what will be done and why. It is important to enlist the patient's explicit consent for the collection of evidence because the patient has just experienced a flagrant disregard for her consent. The clinician must act in a nonjudgmental and noncontrolling fashion because the patient will often have feelings of self-blame. Some patients may want to discuss the events of the rape; others may find it difficult or overwhelming to do so. It is important to be gentle in obtaining the history and to facilitate the patient's ability to tell it. The physician may preface questions either by stating that it may be difficult to talk about the events or by saying that things often occur during the course of an attack that may be difficult or embarrassing to discuss, such as anal or oral penetration. If possible the clinician should inquire into the way the patient dealt with the assault in a manner that supports the patient's adaptive strategies.

B. Medical management

1. **Medical history.** The purpose of the history is to obtain information about potential injuries that require evaluation and treatment. There is a wide range of injuries that may have been sustained, including gunshot or stab wounds, lacerations, bites, contusions of varying severity, and occult dam-

age such as venereal infection and pregnancy. A complete gynecologic history should also be obtained, including:

a. Menstrual history and date of last menstrual period.

b. Use of contraception.

c. History of recent sexual activity before the rape.

d. Whether the patient has bathed, showered, defecated, or douched since the rape; these activities may interfere with the collection of specimens for evidence.

e. The time since the assault.

2. **Physical examination.** This section refers to the examination of a stable patient; patients with life-threatening injuries should be triaged and treated appropriately. The examination should be directed to find and document the following:

a. Outward appearance of clothing, such as rips or stains.

b. Signs of physical trauma (sketches are helpful).

c. A pelvic examination that includes:

(1) A thorough search for signs of vaginal and cervical trauma.

(2) Gonorrhea and chlamydia cultures of all potentially affected areas (including oral and anal cultures if applicable).

(3) Bimanual and rectovaginal examination of the uterus and adnexa.

C. **Documentation and collection of evidence.** Data gathering should be accurate and complete especially since it may ultimately be used as criminal evidence in court. Hospitals usually have standardized protocols for evidence collection, and many states are developing standardized evidence collection kits.

One clinician, preferably at the time of evidence collection, should document the circumstance of the assault including:

1. Sexual acts demanded and performed.
2. Penetration or attempted penetration.
3. Threats, force, and weapons present.
4. Resistance by patient to the assault.
5. Description of reported assailant.

The patient's own words should be used when possible in writing the description of the assault.

Collection of evidence may include but is not limited to the following:

1. Clothing and debris.
2. Fingernail scrapings.
3. Head hair sample and combing.
4. Pubic hair sample and combing.
5. Smears for sperm/acid phosphatase from any orifice involved (vaginal, oral, rectal).

All specimens should be placed in a sealed paper container and given to the appropriate law enforcement agency following the proper legal chain of evidence. With the patient's permission, photographs can be taken to further document physical trauma.

D. **Psychological management.** In addition to the general principles of crisis intervention (see Chap. 2), there are particular issues to bear in mind when treating rape victims:

1. Experience with rape victims who come for emergency care indicates that they want emotional support, help in regaining a sense of control over themselves, and reassurance regarding their physical safety. Rape victims must therefore be approached in a manner that addresses these immediate problems. These patients are often frightened, so it is important for them to know they are safe and protected. Since these patients have just experienced a major loss of control of their own bodies, it is helpful for caregivers to attempt to return a measure of autonomy and control to these patients. Helping the patient identify her needs, mobilize support systems, and solve problems reinforces her self-esteem and her ability to manage her own life. The patient will be faced with decisions in the emergency department—for example, who to tell about the incident and where to stay to feel safe. In an attempt to help the patient, clinicians may inadvertently "take over" and make decisions for the patient, which can encourage regression.
2. For the clinician who is enlisted to provide psychological support, it is not necessary or advisable to document a detailed report of the assault, as this has been done at the time of evidence collection. Documentation of the patient's chief complaint, psychological response, needs, and mental status as well as any clinical interventions are sufficient. One should err on the side of writing too little rather than too much. As the defense strategy is usually to discredit the victim, any inconsistencies in documentation or indications that the patient's character is questionable or unstable may be used against her. Unfavorable aspects of the patient's social history (e.g., divorce, use of recreational drugs) can also be used to discredit the victim. Avoid the use of language that can be construed as judgmental or pejorative. For example, rather than using words such as "alleged" and "refused" use "reported" and "declines." As with any sample of the general population, rape victims present a spectrum of mental health and illness. Patients with a concurrent psychiatric disorder need appropriate intervention. Clinicians need to be aware that an acutely traumatized patient may exhibit symptoms that mimic a major psychiatric illness. Unless psychiatric disturbance is evidenced by history or on examination, inferences about psychiatric diagnosis should be avoided. This is especially important because the emergency department record will likely be entered into evidence in a criminal trial and may be used against the patient.

IV. Treatment and follow-up

A. Medical

1. Any injuries should be treated and tetanus toxoid given if indicated.
2. **Venereal disease.** The risk of developing venereal infection after rape is low. The victim should be given information about prophylactic antibiotics so she can make an informed decision.
3. **Pregnancy.** Postcoital contraception is offered following a detailed menstrual history and after advising the patient of her options. Medication is given if no birth control is being practiced, if intercourse occurred within 48 hours, if pregnancy is likely (i.e., because of the point in the victim's menstrual cycle), and if the victim would be at high risk should a pregnancy occur. Ovral, two tablets stat and two tablets 12 hours later, is usually given.
4. **HIV.** It is not recommended that HIV testing be done in the emergency department or as part of routine sexual assault examination. The patient who is overwhelmed and traumatized by sexual assault needs expert counseling and follow-up to make an informed decision about HIV testing. These referral resources should be given.

5. Patients should be given a follow-up **gynecologic appointment** to allow an appropriate response to culture results, serologic tests, and the presence or absence of pregnancy.

B. Psychological

1. The possible sequelae of the assault should be discussed with the patient, including symptoms of the acute phase and later symptoms such as an exaggerated startle response, repeated reliving of the event, and fearfulness. The patient should also have forewarning that some people develop sexual problems such as aversion to sexual activity, vaginismus, and loss of orgasm. The reason for discussing these possibilities is to emphasize that these are normal reactions to the trauma of sexual assault.
2. It is important for the patient to know that psychological recovery can take months or years and that psychotherapy can help promote the recovery process. The goal of psychotherapy is to restore the victim to a pre-crisis level of functioning. The opportunity to review the events of the assault, the resultant affects, and the adaptive responses can be extremely beneficial to the patient. There is evidence that discussing the rape with family and friends aids in recovery. However, it is important that the patient not be pushed into talking about the rape if she does not feel ready to do so. Patients should be offered follow-up before leaving the emergency department.
3. The patient needs to decide whether to pursue legal charges against the assailant. This is a personal decision, but the clinician can be helpful in clarifying any confusion or providing information for the patient. It is important that the patient be able to enlist the support of friends and family, which may include their presence during legal proceedings. In some areas personnel from rape crisis centers are available to help the victim through the legal process. Some states also have victim-witness advocacy programs.
4. A benzodiazepine may help calm the patient who is extremely anxious or in a state of panic. Lorazepam (Ativan), 1–2 mg, or diazepam (Valium), 5–10 mg PO stat and then twice daily and at bedtime, may be helpful.
5. A written handout or information sheet should be provided for the patient. This should include medical, psychological, and legal resources and referrals. Information about the psychological reactions to sexual assault for the patient and family and friends should also be included.

Selected Readings

Beebe, D. Emergency management of the adult female rape victim. *Am. Fam. Physician* 43:6, 1991.

Burgess, A. W., and Holstrom, L. L. *Rape: Crisis and Recovery*. Bowie, MD: Robert J. Brady Co., 1979.

Burgess, A. W., and Holstrom, L. L. Rape trauma syndrome. *Am. J. Psychiatry* 131:981, 1974.

McComber, S. (ed.). *The Rape Crisis Intervention Handbook*. New York: Plenum, 1980.

Notman, M., and Nadelson, C. The Rape Patient. In F. Guggenheim and M. Weiner (eds.), *Manual of Psychiatric Consultation and Emergency Care*. New York: Jason Aronson, 1984.

Sexual Assault Evidence Collection Kit Training Manual. Commonwealth of Massachusetts, 1988.

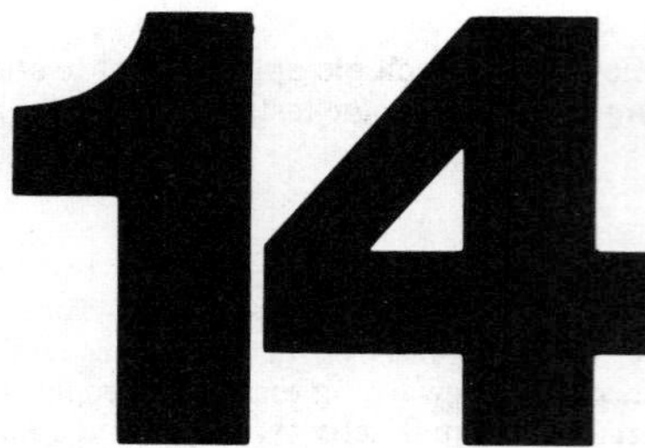

14 Homelessness and Psychiatric Emergencies

Michael F. Bierer
George E. Tesar

I. Homelessness is a socioeconomic problem that has become increasingly prevalent in the United States over the past decade.

A. A widely held assumption is that deinstitutionalization of the mentally ill, which began in the 1960s, is a significant cause of the increase in homelessness. Epidemiologic data, however, indicate that a minority of the homeless suffer from disabling major psychiatric disorders, suggesting that deinstitutionalization, though important, is not the only determinant of homelessness. Economic problems are of paramount importance.

B. The prevalence of psychiatric disorders among homeless adults is nonetheless substantial, and these individuals merit special consideration because of the unique problems and challenges they present to medical and psychiatric practitioners. For example:

1. **Diagnostic problems** arise as a result of the complex interaction between symptoms of mental illness and the state of homelessness.

2. **Substance abuse** is a prevalent and confounding problem in up to 50% of the homeless mentally ill.

3. The lack of stable shelter, a strong social network, and family connections complicates both treatment planning and **disposition.**

4. The **clinician's emotional response** to homelessness and to concomitant psychiatric illness may interfere with adequate delivery of care.

C. The purpose of this chapter is to familiarize the clinician with the clinical characteristics of homeless individuals who suffer from psychiatric illness so as to promote effective care of this comparatively difficult to treat population.

II. Epidemiology

A. Methodologic issues. Several problems interfere with the ability to make generalizations based on epidemiologically derived data from studies of the homeless.

1. The **definition of homelessness** is problematic. Housing status, which occurs along a continuum, does not adequately define homelessness. For example, both the street dweller as well as the person without a mailing address who moves among relatives, friends, and/or acquaintances can be considered homeless.

2. The homeless are a **diverse population.** Historically, the homeless population has been predominantly male but has grown to include families, single women, women with children, runaway youth, and battered wives.

3. The homeless **congregate in no single area.** Some populate shelters, others jails, and still others the streets. Many are intermittently homeless. Different regions of the country have distinctly different types of people becoming homeless, depending on diverse factors (e.g., the climate, the local housing market).

B. **Characteristics of the homeless.** The exact number of homeless individuals in the United States is uncertain. It has been estimated that at least 600,000 are homeless at any one time.

1. The majority are **single adults** in their thirties, unemployed, and without family contact.
2. The fastest growing segment of homeless individuals, though still a minority, are **children in families.**
3. As many as one-third of homeless people are **military veterans.**
4. Approximately two-thirds of homeless men and one-third of homeless women have **arrest histories.**
5. Methodologically sound studies of this population have reached similar conclusions: the homeless exhibit a higher rate of **substance abuse and psychiatric and physical disorders** than the general population.

C. **Psychiatric disorders**

1. Approximately one-third of homeless individuals suffer from a psychiatric disorder; depending on the study and the population the range of prevalences is 20–91%. In one sample, approximately one-fourth of men and one-third of women had been admitted within the prior year to a psychiatric inpatient unit.
2. The majority of psychiatric morbidity is due to personality disorders (especially antisocial personality disorder), depressive disorders, and anxiety disorders.
3. Schizophrenic and bipolar disorders are less prevalent. However, the ratio of schizophrenic and bipolar individuals who are homeless to those who are housed is far greater than the ratio of homeless individuals with less severe disorders to their domiciled counterparts. This inordinate concentration of disabling psychotic disorders among the homeless mentally ill may contribute to the erroneous impression that psychotic illness is almost synonymous with homelessness.

D. **Substance abuse.**

1. **Alcohol** is the most common substance abused by homeless individuals. As many as two-thirds of homeless men and one-third or more of homeless women are known to have abused alcohol (Breakey, et al. 1989). A smaller but still significant number suffer from alcohol dependence. The preferred substance may vary with age and ethnicity.
2. A smaller number meet criteria for a diagnosis of abuse of or dependence on drugs other than alcohol, with little difference between the sexes.

E. **Comorbidity**

1. The rate of comorbid substance use disorders and psychiatric disorders among the homeless is high. In a sample of homeless Baltimore men with a major mental illness, 60% also had an alcohol abuse disorder and 24% a drug abuse disorder; the rates among homeless women with a major psychiatric disorder were somewhat lower (i.e., 46% and 20%, respectively) (Breakey, et al., 1989).
2. Of homeless substance abusers, approximately one-third have a corresponding psychiatric disorder. In the Baltimore study, among those with lifetime alcohol use disorders, 38% of men and 32% of women had a major mental illness (Breakey, et al., 1989).

F. A small group of the homeless manifest **cognitive impairment** in the absence of other psychiatric or substance use disorders. In a Los Angeles sample, nearly

2% had a primary cognitive disorder, a rate that was nearly five times that measured in the general population (Koegel, et al., 1988).

G. Environmental exposure and poor self-care contribute to substantial **medical problems** in the homeless. Mouth and dental problems are common as are gynecologic, circulatory (e.g., lower extremity venous stasis), endocrine, gastrointestinal, musculoskeletal, respiratory (e.g., tuberculosis), and neurologic disturbances.

III. **The interaction of homelessness and psychiatric illness.** Epidemiologic data suggest a relationship between psychiatric illness and homelessness. The interaction of these two phenomena is complex and bidirectional.

A. **Psychiatric illness as a cause of homelessness.** Psychiatric illness is a precursor of homelessness to the extent that it interferes with an individual's ability to compete for scarce housing. The downward drift hypothesis of schizophrenia may be of heuristic value here. In contrast to the assumption that poverty is a cause of schizophrenia, the downward drift hypothesis suggests that schizophrenia's disabling effects cause progressive downward social mobility. Homelessness can be viewed as a potential consequence of such mental and behavioral deterioration. Among homeless people in Los Angeles with a history of major depression, for example, the first depressive episode preceded homelessness in 71% (Koegel, et al., 1988).

B. **Homelessness as a precipitant of psychiatric illness.** Given a hereditary or at least familial basis for many major psychiatric disorders, the stressors of homelessness probably serve as precipitants and contributors rather than causes of illnesses such as schizophrenia, personality disorders, affective disorders, and anxiety disorders. Typical stressors faced by the homeless include the crowded and occasionally frightening shelter environment, adverse weather conditions, poor nutrition, and sleep deprivation. The shelter existence is characterized in general by lack of privacy, crowding, long waiting periods for basic human necessities, the constant threat, if not occurrence, of physical violence, and an overarching sense of powerlessness. These factors can trigger or exacerbate suspiciousness, irritability, anxiety, mood disturbance, and, likely, relapses of chronic psychotic disorders.

IV. **Evaluation**

A. **General approach**

1. **Attend to the patient's priorities.** Command hallucinations may be less bothersome to the homeless patient than ill-fitting shoes or gnawing hunger. Once the patient's basic needs have been addressed, attention can shift more easily to the important psychiatric issues. Perception of the clinician as an ally in pursuit of important proximate goals will enhance trust and the potential for effective intervention.

2. **Corroborate information.** Often, the homeless person's closest contact is a service provider. A food pantry worker or a shelter counselor, for example, can be called on to provide or confirm information about the homeless person when necessary. The local bureau of missing persons may also assist in the identification of some patients.

3. **Maintain confidentiality.** Homeless people lead a public existence, their personal histories in bureaucratic files and their lives visible to the public eye. As a result, homeless patients often require the assurance that confidentiality will be maintained to the extent permitted by clinical circumstances. During the clinical encounter, the issue of confidentiality should be addressed directly and sensitively. It may be helpful to review the definition of confidentiality with the patient.

4. **Know street drugs.** Since there is a high risk of substance abuse in homeless individuals, knowledge about the local mix of street drugs and street

terminology may be valuable. Local police often serve as a ready source of information (e.g., about patterns of drug use, drug potencies). Clinician awareness of an unusually potent batch of street drug may save critical time in treating overdoses. The clinician's knowledge of street terminology not only facilitates history taking; for the patient it may also be a reassuring indication of the clinician's familiarity with the circumstances of homelessness.

5. **Attend to medical problems.** Greater than average vigilance should be maintained for medical problems in homeless patients. Contact with physicians may be rare and certain important medical conditions are prevalent among homeless adults. The incidence of pulmonary tuberculosis (TB), for example, has been increasing among shelter dwellers. It is prudent to inquire of every homeless patient about TB skin testing and to skin test asymptomatic patients or obtain a chest radiograph for anyone with pulmonary symptoms. Anticipated transfer of a potentially infected patient to an inpatient unit makes these measures imperative.

6. **Foot care.** Screening for foot problems is important because (1) they are common in the homeless, (2) early infection is easily treatable, and (3) the consequences are preventable. Every patient should have his or her feet inspected. Patients with peripheral neuropathy (e.g., from HIV infection, alcohol abuse, or frostbite) may have an asymptomatic foot infection.

B. **Diagnostic problems and considerations.** The assessment of psychiatric symptoms in the homeless can be confusing since the symptoms are either the consequences of life on the street, the manifestations of an identifiable psychiatric disorder, or both. Indeed, the circumstances of homelessness produce symptoms easily confused with bona fide psychiatric disorders.

1. **Depression.** Depressed mood is an obvious sequela of the inevitable frustrations, disappointments, and rigors associated with being homeless. In addition, homeless individuals frequently report symptoms that are consonant with the homeless lifestyle and that also suggest depressive illness.

   a. **Sleep disturbance.** Poor sleep is the rule, especially for patients sleeping outside or on the street. Often, sleep is possible only in brief intervals during daylight hours, or when a partner is present who can maintain watch. The ambience of most shelters and missions provides for little peace or privacy.

   b. **Fatigue or anergy.** Diminished energy may be secondary to disrupted sleep, inadequate nutrition, and the rigors of the homeless lifestyle.

   c. **Weight loss.** It is important to distinguish anorexia from lack of available food when inquiring about appetite and the cause of weight loss.

   d. **Psychomotor changes.** Factors other than clinical depression can produce restlessness, irritability, agitation, or psychomotor retardation. These include sleep deprivation, inadequate food, frustrating circumstances (e.g., long lines, lack of available resources), the ever-present threat of assault, and exposure to the elements.

2. **Paranoia.** Hypervigilance and suspiciousness, which might be mistaken for paranoia, are often appropriate and adaptive characteristics in homeless individuals. Frequently, all possessions are kept in one or more bags at the homeless person's side. Robbers have been known to cut off a sleeping individual's clothes in order to steal pocket contents. Without privacy and security, homeless people are frequently the victims of sexual or physical assault. Often there are outstanding warrants for them or other problems the patient may want to conceal.

3. **Antisocial personality features.** The diagnostic criteria for antisocial personality disorder (ASPD) in the *Diagnostic and Statistical Manual of Mental*

Disorders, Fourth Edition, Draft Criteria (DSM-IV) are unreliable in homeless individuals, since the circumstances of homelessness can create a clinical impression of ASPD. Homelessness is a potential consequence of ASPD, but being homeless can also beget circumstances that suggest ASPD—for example, prolonged unemployment, transience, and criminal behavior (Koegel and Burnam, 1992).

4. **Psychoactive substance abuse.** Substance abuse frequently complicates the evaluation of emergency psychiatric patients. The clinician must resist making a psychiatric diagnosis until after the patient is reevaluated in the sober state. Often, a definitive diagnosis requires prolonged abstinence from the offending psychoactive substance.

5. **Physical or sexual abuse.** As a group the homeless experience a high rate of sexual and physical abuse causing symptoms of either acute or chronic posttraumatic stress disorder.

V. Barriers to effective care and treatment

A. Health care access. In addition to poverty, nonfinancial factors limit the homeless person's access to health care. Scheduled clinic appointments may be difficult to keep if it is necessary to wait long periods for basic necessities (e.g., food, shelter, and clothing) at sites distant from the clinic. The distance between shelter and clinic may be daunting for those on foot. Being dissheveled or unwashed may make the person reluctant to sit with others in a clinic waiting room.

B. Reluctance to use services. For these and other reasons, homeless people, especially those with psychiatric problems, are inclined to use emergency departments and walk-in clinics rather than scheduled outpatient clinic and mental health services. Ironically, waiting times at such services are often long and the likelihood of being subjected to restraining procedures is great depending on the nature of the presenting problem and on the design and safety of the emergency facility. If hospitalization is deemed necessary, transfer to a psychiatric hospital (particularly a public psychiatric hospital) can be delayed for hours, and in some areas of the country, for days. Irregular follow-up and monitoring contribute to inadequate treatment either of the underlying illness or of medication side effects. Consequently homeless adults often develop aversion to medical and psychiatric treatment.

C. Medications

1. One's prescribing practice should account for the special needs and circumstances of homeless individuals. For example:
   a. The **need to remain alert** and aware of the surroundings.
   b. The high likelihood of ongoing or remitted **substance abuse.**
2. **Sedating medications** may reduce survival where vigilance is required. Benzodiazepines and antidepressants with sedative properties (e.g., the tertiary amine tricyclic antidepressants imipramine (Tofranil), amitriptyline (Elavil), and doxepin (Sinequan) should be prescribed cautiously, with treatment initiated at low doses (e.g., 10–25 mg). Another reason for the judicious prescription of benzodiazepines is the relatively great risk of polysubstance abuse in this population.
3. Homeless people often do not have a **safe place** to keep medications. Medicines are frequently stolen and many have a street value; selling them may be more consistent with the patient's priorities.
4. The likelihood of **noncompliance** with prescribed medication regimens is comparatively great. Not only does the homeless lifestyle make it difficult

to maintain regular schedules, but a wristwatch can be an unaffordable luxury, making it more difficult to abide by a multidose medication regimen. The simpler the dosage schedule, the greater the likelihood of compliance. When possible, single or twice daily dosing is preferable.

5. Ensure **access** to medications, if possible. Patients who cannot afford medication often will underdose to prolong their supply.

D. Clinician reactions

1. A clinician's negative response to the patient can interfere with the delivery of effective care.
2. For several reasons treatment of the homeless is likely to arouse negative emotional reactions in caregivers. Relevant factors include:
   a. **Homelessness itself.** Some may regard homelessness as a sign of weakness or moral depravity.
   b. **Personality disorders.** The homeless have a high rate of personality disorders. Needy but help-rejecting individuals who have poor interpersonal relationships can confound the most patient and understanding clinicians.
   c. **Substance abuse.** Intoxicated individuals who are irritable, agitated, and/or self-destructive may in turn anger emergency department personnel entrusted with their care. Even experienced clinicians are prone to blame and judge such patients.
   d. **Poor personal hygiene and appearance.** A dirty, malodorous, or disheveled individual may elicit aversive responses from the care provider.
3. Visceral reactions to these attributes are neither wrong nor avoidable. It is important that the clinician monitor these reactions in himself or herself to ensure that they do not interfere with the delivery of dignified and appropriate care.

E. Follow-up. Many homeless people do not stay in one place. Contacting the patient may be difficult. The use of aliases further complicates the picture. Often patients have no mailing address.

VI. Disposition

A. Community services

1. Currently, there are 110 federally funded **Health Care for the Homeless** (HCH) programs in the United States. These programs provide networks of medical and nursing care for homeless people. They also provide necessary outreach and help to coordinate psychiatric services for those who need them. Information on local networks should be available from emergency department administration.
2. Emergency personnel should maintain active communication with area **shelters** and their representatives. Knowledge about a particular shelter's capacity to monitor medical and psychiatric treatment will permit caregivers to address patient problems appropriately. Compliance with or response to prescribed medication, for instance, can often be monitored by shelter nursing staff.

B. Hospital social services. Referral to the hospital's social service is indicated for the management of the many financial barriers encountered by homeless people. Knowledge about benefits and entitlements may help the patient acquire otherwise inaccessible health care or medications.

C. Detoxification and rehabilitation facilities. When substance abuse is the primary problem, referral to an inpatient or outpatient detoxification and treatment center is indicated. Specialty centers are capable of caring for patients with a "dual diagnosis"—that is, simultaneous occurrence of both a psychiatric disorder and a substance abuse disorder.

D. Communication with other providers

1. If the patient resides at a shelter or mission, it is important to notify shelter personnel of the assessment and plan. It may also be important to reassure shelter staff of the safety of a patient who will be returning to the shelter.
2. Many shelter-clinics dispense medications and can help in the care of the patient.
3. Some laboratory tests (e.g., blood levels) can be performed at shelters or through HCH in coordination with the emergency clinician.

E. Involuntary hospitalization

1. In most states, the decision to commit a psychiatric patient to involuntary hospitalization is based on the **dangerousness criterion.**
2. The **inability to care for self** can also pose a risk of danger, but the degree of risk and the grounds for commitment are often less clear. Some may consider homelessness itself as prima facie evidence of impaired self-care. Given this view one might predict a greater incidence of involuntary psychiatric hospitalization of the homeless (M. Bierer, unpublished data, 1990).
3. In contrast, adaptation to homeless circumstances can be viewed as a sign of resilience. Survival on the streets requires considerable resourcefulness, shrewdness, and adaptive strength.
4. Homelessness, therefore, is not in and of itself a criterion for enforced hospitalization. Rather the important determinants include:
   a. **Recent development of homelessness.** Recent homelessness should alert the clinician to the possibility of an acute or reversible medical or psychiatric process. If adequate follow-up evaluation and treatment cannot be assured, then hospitalization may be necessary.
   b. **History of dangerousness.** An otherwise unstable and dangerous patient may present a picture to emergency department staff of behavioral calm, emotional control, and cognitive clarity. If the history is even suggestive of dangerousness, every effort should be made to acquire the independent observations of a third party (e.g., shelter worker). The application for involuntary commitment can be made on history alone.
   c. **Inadequate social support.** A lack of social support is an important factor that may account for the frequent psychiatric hospitalization of homeless patients. A failure of self-care is less likely to require hospital treatment if the patient can be safely returned to a supportive family network. Contrary to the hopes and expectations of emergency personnel, the typical shelter environment can provide this supportive function only rarely.
   d. **Untreated serious or life-threatening medical conditions.** An incompetent patient can be forced to undergo necessary medical treatment. However, unconventional alternatives to hospitalization do exist. If the network of medical care providers is sufficiently resourceful and well-organized, it may be possible to provide outpatient treatment for conditions that would otherwise require hospitalization. It has been our experience that relatively severe cellulitis, even in diabetics, can occasionally be safely treated with oral or even intramuscular antibiotics administered in the shelters, soup kitchens, or wherever the patient moves throughout the day. Success depends on close collaboration in the network of caregivers. In general, it is worth attempting the least restric-

tive method of medical treatment before enforcing it through involuntary commitment.

Selected Readings

Breakey, W. R. Mental Health Services for Homeless People. In M. J. Robertson and M. Greenblatt (eds.), *Topics in Social Psychiatry: Homelessness—A National Perspective*. New York: Plenum, 1992.

Breakey, W. R., et al. Health and mental health problems of homeless men and women in Baltimore. *J.A.M.A*. 262:1352, 1989.

Committee on Health Care for Homeless People, Institute of Medicine. *Homelessness, Health, and Human Needs*. Washington, D.C.: National Academy Press, 1988.

Fischer, P. J., et al. Mental health and social characteristics of the homeless: A survey of mission users. *Am. J. Public Health* 76:519, 1986.

Koegel, P., and Burnam, M. A. Problems in the Assessment of Mental Illness Among the Homeless: An Empirical Approach. In M. J. Robertson and M. Greenblatt (eds.), *Topics in Social Psychiatry: Homelessness—A National Perspective*. New York: Plenum, 1992.

Koegel, P., Burnam, A., and Farr, R. K. The prevalence of specific psychiatric disorders among homeless individuals in the inner city of Los Angeles. *Arch. Gen. Psychiatry* 45:1085, 1988.

Koegel, P., and Sherman, D. Assessment and Treatment of Homeless Mentally Ill Adults. In D. Wood (ed.), *Delivering Health Care to Homeless Persons: The Diagnosis and Management of Medical and Mental Health Conditions*. New York: Springer, 1992.

Wright, J. D., and Weber, E. *Homelessness and Health: Health, Health Policy, and the Nation's Homeless*. New York: McGraw-Hill, 1987.

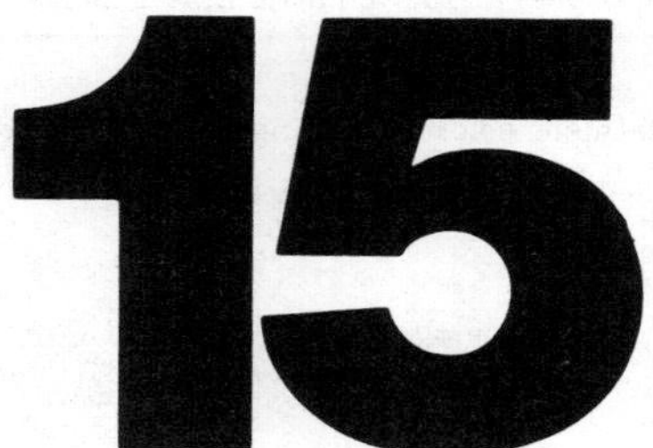

The Patient with Mental Retardation

Mark J. Hauser
John J. Ratey

I. **Mental retardation** (MR) refers to deficits in cognitive and adaptive functioning with onset during development. MR is not a specific diagnosis; there are diverse etiologies and in many cases the etiology is not known. MR is a persistent condition and therefore is not, by itself, a cause of emergency department visits. However, the presence of MR may make individuals vulnerable to environmental disruptions, and it complicates evaluation, management, and treatment planning whatever the acute intercurrent condition. When individuals with MR come to the emergency department there are special considerations to take into account, which are addressed in this chapter.

A. **Diagnosis.** In general, the mentally retarded person has substandard cognitive functioning as measured by an IQ test and substandard adaptive functioning in such spheres as interpersonal relationships, daily living skills (grooming, hygiene, dressing, self care, safety and self preservation), managing vocational and/or recreational aspects of life. Three criteria must be met for a **diagnosis of mental retardation.**

1. IQ (a measure of cognitive function based on verbal and performance measures) of 70 or below.
2. Deficits in adaptive functioning.
3. Onset of the disorder before age 18.

B. **Severity** is judged by the degree of cognitive dysfunction as measured by IQ.

1. Borderline intellectual functioning: IQ greater than 70.
2. Mild MR (85% of cases): IQ 50–55 to 70.
3. Moderate MR (10%): IQ 35–40 to 50–55.
4. Severe MR: (3.5%): IQ 20–25 to 35–40.
5. Profound MR (1.5%): IQ below 20–25.
6. Unspecified MR: Severity undetermined.

C. **Epidemiology**

1. **Prevalence.** Depending on whether mild MR is included, 1–3% of people have MR.
2. **Sex ratio.** MR is approximately 1.5 times more common in males than in females, possibly due to X-linked genetic conditions.

D. **Etiology**

1. There are over 250 known causes of retardation.
2. In only approximately 25% of people with MR is there a known biological cause; in the other 75% of cases, the cause is unknown or due to factors other than biological ones, such as psychosocial factors.

3. **Known etiologic factors** include:
   a. Chromosomal abnormalities.
   b. Genetic defects.
   c. Perinatal factors (e.g., anoxia).
   d. Acquired childhood diseases.
   e. Environmental factors (e.g., lead toxicity, psychosocial factors).

II. Approaching the patient with MR

A. There are many **misconceptions** about individuals with MR that may adversely affect care.

1. It is sometimes believed that people with MR cannot have mental illness; in fact they are vulnerable to the full range of mental illnesses.

2. Too often individuals with MR are treated as if they do not have normal feelings and emotions. Of course they do; they are capable of the full range of human emotions. They can be vulnerable and sensitive, and in the emergency setting they can be frightened.

3. It is sometimes thought that individuals with MR are not affected by changes in their environment. In fact, with a diminished capacity to understand what is happening to them, people with MR may have heightened reactions to such events as staff turnover or other changes in their residential or vocational programs, new housemates, or illnesses in family members. These are all stressors that can precipitate behavioral decompensation. Indeed, being evaluated in the emergency department is itself an event that can have dramatic behavioral consequences.

4. It may not be recognized that people with MR may have substance abuse problems, particularly with alcohol.

5. There is controversy over the use of antipsychotic drugs (neuroleptics) in people with MR. Some caretakers believe that these drugs should never be used. Of course antipsychotic drugs have serious side effects and their misuse or overuse (e.g., as a substitute for potentially effective psychosocial interventions) is poor practice. However, when prescribed appropriately (e.g., for psychotic disorders or for severe behavioral disturbances that fail to respond to less restrictive treatment modalities), antipsychotic drugs may have significant beneficial effects.

B. General approach to the patient and the patient's regular caregivers

1. Conducting the evaluation

a. **Evaluate the patient in a safe, private, quiet place.** Being observed and overheard by other patients and staff in the emergency department can be frightening, distracting, or overstimulating. Some individuals enjoy the attention they get for disruptive behaviors (e.g., throwing a tantrum), especially when other patients, families, and staff comprise an audience. Using a quiet and private place will enhance the evaluation. While noise and distractions are inevitable in the emergency setting, they complicate the assessment.

b. **Conduct the evaluation promptly.** The patient with MR may have a diminished capacity to cope with waiting. Having to wait may cause additional behavioral deterioration, which may make the subsequent evaluation and any intervention more difficult.

c. When possible, **invite familiar staff or family to keep the patient company;** their presence is likely to facilitate the evaluation. MR patients benefit from predictability; the presence of a familiar staff member may foster this. Even more important, the patient's regular caregivers will be needed to provide history.

d. Explain any procedures simply and clearly.

2. **Role of the psychiatrist**

a. In the approach to the patient with MR, the psychiatrist must use his or her training in both medicine and psychiatry. This is because **people with MR brought to the emergency department because of a behavioral disturbance or change in mental status may actually have an underlying medical or surgical problem** that has not previously been identified. The psychiatrist must then make appropriate medical or surgical referrals. However, a further role is often warranted: The psychiatrist may have to act as a representative for the patient—for example, helping other physicians understand the patient's behavior—so that the patient receives appropriate evaluation and treatment.

b. When the problem is behavioral rather than medical, it must be ascertained whether the patient has a primary psychiatric disorder or whether the problem has resulted from a change in the patient's environment. For example, if a patient is profoundly upset over placement with a new roommate, effective intervention requires attention to the living situation rather than simple administration of a sedative.

c. Whether the recommendation involves administration of a psychotropic medication, a change in the patient's living arrangement, or some other psychosocial intervention, the psychiatrist must not only take the acute problem into account but also the patient's relationship to long-term caregivers. Thus the psychiatrist must use an interdisciplinary team model, which is the model for most long-term care of individuals with MR.

3. **The concerns of the referring caregiver must be taken into account.**

a. It is useful to consider the context of the decision to seek emergency department consultation. Often, the decision is made when caregivers are "at the end of their rope" and feel as if they can no longer cope with the patient. Often the last thing that caretakers of mentally retarded individuals want is to involve medical personnel or a hospital in their client's care. They often have put an evaluation off until the problem is far advanced, and they come in grudgingly.

b. Despite their distrust of physicians and hospitals, caregivers may also have the expectation that the emergency department staff has miracle workers who will solve the problem, either by taking the patient off their hands or by telling them what to do. Such mixed feelings may lead to hostility and disappointment in the caregivers when problems are not magically solved. The psychiatrist must be aware of the possibility of such feelings and therefore avoid playing the role of magical rescuer. Even worse is saying that nothing can be done to help.

c. Long-term caregivers generally refer to individuals as clients rather than patients. It may be helpful to respect their terminology.

d. Although it is dangerous to generalize, **some characteristics of the caregivers who may be bringing in the patient are:**

(1) They have a deep involvement in the client's life and care a great deal about that client.

(2) They often have a philosophical (or ideological) perspective that medication is toxic and even poisonous.

(3) They may mistrust doctors.

(4) Often, their entire career—their *raison d'être*—is based on the desire to help their clients **without** medication and **without** involving psychiatry.

e. Some individuals with MR have been cared for by families rather than professional staff. Such individuals may need referrals for appropriate services.

III. The emergency evaluation

A. People with MR are brought to the emergency department for a variety of reasons:

1. A change in mental status—for example, confusion, agitation, or psychotic symptoms.
2. A change in mood, energy, or sleep patterns.
3. A change in behavior, such as a new onset of aggressive behavior toward others or self-destructive thoughts or behavior (e.g., head banging).
4. New physical complaints, such as pain, or behaviors, such as agitation, that might signify physical illness. Sorting out such problems can be extremely challenging. A normal person might say, "My stomach hurts," whereas a retarded person might become irritable and attack the staff when he or she has abdominal pain.

B. The "disappearing" problem. Often, the patient's behavior changes when brought to the emergency department. For example, if the patient was aggressive in his residence, by the time he arrives at the emergency department he might have calmed down. It is obviously difficult for the clinician to evaluate a behavior that is no longer in evidence. Indeed, in a busy emergency department, only acute problems get serious attention. The emergency staff may say, "Well, he's not aggressive anymore, so take him home." The regular caregivers may fear a return of the aggression, however. It is therefore important to assist these caregivers by evaluating the underlying problem, assessing the likelihood of a recurrence, and suggesting appropriate interventions.

C. Assessment of the problem

1. **A thorough history must be obtained,** including history from caregivers. Information must be obtained not only about the current problem and the events leading up to it but also about the patient's usual level of functioning.
2. **Medical illness must be ruled out.** This is especially important in mentally retarded individuals because of limitations in their capacity to communicate. However, people with MR frequently communicate by their behavior, such as increased irritability or impulsivity, or outbursts of aggression. Such behavioral change may represent constipation (perhaps the most common medical cause of agitation), a dental problem, a urinary tract or other infection, or other medical problem.
3. It is important to consider medication side effects as a possible cause of behavioral deterioration.

a. Benzodiazepines are commonly used as sedatives and hypnotics. Benzodiazepines with long half-lives (see Appendix III) may accumulate, especially in older individuals, and cause drowsiness and mental clouding. Short-acting benzodiazepines may cause interdose rebound symptoms, with marked worsening of anxiety just prior to scheduled doses (see Chap. 18). Inarticulate individuals with such side effects may cause a very confusing picture. In autistic individuals, benzodiazepines may cause ataxia.

b. **Anticonvulsants** may produce excessive sedation. Phenobarbital may be sedating; occasionally it may have paradoxical disinhibiting effects.

c. **Antipsychotic drugs.** Individuals with MR are prone to the same side effects as anyone else, such as parkinsonism and akathisia. It is particularly important to recognize akathisia because it can present as worsening agitation and lead to an unnecessary extensive workup. Even worse, misdiagnosis of akathisia may lead to an inappropriate increase in the neuroleptic dose. As with all patients, excessive doses of antipsychotic drugs can interfere with alertness and overall performance. Therefore it is important to maintain individuals with MR on the lowest possible dose of antipsychotic medication to control psychotic symptoms or target behaviors. Reducing dosages can lead to problems such as agitation, behavioral deterioration, and worsening of abnormal involuntary movements, which may represent transient withdrawal dyskinesias. Therefore dosage reductions must be slow and careful.

d. **Other medications,** easily forgotten in the history, may cause psychiatric symptoms. These include antihypertensive drugs, eyedrops for glaucoma (often beta-adrenergic blockers), and allergy medications (almost all anticholinergic).

4. It is important to conduct a **full physical examination.** This must be performed systematically and patiently. The presence of familiar staff may help calm the patient. In some emergencies, when a patient cannot comply with examination, sedation may be necessary.

5. Appropriate laboratory tests depend on the differential diagnosis.

IV. Treatment and disposition planning

A. Acute treatment considerations

1. Consider a need for changes in the patient's immediate environment. Are there addressable stressors that triggered the decompensation?

2. Assess the need for increased supervision of the individual's activities.

3. If necessary, suggest a consultation for behavioral management strategies; these are often designed to guide the actions of the staff.

4. Whatever psychosocial treatment recommendations are made, it is critical to promote consistency of staff behavior toward the patient and consistency of the patient's environment.

5. **Psychopharmacologic treatment** should be reserved for appropriate target disorders and syndromes.

   a. Medications should not be administered to the patient simply to diminish staff anxiety. In such cases skillful management of staff expectations are needed. For example, the clinician can acknowledge that it would be ideal to have a medication that would effectively treat these symptoms without producing serious side effects, but such a medication does not exist. It is important to address possible environmental causes of problem behaviors. This will help the staff recognize the context in which such behaviors occur and make appropriate adjustments rather than demanding inappropriate prescription of antipsychotic drugs.

   b. **The danger of prescribing antipsychotic drugs** for nonspecific sedation is that they will be continued indefinitely, resulting in serious side effects for the patient. If nonspecific sedation is clearly needed, short-term administration of a benzodiazepine is a better choice.

   c. Medications are often needed for longer-term treatment of depression, obsessive-compulsive disorder, psychotic disorders, and attention deficit disorder. In addition, pharmacologic treatment may be useful in treating certain symptoms that have not responded to reasonable environmental interventions. These circumstances include short-term treatment of sleep disturbances (e.g., with a benzodiazepine), treatment of impulsivity or aggression (e.g., with a series of empirical trials with buspirone, beta-adrenergic blockers, or carbamazepine), treatment of agitation (e.g., with a benzodiazepine), and treatment of self-injurious behavior. **In general, doses of medications for individuals with MR are no different from doses used for other individuals of the same size and age.**

B. Determination of responsibility for subsequent care. Most patients are already part of an existing caretaking system to which they can return. At times, the existing caretakers are not capable of caring for the person during the acute episode, so the emergency staff must help develop an alternative plan. Such a plan may include temporary acute hospitalization. However, appropriate acute treatment coupled with long-term treatment recommendations may make it possible for the individual to return to his or her prior environment.

1. Create a data collection mechanism to assist the patient's regular caregivers in observation, recording, and communication of pertinent information.
2. Recommend any additional appropriate tests.
3. Articulate triggers for follow-up either by telephone or a repeat visit to the emergency department.
4. If appropriate recommend a meeting with other clinicians involved in the person's care—for example, the primary care physician, residential caregivers, vocational and/or day program staff, medical specialists, and behavioral specialists.

V. Legal issues

A. Informed consent. The diagnosis of MR does not by itself imply that the retarded person cannot consent to his or her own treatment (see Chap. 10). However, in many cases the competence of the individual to consent may be impaired; in such cases there may already be a guardian or the establishment of guardianship may have to be considered. Competence must be assessed on a case by case basis. In the emergency setting, life-threatening problems warrant emergency treatment, even in the absence of informed consent. If someone is obviously not competent, a long-term caregiver or family member should be asked to consent to the evaluation and treatment.

B. Guardianship. When there is a legal guardian, authorization for evaluation and treatment must be obtained from the guardian except in the case of life-threatening emergencies.

C. Mandated reporting of abuse of disabled persons. Many states have statutes that require medical personnel to report a suspicion of abuse. Clinicians should become familiar with their own state's requirements, laws, guidelines, and standards of practice.

D. Consent decrees. Many states have entered into binding legal agreements as a result of lawsuits initiated by plaintiffs who wanted to improve the quality of care delivered to people with MR. These consent decrees may mandate specific degrees of quality of treatment. Again it is useful to become familiar with state requirements, laws, guidelines, and standards of practice.

Selected Readings

Gualtieri, C. T. *Neuropsychiatry and Behavioral Psychopharmacology.* New York: Springer, 1991.

Ratey, J. J. (ed.). *Mental Retardation: Developing Pharmacotherapies.* Washington, D.C.: American Psychiatric Association Press, 1991.

Sovner, R. (ed.). *The Habilitative Mental Healthcare Newsletter.* Psych-Media Inc.

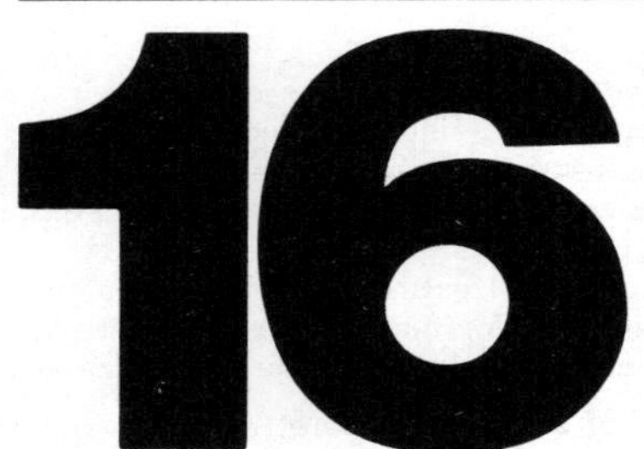

Psychiatric Emergency Repeaters

George E. Tesar

I. Repeat users of emergency services are well-known to both general and psychiatric emergency personnel.

A. Repeat users are glibly referred to as "regulars" or "frequent fliers," and the mention of a repeater's name often elicits eye-rolling, smirking, sighs of frustration, or unrestrained disparagement from clinicians familiar with the patient. Emergency or crisis staff focused on rapid evaluation, treatment, and referral of patients who are acutely ill or in crisis may find the repeater troublesome, particularly if the patient is hostile or help-rejecting. Frustration and resentment develop not only because the repeater seems to confound basic service goals but also because of the perception that repeaters consume more than their fair share of limited time, space, and personnel resources.

B. In fact, emergency psychiatric repeaters constitute a heterogeneous population composed of (1) patients in treatment who periodically need psychiatric emergency services, (2) patients beginning treatment for a new or recurrent episode of illness, (3) patients not in regular treatment who frequent the crisis center during time-limited crises, and (4) patients who seem to use the service as part of their social network. The purpose of this chapter is to assist the clinician in dealing with this diverse and sometimes difficult group of emergency psychiatric patients.

II. Definition. Most of the available data on emergency psychiatric repeaters have been gathered from studies that define repeaters as patients returning to a service more than once every 6–12 months (Ellison, et al., 1986); only a few studies have looked selectively at patients who repeat more frequently (Ellison, et al., 1989). Repeaters constitute 7–18% of emergency psychiatric patients and account for as many as one-half of total psychiatric emergency visits.

III. Characteristics. In general, repeaters are distinguished by a lack of social supports, chronic illness, past psychiatric treatment, and severe illness. These characteristics are associated with greater resistance to treatment and more difficulty tolerating or sticking with usual treatment methods. Current treatment status, visit frequency, and the primary service to which the repeater presents (i.e., either psychiatric or non-psychiatric) influence repeater characteristics and the types of problems repeaters present to the emergency department.

A. Treatment status

1. **Repeaters initiating treatment.** Some repeaters make frequent and generally appropriate use of an emergency department during initiation of treatment for either the first or a recurrent episode of illness. If the patient is not already in established outpatient treatment, then both scheduled and unscheduled visits to the crisis clinic can be used for stabilization until the first outpatient evaluation.

2. **Repeaters in treatment.** Patients in established outpatient psychiatric treatment typically require acute psychiatric services at the beginning or termination of treatment, when the therapist is unavailable, when there is

a change in the treatment plan, when the treatment is ineffective, or at the emergence of unbearable transference feelings.

a. When patients involved in outpatient psychotherapy present to the emergency department, the clinician should assume some disturbance of the psychotherapeutic relationship. In many instances, the outpatient therapist has become the single most important person in the patient's life.

b. When transference reactions overwhelm the coping abilities of a patient in regular psychodynamic psychotherapy, profound loneliness, guilt, anxiety, affective instability, dysfunctional behavior, and either suicidal or homicidal impulses may require acute psychiatric intervention. Therapist absence, empathic failure, negative countertransference reactions, or an unexpected adjustment of treatment may have precipitated the crisis. Such patients typically are being treated for either borderline, hystrionic, or narcissistic personality disorder (see Chap. 22) and are probably the highest-frequency users of walk-in and emergency psychiatric services.

c. Patients on psychotropic medication may present either for prescription refill or reevaluation of pharmacologic treatment. Repeated visits suggest either substance abuse (e.g., if the patient is in search of anxiolytic or analgesic medication), a ruptured outpatient therapeutic alliance, or inadequate or incorrect treatment. For example, the medicated schizophrenic who presents repeatedly in an agitated state may be suffering from unrecognized akathisia or may be receiving an inadequate dose of antidote (e.g., a benzodiazepine, beta-blocker, or anticholinergic agent). Similarly, the patient who returns repeatedly complaining of anxiety despite apparently therapeutic benzodiazepine treatment may be suffering from an atypical depression rather than an anxiety disorder.

3. Repeaters not in treatment. This subgroup of repeaters is perhaps the most troublesome for crisis and emergency clinicians.

a. Despite persistent efforts to engage these individuals in ongoing treatment, they either rely solely on the emergency department for their care (usually during crises), or are brought to the department involuntarily when they become dangerous to themselves or others.

b. These individuals are often victims of early and severe deprivation and abuse, or are compromised by cognitive dysfunction and impaired reality testing. They often have a history of severe interpersonal difficulties and engage in a sustained pattern of self-destructive behavior such as self-mutilation, low-risk suicide attempts, or chronic substance abuse.

c. Commonly characterized as help-rejecting, obnoxious, or demanding and prone to hostile interactions with caregivers, these patients test the patience, compassion, and skills of the most gifted clinicians. Typically, they pass from one treatment center to another, exhausting their welcome and their caregivers wherever they go.

B. Frequent visits. Ellison and colleagues identified **anxiety and impulsivity** as the predominant characteristics of repeaters who were seen six or more times during a six-month period in a busy urban psychiatric emergency service (Ellison, et al., 1989). Vulnerable to episodes of unbearable anxiety, these frequent repeaters used emergency visits, self-injury, alcohol abuse, or anxiolytic medication to discharge painful affect.

C. Primary service. Psychiatric emergency department repeaters differ in several respects from repeaters to nonpsychiatric emergency services. The nonpsychiatric repeaters are more often male and intoxicated or alcoholic, and less often hospitalized (Purdie, et al., 1981). Psychiatrists can become secondarily involved in the care of these patients when called to see an intoxicated individual who has made a suicidal threat or to see someone who has a concurrent psychiatric disorder.

D. Factors not related to repeater status. Although systematic studies of repeaters have found that homelessness, dangerousness (i.e., suicidality or homicidality), or substance abuse do not distinguish repeaters from one-time users of emergency psychiatric services, these characteristics may complicate the evaluation, treatment, and disposition of repeaters, leaving a lasting, often negative impression on the caregivers.

IV. Evaluation and treatment

A. General approach

1. For several reasons the clinician evaluating the repeater must guard against the tendency to perform a hurried and incomplete evaluation. Familiarity with an abusive patient may breed not only contempt, but complacence as well, resulting in failure to detect an acute injury, illness, or important change in the patient's usual mental state, especially if the patient is uncooperative, disorganized, or help-rejecting.

2. Ironically, clinicians quite familiar with the patient are often unfamiliar with his or her medical and psychiatric history. Fear of "opening Pandora's box," the need to limit visits in compliance with a strict treatment protocol (see sec. **C**), or being absorbed in the immediate clinical circumstances account for this phenomenon. "Problem patient rounds" (see sec. **E**) is one method of pooling information and familiarizing all caregivers with illuminating and relevant aspects of the patient's history. A brief, typed outline of this important data can be stapled to the back of the chart for easy reference.

3. A careful mental status examination, focusing on the performance of cognitive and executive functions, should be performed. Some patients (e.g., negative-symptom schizophrenics and patients with prefrontal cortical dysfunction) may have trouble maintaining regular contact with a therapist because of impaired attention, motivation, and planning skills. The clinician should perform tests that examine the patient's fund of information, abstraction ability, and mental flexibility (i.e., the ability to shift from one conceptual set to another). Useful clinical tests include having the patient draw a clock, having the patient perform an alternating sequence of movements such as the fist-side-palm test (ask the patient to repeatedly strike a surface, first with a fist, then with the side of the hand, and then with an open palm, repeating the sequence several times), or having the patient perform a visual pattern completion test. Formal neuropsychological testing may be indicated for those who exhibit perseveration or poor planning.

4. Every effort should be made to obtain potentially valuable and clarifying information from family members, associates, pharmacists, police, and other providers.

B. Crisis intervention with patients in treatment (see Chap. 2). For selected patients, the psychiatric emergency service can provide an important adjunct to the usual network of care. When the patient's needs outstrip the capabilities of the usual caregiver(s), the emergency service is available for 24-hour back-up care.

1. In the more neutral setting of the crisis clinic, a patient may find it easier to acknowledge intense feelings toward the outpatient therapist. The emergency psychiatric clinician can play an important supportive role by helping to defuse negative transference, clarifying distortions, and treating intense anxiety. Telephone consultation between the emergency clinician and the primary therapist can help clarify the nature of the transference or the

extent to which negative countertransference contributes to a therapeutic impasse.

2. When the patient experiences imminent loss of control or dangerous, suicidal, or homicidal impulses, the crisis service can serve as a protective holding environment. Temporary mechanical restraint may help the patient regain a sense of safety and control.

C. A **treatment protocol** may be necessary for the care and management of repeaters who are manipulative, help-rejecting, or violent or for patients who overuse the service for nonurgent or social reasons. Clinicians should be careful not to enforce protocols in a punitive or judgmental fashion, although one of the important goals and benefits of treatment protocols is the mitigation of clinician frustration and patient-directed rancor.

1. In general, treatment protocols help shape or modify inappropriate behavior by specifying the guidelines and limits of treatment. This is particularly useful for patients whose behavior is either threatening or disruptive. The patient's failure to abide by the protocol's guidelines results in predetermined consequences such as discharge from the service, termination of all care, or immediate hospitalization. For example, the patient who insists on carrying a weapon (e.g., a knife) may be required by protocol to leave all weapons at the hospital's security office before presenting for psychiatric evaluation; failure to do so would result in forfeiture of the right to be seen that day. Patients who are repeatedly physically or verbally threatening may be required to submit to mechanical restraints during any and all interviews.
2. A clearly written protocol available to all staff members standardizes and unifies the approach to patients who, through manipulation or the defense of splitting, elicit a fragmented approach to their evaluation and care.
3. The treatment protocol also helps focus the disorganized or circumstantial patient and minimize expectations for unlimited treatment.
4. For the patient who presents repeatedly with unfocused requests, one approach is to permit no more than 15–20 minutes per visit and no more than one visit per day. The patient's failure to comply with the protocol can be interpreted as signifying a need for more intensive care on either an inpatient or crisis stabilization unit.
5. By defining and clarifying the type of treatment to be dispensed, the treatment protocol minimizes the likelihood of disappointment and frustration for both the patient and the clinician.

D. While the thrust of most treatment protocols is to make crisis evaluation and treatment contingent on appropriate behaviors, there are some patients who are simply unable to comply without endangering or compromising their health status.

1. In those unusual circumstances where all other approaches, including hospitalization, treatment protocols, and therapeutic limit setting, have failed to control inappropriate or dangerous behavior, the crisis center may be the only place capable of administering necessary treatment to the repeater.
2. It is important that latent frustration and anger at such patients be dealt with in a professional manner. Adopting an attitude of resignation and acceptance may help caregivers tolerate and acquiesce to the care of such patients.
3. Presumably unable to tolerate the closeness of a regular therapeutic relationship, these patients are best dealt with in a simple, concrete, problem-solving manner.

E. As noted above, another method of unifying the approach to care of repeaters is **problem-patient rounds** (Santy and Wehmeier, 1984). Conducted on a regular or ad hoc basis, such an approach allows caregivers to develop a uniform care plan and to ventilate their feelings of frustration and anger at noncompliers, hypochondriacs, dependent patients, malingerers, and entitled demanders who frequent the service.

F. Communication with other caregivers is essential when repeaters use multiple services. Interagency communication reduces the confounding effects of splitting, distortion, and lying and increases the likelihood of rapid and accurate problem formulation.

Selected Readings

Bassuk, E., and Gerson, S. Chronic crisis patients: A discrete clinical group. *Am. J. Psychiatry* 137:1513, 1980.

Ellison, J. M., Blum, N., and Barsky, A. J. Repeat visitors in the psychiatric emergency service: A critical review of the data. *Hosp. Community Psychiatry* 37:37, 1986.

Ellison, J. M., Blum, N., and Barsky, A. J. Frequent repeaters in a psychiatric emergency service. *Hosp. Community Psychiatry* 40:958, 1989.

Mannon, J. M. Defining and treating "problem patients" in a hospital emergency room. *Medical Care* 14:1004, 1976.

Munves, P. I., Trimboli, F., and North, A. J. A study of repeat visits to a psychiatric emergency room. *Hosp. Community Psychiatry* 34:634, 1983.

Purdie, F. R. J., Honigman, B., and Rosen, P. The chronic emergency department patient. *Ann. Emerg. Med.* 10:292, 1981.

Raphling, D. L., and Lion, J. Patients with repeated admissions to a psychiatric emergency service. *Community Ment. Health J.* 6:313, 1970.

Santy, P. A., and Wehmeier, P. K. Using "problem patient" rounds to help emergency room staff manage difficult patients. *Hosp. Community Psychiatry* 35:494, 1984.

Slaby, A. E., and Perry, P. L. Use and abuse of psychiatric emergency services. *Int. J. Psychiatry Med.* 10:1, 1980–81.

Ungerleider, J. T. The psychiatric emergency. *Arch. Gen. Psychiatry* 3:593, 1960.

Emergency Evaluation and Treatment of Major Psychiatric Disorders

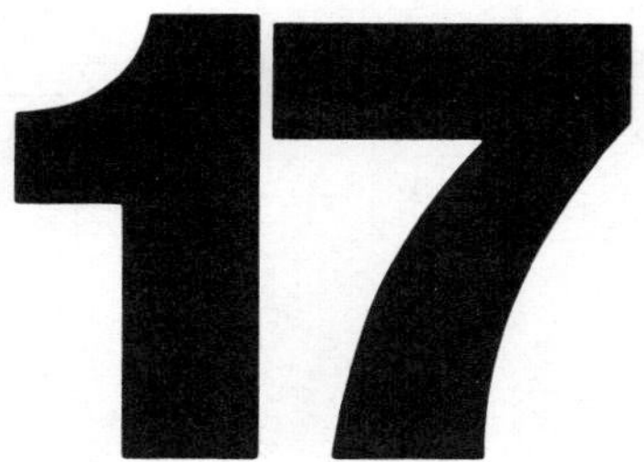

Depression

Paul J. Barreira

I. **Depression** is among the most common conditions clinicians have to evaluate in emergency settings. When a patient who is depressed also experiences suicidal impulses, a life-threatening crisis may result. The distinction between sad mood and clinical depression is not always clear. The clinician must be able to distinguish depression from normal sadness, response to loss, disappointment, normal grief, drug reactions, and response to a chronic illness. The distinction is important because depression, if left untreated, is associated with significant morbidity and mortality and is frequently recurrent. **Major depression** refers to a psychiatric syndrome characterized by depressed mood and neurovegetative symptoms and signs of significant duration. The clinician's task in the emergency department is to determine whether depression or another major psychiatric disorder is present and to initiate appropriate treatment based on that assessment. Of particular importance in emergency assessment is the need to distinguish between primary mood disorders and organic mood syndromes and disorders. Assessment and diagnosis of depression is made by evaluating the following:

   A. Clinical presentation (including mental status).

   B. History of the present illness.

   C. Past psychiatric history (diagnoses, if properly made, are stable over a lifetime).

   D. Family history (including both a history of psychiatric illness in biological relatives and an evaluation of the family's ability to care for the patient).

   E. Medical history (including use of prescribed and nonprescribed drugs).

   F. Physical examination and appropriate laboratory studies.

II. **Clinical presentation.** Although opinion varies about the subclassification of depressions, there is general agreement about the signs and symptoms that characterize depression (Table 17-1).

   A. **Symptoms.** The most common symptoms of a depressive disorder are depressed mood, loss of interest in usual pursuits, and anxiety. The next most common are sleep disturbance, loss of appetite, lack of energy, and inability to concentrate. As the depression becomes more severe, feelings of guilt, suicidal thoughts, and psychotic symptoms (delusions or hallucinations) may appear. Some clinicians prefer the term *dysphoric mood* to *depressed mood* because patients often complain of feeling irritable, fearful, worried, discouraged, or frustrated rather than sad or despondent. Some patients will not even identify mood change as the primary problem but will focus on disturbances in behavior or thought such as memory loss, inability to concentrate, lack of self-confidence, or lack of self-esteem. Some patients will focus on physical complaints such as low energy, poor sleep, or a variety of somatic complaints such as headache, abdominal pain, or joint pain; such complaints are common in the elderly. In general, symptoms are more severe, more numerous, and of longer duration as the depression worsens.

Table 17-1. Clinical presentation of depression

Psychologic symptoms
Depression, feeling sad or blue
Anxiety
Irritability
Loss of interests
Anhedonia
Withdrawal from friends and family
Guilt
Hopelessness
Feelings of helplessness or worthlessness
Hypochondriacal preoccupations
Rumination, obsessive thoughts
Poor concentration
Poor memory
Suicidal thoughts
Psychotic thoughts such as delusions or hallucinations
Vegetative symptoms
Decreased energy
Sleep disturbance
Appetite disturbance
Decreased libido
Diurnal variation in mood
Constipation
Signs
Depressed affect
Tearful, sad, or anxious expression
Slowed speech, no spontaneous comments, prolonged lag before responding
Psychomotor retardation
Psychomotor agitation such as pacing, wringing hands, picking at self

B. Signs of depression. The major sign of depression is a depressed affect. This may be subtle and at times noticed by the clinician only because he or she begins to feel sad while talking to the patient. As depression worsens there may also be psychomotor changes, usually retardation, with slow movements, slow speech, and a long latency before the patient answers questions. Conversely, some patients may be agitated, with motor restlessness and rapid speech. These patients are usually anxious and irritable rather than sad.

C. Laboratory tests. There are no tests sensitive or specific enough to be useful in routine clinical diagnosis. Approximately 50% of patients with a major depressive syndrome will have abnormal responses to 1 mg of dexamethasone (a 4 P.M. or 11 P.M. serum cortisol > 5 μg/100 ml after receiving 1 mg of dexamethasone at 11 P.M. on the previous night). This test takes 2 days to complete and is normal in half of the patients who have major depression; therefore it is not generally helpful in decision making.

D. Suicide is a danger in patients with depression; thus, the clinician must evaluate all depressed patients for their risk of suicide (see Chap. 4). Suicidal intent may come on acutely, especially if the patient is psychotic, but patients will usually first describe feeling that life is not worth living. Then they may wish that they would never wake up or that they would die in an accident. Eventually they become preoccupied with death and begin to think of suicide. It appears that the period of risk for individuals with an acute depressive episode continues for weeks to months after their depressive symptoms begin to improve. Among

Table 17-2. Classification of mood disorders

Mood disorders
- Bipolar disorders
  - Bipolar disorder
  - Cyclothymia
  - Atypical bipolar disorders
- Depressive disorders
  - Major depression
    - Single episode
    - Recurrent depressive episodes can be characterized as:
      - Mild, moderate, or severe with psychotic features
      - Seasonal pattern
  - Dysthymia (depressive neurosis)
  - Atypical depressive disorders

Organic mental disorders
- Organic mood disorders

Adjustment disorders
- Adjustment disorder with depressed mood

Conditions not attributable to a mental disorder
- Uncomplicated bereavement

patients who are bipolar, there is greater risk during the period of switching from mania to depression. Other characteristics associated with high suicide risk include advanced age, male sex, white race, widowed or divorced, poor physical health, alcoholism, social isolation, previous suicide attempts, and a family history of suicide. The lifetime suicide rate is 15% in patients with recurrent depressions.

E. **The role of precipitating stressors** in the pathogenesis of depressed episodes is controversial. Apart from grief reactions and adjustment disorders, which are, by definition, precipitated by a stress, it is not clear if stressors play a significant role in the onset of major depressive episodes. Depressed patients may or may not identify events they consider to be precipitants for their illness. When a presumed precipitating event is described, it often seems minor. Moreover, careful questioning may show that the alleged precipitating event was preceded by symptoms of depression that were unrecognized. Therefore the clinician should not depend on the presence or absence of a precipitating event to determine the etiology of a major depressive disorder.

III. **Subtypes of depression.** Once the presence of a depressive syndrome is identified, a more specific diagnosis should be made. Significant controversy exists regarding classification of depression, and no single classification system is universally recognized. The current standard for classification in the United States is the *Diagnostic and Statistical Manual of Mental Disorders, Fourth Edition, Draft Criteria* (DSM-IV). Its classification of depressive syndromes is summarized in Table 17-2. The mood disorders are functional psychiatric disorders (i.e., disorders with no apparent organic cause), which are divided into two main groups: bipolar disorders and depressive disorders. Depressions judged to stem from organic brain disease are placed in a separate category of organic mood disorders. A reactive depression that seems to be attributable to a particular stressor and that remits in response to resolution of the stress is termed an adjustment disorder with depressed mood. (This should be considered a diagnosis of exclusion.) Finally, DSM-IV makes provision for a diagnosis of uncomplicated bereavement. The following is a guide to diagnosing depressive syndromes:

A. Major depression

1. Clinical manifestations

a. As outlined above, dysphoric mood is a characteristic feature of this syndrome. The dysphoric mood is usually described as depressed, sad, or blue, but may be characterized as not caring anymore or a lack of pleasure. Other symptoms may include irritability, anger, or anxiety. These affective symptoms dominate the clinical picture and are relatively persistent.

b. DSM-IV requires the presence of at least five of the following nine symptoms including at least one of the first two for a period of at least 2 weeks; symptoms must be present nearly every day.

(1) Depressed mood.

(2) Decreased interest or pleasure.

(3) Significant weight change without dieting.

(4) Insomnia or hypersomnia.

(5) Psychomotor agitation or retardation.

(6) Fatigue or loss of energy.

(7) Feelings of worthlessness or extreme guilt.

(8) Decreased ability to think or concentrate.

(9) Suicidal ideation.

c. The diagnosis of organic affective disorders, adjustment reaction, bereavement, and other psychotic disorders must be ruled out.

d. Patients may have delusions, hallucinations, or bizarre behavior. If these symptoms are present in the absence of mood disturbance, however, another diagnosis, such as schizophrenia, should be entertained.

e. The presence or absence of a presumed precipitating event is not critical to the diagnosis.

f. The onset of a major depressive episode is variable; symptoms usually develop slowly over weeks to months but may develop suddenly.

g. In women there may be increased risk within 6 months postpartum or in the perimenopausal period.

h. Major depression is more common in women than in men.

i. It is crucial to obtain a history of any medications the patient has been taking (see sec. **III.A.5**). The physician has to be mindful of the side effects of neuroleptics. Neuroleptic-induced akinesia and akathisia may be clinically indistinguishable from the psychomotor changes of depression.

2. Past psychiatric history

a. Since it is estimated that approximately 50% of individuals with a single major depressive episode will experience a second episode, a history of prior depression helps confirm the diagnosis.

b. Major depressive episodes appear to occur more often in individuals with a history of drug dependence, cyclothymic and dysthymic disorders, anxiety disorders (especially those with panic attacks), and chronic physical illness.

3. Family history

a. Patients with family histories positive for major depression or bipolar

Table 17-3. Organic etiologies of depression

Drug-induced	Neurologic disorders
Reserpine	Multiple sclerosis
Beta-adrenergic blockers	Subdural hematoma
Methyldopa	Frontal tumors
Guanethidine	Parkinson's disease
Levodopa	Syphilis
Oral contraceptives	Stroke
Corticosteroids	Epilepsy
Alcohol	Huntington's disease
Anticholinesterases	Early dementias
Benzodiazepines	Infections
Neuroleptics	Mononucleosis
Ranitidine, cimetidine	Hepatitis
Endocrine disorders	Influenza
Hypo- and hyperthyroidism	Nutritional disorders
Hypo- and hyperadrenocorticalism	Vitamin B_{12} deficiency
Hyperparathyroidism	Folate deficiency
Diabetes mellitus	Pellagra
Tumors	Electrolyte disturbances
Carcinoma of pancreas and lung	Hyponatremia
Brain tumors	Hypokalemia
	Hypercalcemia
	Other disorders
	Turner's syndrome
	Psychostimulant withdrawal

disorder have an increased incidence of major depression. There is some evidence that familial major depression is associated with onset early in life.

b. Other risk factors for depression apparently include early parental death and childhood experiences in a chaotic and generally negative environment.

c. Alcoholic patients often develop secondary depression, but current evidence suggests that familial depression and familial alcoholism are genetically distinct.

4. **The mental status examination** is usually remarkable for depressed mood and affect; thoughts of guilt, helplessness, worthlessness, and hopelessness may be present. There is often somatic concern; there may be suicidal ideas and urges. There may be psychomotor retardation or agitation.

5. **Medical history and physical examination.** The diagnosis of major depression should be made only after other known medical causes of depression have been ruled out (Table 17-3).

B. Bipolar disorder, depressed phase

1. **Clinical manifestations.** There are no differences in the clinical presentation of a depressed episode between unipolar and bipolar patients.

   a. A large number of these patients will describe a hypomanic or manic period immediately preceding the development of a major depressive episode.

   b. In contrast to major depression, bipolar disorder is equally common in men and women.

2. **Past psychiatric history.** By definition, patients with bipolar disorder who have a major depressive episode have a previous history of at least one manic episode (see Chap. 20 for the necessary criteria to diagnose a manic episode).

3. **Family history.** Individuals with bipolar disorder have a high rate of first-degree relatives with either bipolar disorder or unipolar depression compared with the general population.

4. **Mental status examination**

   a. Mental status is indistinguishable from patients with unipolar major depression.

   b. One particularly difficult differential diagnostic problem occurs in distinguishing a major depressive episode with psychomotor agitation from what is called *dysphoric mania* (a stage of mania in which the patient is no longer euphoric but instead is predominantly irritable, paranoid, or frightened). This differentiation is not always possible to make on the basis of mental status alone. Usually, however, the physician can make the diagnosis on the basis of the course of the episode. The dysphoric manic patient often gives a history of progression of symptoms from typically euphoric hypomania or mania to a state of increased agitation, dysphoric mood, and paranoia. The distinction is a crucial one, because the administration of antidepressants to any manic patient may worsen symptoms markedly.

5. **Medical history and physical examination.** As for unipolar depressives, a major depressive episode should be diagnosed only after known medical causes have been ruled out (see Table 17-3).

C. **Dysthymic disorder** has previously been called neurotic depression or depressive personality. It is important to distinguish these patients from those with major depression because they are less likely to respond to any pharmacologic interventions unless an episode of major depression is superimposed on the more chronic disorder.

1. **Clinical manifestations**

   a. Individuals with dysthymic disorder have depressive symptoms that are not of sufficient severity or duration to meet the criteria for a major depressive episode.

   b. Psychotic symptoms are absent in dysthymic disorder.

   c. As defined by DSM-IV, dysthymic disorder is a chronic condition that has been present for at least 2 years. Individuals describe persistent depressed mood or loss of interest or pleasure in almost any activity, although there may be short periods of normal mood lasting a few days to weeks. The diagnosis should not be made if the chronic course has been interrupted by a period of normal mood lasting more than a few months.

   d. Individuals usually describe mild to moderate impairment in social and occupational functioning due to the chronicity rather than the severity of the depressive symptoms. Frequently individuals come to the physician or emergency department because of significant stress in their personal or work life that exacerbates the depressed feelings. Substance abuse may also lead to a crisis.

   e. Onset of symptoms is usually early in adult life. Women are affected more often than men.

   f. At times, the severity and duration of the depressive symptoms meet criteria for a major depressive episode. In that case, both diagnoses may be entertained.

2. **Past psychiatric history**

   a. Individuals with dysthymic disorder may describe a history of a conduct disorder in childhood or attention deficit disorder in childhood or adolescence.

   b. Patients may give histories of chronic feelings of inadequacy, low self-esteem, emptiness, or boredom.

3. **Family history**

   a. In contrast to major depression and bipolar disorder, there is little evidence that this disorder is familial.

   b. Individuals may report loss of parents at an early age, multiple losses, and a hostile family environment.

4. **The mental status examination** may reveal depressed mood and affect, thoughts of helplessness, worthlessness, and hopelessness. These patients may express suicidal ideation. They do not have psychomotor changes or psychotic symptoms unless there is a superimposed disorder or intoxication.

D. **Cyclothymic disorder** resembles bipolar disorder, but the mood swings are less severe. Patients with this disorder may benefit from an extended trial of lithium carbonate, but lithium does not work rapidly enough to be useful in emergency situations.

1. **Clinical manifestations**

   a. Individuals with cyclothymic disorder show a chronic mood disturbance characterized by numerous periods of depression and elevated mood, but not of sufficient severity or duration to meet the criteria for major depressed or manic episodes.

   b. Psychotic symptoms are not present with cyclothymic disorder.

   c. Substance abuse is a frequent problem and may confuse the evaluation of symptoms.

   d. The disorder usually begins early in adult life. DSM-IV requires that symptoms be of at least 2 years' duration with no more than 2-month periods of remission.

   e. Individuals may describe impairment of social and work functioning.

   f. Periods of depressed and elevated mood may be separated by periods of normal mood lasting from several weeks to two months.

2. **Past psychiatric history.** There is no clear association with other psychiatric syndromes.

3. **Family history.** Bipolar disorder and major depression are more common among family members of individuals with cyclothymic disorder than in the general population.

E. **Atypical depression** or depression not otherwise specified is a residual category for individuals with depressive symptoms who cannot be diagnosed as having any specific affective syndrome or adjustment disorder.

F. **Organic affective illness** (see Table 17-3).

1. **Clinical manifestations**

   a. Symptoms and mental status are characteristic of major depression and may even include psychotic symptoms.

   b. Symptoms of delirium and dementia are usually absent.

c. The characteristics of the history vary with the causative factors. For example, in the case of depression caused by a drug, the onset of symptoms is temporally related to the use of the medication. In some cases, however, such as with methyldopa (Aldomet), depressive symptoms may occur weeks to months after initiating the drug.

d. The onset of depressive symptoms caused by medical illness (e.g., pancreatic cancer) may be insidious; the depressive symptoms may even dominate the early clinical picture.

e. When depression is due to an endocrine disorder, other endocrine symptoms are usually present, although they may be subtle (as in thyroid disorders in the elderly).

2. **Past psychiatric history.** Whether individuals with a history of functional affective disorders are more vulnerable to depression of organic etiologies is unknown. If correction of suspected organic factors does not result in the remission of the depressive syndrome, antidepressant therapy should be strongly considered.

3. **Mental status** may not differ from functional depression.

4. **Medical history and physical examination.** In most cases of organic affective disorders it is possible to identify the etiologic event from the history, physical examination, or laboratory tests (see Table 17-3). Every patient should receive a physical examination; laboratory tests should be ordered when the history or physical examination suggests a possible organic condition.

G. **Uncomplicated bereavement** (see Chap. 6, sec. **III**)

1. **Clinical manifestations**

a. A normal grief reaction often has symptoms identical to those of a major depressive episode.

b. Guilt associated with bereavement usually focuses on things not done by the survivor for the deceased.

c. Thoughts of death focus on a wish to join the person who died or the wish to have died in his or her place.

d. Most bereaved individuals have fewer symptoms than patients with major depression.

e. Patients with normal grief do not experience psychotic symptoms.

2. **Past psychiatric history.** An apparently abnormal grief reaction may be associated with a past history of a major psychiatric disorder.

H. **Adjustment disorder with depressed mood**

1. **Clinical manifestations**

a. Patients usually exhibit a depressed mood associated with feelings of hopelessness, helplessness, worthlessness, and anxiety. Sleep and appetite disturbances are often present. Although the symptom picture does not usually meet criteria for major depressive disorder, the initial clinical presentation may be quite similar to major depressive disorder

b. Symptoms are severe enough to interfere with work and social functioning. Psychotic symptoms are not present.

c. During the interview these patients frequently respond well to reassurance.

d. By definition, symptoms occur within 3 months of a clearly definable stress. Stressors may include marital discord, divorce, business crisis, illness, or retirement.

e. The severity of the stress often does not predict the severity of the reaction.

f. The duration of symptoms is usually weeks to months. The maladaptive reaction improves either when the stressor is removed or the individual finds a better coping mechanism.

2. Past psychiatric history. Individuals with other major psychiatric disorders (including personality disorders and substance abuse) may be more vulnerable to stress.

IV. Emergency management of depression. Once a depressive episode has been identified and a more specific diagnosis has been made, the clinician must initiate appropriate treatment. This section is essentially intended to aid in the care of the more severely depressed patients—those who will almost certainly satisfy the diagnostic criteria for major depression or bipolar disorder (depressed phase). Patients with dysthymic disorder, the depressed phase of cyclothymic disorder, and adjustment reactions should also be managed according to the principles set out in secs. **A** and **C.** However, they are not likely to require medication while in the emergency department and are likely to need hospitalization only if they express serious thoughts of suicidality or self-destructiveness. All patients with major depression require treatment beyond the emergency visit. Although therapeutic approaches should be individualized for each patient, the major issues in emergency management include: psychologic management, medication, and disposition.

A. Psychologic management. All patients suffering from a major depressive episode, regardless of diagnostic type, require careful psychologic management. The clinician should communicate with the patient in a clear, empathic, and hopeful manner. Many patients will feel some relief when the clinician successfully communicates that he or she understands the patient's problem and the patient realizes that help is forthcoming. Patients may express the feeling that they do not deserve help or that they are reluctant to accept help. This attitude is a frequent symptom of depression. During the interview the clinician should try to establish a trusting relationship that will facilitate the patient's cooperation in participating in the proposed treatment.

1. Since many patients suffering from depression experience significant stresses prior to the evaluation, it may help the patient to identify these stresses and provide realistic reassurance that they are manageable. Particularly with depressed patients who do not meet diagnostic criteria for major depression, supportive psychotherapy can be the most useful intervention. The tasks of supportive psychotherapy include identifying the problem, maintaining an attitude of interest and concern, offering explanations and advice, and setting realistic goals. Although supportive therapy usually requires a number of sessions, many patients significantly improve in a single interview with clarification of the problem and the identification of specific options to resolve the problem.

2. It often helps to remind patients who, in the midst of their depression, feel as if the depression will never end, that, in fact, within a reasonable time they will feel better.

3. If a patient is severely depressed, agitated, or psychotic, it may be impossible to have a conversation. In this case the clinician must take charge and present to the patient a well-organized plan that has family support.

4. Whenever possible, family members or friends should be included both in the assessment of the patient and the treatment. Families often present more detailed and accurate historical information than the depressed patient because the latter may be too forgetful, agitated, or psychotic to give

a good history. It is also critical to disposition planning for the clinician to obtain an impression of the family's ability to support, supervise, and encourage the patient if he or she returns home. The decision to hospitalize a patient is often based on the quality of support available to the patient at home rather than solely on the severity of symptoms. Even patients with some psychotic or suicidal symptoms can be managed at home if the family is supportive, consistent, nonthreatening, and reliable. Finally, the clinician may identify conflicts in family members that are exacerbating, if not causing, the patient's depression. Patients who live alone or who are involved in hostile relationships are more likely to require hospitalization since they lack a source of social support and encouragement.

5. If the patient is already in treatment, the therapist should be contacted. The therapist may have important information about the patient's clinical status, need for medication, and past treatment history.

B. Somatic treatments

1. Antidepressants (see Appendix II). Although antidepressant medication is effective in the treatment of major depression, the delayed onset of therapeutic response and significant side effects limit its use in emergency management of depression. The problems with side effects are particularly marked with elderly patients, who are sensitive to anticholinergic toxicity (e.g., confusion or urinary retention: see Chap. 24) and orthostatic hypotension, even on low doses of tricyclic antidepressants. In addition, because of the potential for a lethal overdose if the patient is suicidal, close supervision of the patient by the physician is necessary. Despite these limitations, a large number of antidepressants are available to treat major depression. Given these limitations, however, especially the possibility of overdose, antidepressants should be started only with the knowledge and consent of the physician who will be following the patient. These drugs should never be prescribed unless reliable follow-up can be arranged. In addition, in emergency situations, only the number of pills required until the next appointment should be prescribed.

Efficacy, side effects, and potential lethality are the critical factors in choosing an antidepressant agent. In general, most of the commonly used antidepressants have similar efficacy in treating major depression. The most important side effects to consider include anticholinergic effects, postural hypotension, sedation, decreased seizure threshold, dietary interactions (such as with monoamine oxidase inhibitors [MAOIs]) and cardiac toxicity. The cyclic antidepressants vary in their ability to cause sedation, postural hypotension, and anticholinergic activity (see Appendix II). In contrast, all tricyclic and related cyclic antidepressants appear to possess equivalent cardiac toxicity at therapeutic doses. Acute overdoses of more than 1 g of tricyclic and related cyclic antidepressants are usually toxic and may be lethal due to central nervous system toxicity, cardiac arrhythmias, or hypotension.

Newer antidepressants unrelated to the tricyclics or MAOIs offer significantly different side effect profiles. Fluoxetine (Prozac), sertraline (Zoloft), and paroxetine (Paxil)—highly selective serotonin reuptake inhibitors (SSRIs)—produce no cardiac toxicity, usually are not sedating, and have minimal anticholinergic or postural hypotension effects. Fluoxetine, the most widely used of these compounds, may cause agitation, insomnia, nausea, headache, and diarrhea. One significant advantage of the SSRIs are their low lethality even when large quantities are ingested acutely. Bupropion (Wellbutrin), a phenylethylamine compound, has been reported to possess stimulatory effects, presumably due to its structural similarity to amphetamine. It does not significantly affect cardiac conduction, nor does it possess significant anticholinergic properties or a tendency to produce postural hypotension. Bupropion has been associated with a significant risk of seizures, 0.4% compared to 0.1% for other antidepressants. Due to the seizure risk, daily doses of bupropion should not exceed 450 mg per day, with individual doses not to exceed 150 mg every 6 hours. Bupropion must be considered highly lethal if taken as an overdose due to its significant seizure potential. At present the only other antidepressant agent that might be prescribed in an emergency department is trazodone (Desyrel). Trazodone may cause sedation, postural hypotension, nausea, and vomiting. It has little anticholinergic activity and minor effects on cardiac conduction. Unlike other antidepressants, trazodone has caused priapism. Trazodone has the advantage of being relatively safe even if taken in overdose. However, there is no consensus among clinicians that trazodone is as effective as other agents. Because of the complexity of their use, MOAIs should not be started in an emergency department.

2. **Benzodiazepines** have a role only in the acute treatment of anxiety and insomnia associated with depression. They should be prescribed only for a short time. One must be alert to the possibility of drug dependence. Alprazolam is a benzodiazepine that may have antidepressant properties, but it is associated with both physical and psychologic withdrawal syndromes that are more frequent and severe than those following treatment with other benzodiazepines. Other benzodiazepines have the potential for exacerbating depressive symptoms.

3. **Neuroleptics** are used in the treatment of major depressive episodes that are accompanied by delusions and hallucinations. They are used in such settings in combination with tricyclic antidepressants. In the emergency setting the neuroleptic may be started first in patients who are delusional and agitated. Since antidepressants will also be required, the clinician should choose a neuroleptic with a low level of anticholinergic effects, such as haloperidol.

4. **Electroconvulsive therapy** (ECT) should be considered for patients suffering from serious depressions characterized by refusal to eat, severe agitation or retardation, mutism, or severe suicidality; for patients with medical contraindications to antidepressant medications (especially cardiac conduction disturbances); and for patients who have failed to respond to adequate trials of antidepressant medications. Despite its unfavorable reputation with the general public, ECT may be the most effective and safe form of treatment for depression. Temporary short-term memory loss is the most troublesome side effect; this can be minimized by delivering unilateral shock to the nondominant cerebral hemisphere. The only absolute contraindication to ECT is increased intracranial pressure. Patients who require ECT should usually be hospitalized.

C. **Disposition.** In most cases the resolution of a major depressive episode, even with the administration of antidepressants, takes weeks. Therefore the clinician must plan for treatment beyond the emergency visit. Usually the first decision the clinician makes is whether the patient should be treated as an outpatient or in a hospital. If, for example, the patient is already followed by a psychiatrist who agrees to continue seeing the patient and a supportive social environment exists, the patient can be discharged home. If, however, a patient has a chronic, unresponsive depression and the family and patient feel demoralized and frustrated, hospitalization may be indicated.

1. Indications for **hospitalization** include

   a. A high risk of suicide (see Chap. 4).

   b. Lack of reliable social supports (if the depression is severe).

   c. History of previous poor response to treatment.

d. Symptoms so severe that the patient requires constant observation and nursing care.

e. Depression with psychotic symptoms, especially if associated with suicidal ideation or attempt.

If the patient is judged to be suicidal but denies it or refuses treatment, civil commitment may be necessary.

2. If the patient is not admitted to a hospital, the clinician must arrange for **follow-up care.** This should include a confirmed appointment within a short time after the emergency evaluation and referral to a psychiatrist for follow-up psychopharmacology if the patient has a therapist who is not a physician. It is always best to be able to give the name of the person and the time of the appointment to the patient and the family.

Selected Readings

American Psychiatric Association Task Force on DSM-IV. *Diagnostic and Statistical Manual of Mental Disorders, Fourth Edition, Draft Criteria:* 3/1/93. Washington, D.C.: American Psychiatric Association.

Arana, G. W., and Hyman, S. E. *Handbook of Psychiatric Drug Therapy* (2nd ed.). Boston: Little, Brown, 1991.

Goodwin, D. W., and Guze, S. B. *Psychiatric Diagnosis* (4th ed.). New York: Oxford University Press, 1989.

Keller, M. B., Lavori, P. W., Rice, J., et al. The persistent risk of chronicity and recurrent episodes of non-bipolar major depressive disorder: A prospective follow-up. *Am. J. Psychiatry* 143:24, 1986.

Weissman, M. M., Leaf, P. J., Bruce, M. L., et al. The epidemiology of dysthymia in five communities: Rates, risks, comorbidity, and treatment. *Am. J. Psychiatry* 145:815, 1988.

Winokur, G., Black, D. W., and Nasrallah, A. Depressions secondary to other psychiatric disorders and medical illnesses. *Am. J. Psychiatry* 154:233, 1988.

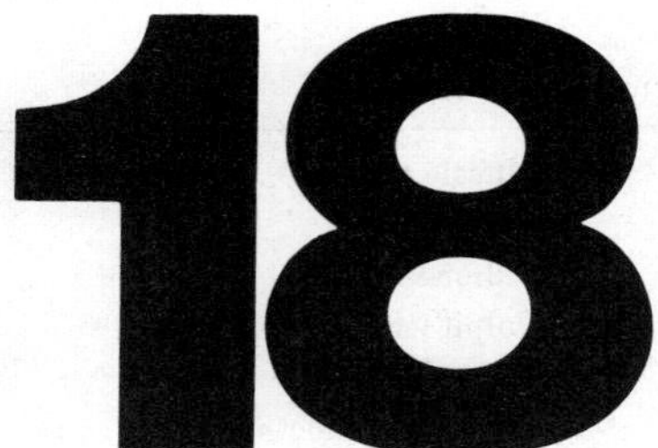

The Anxious Patient

George E. Tesar
Jerrold F. Rosenbaum

I. Anxiety is a nonspecific symptom that has diverse causes as well as diverse clinical manifestations.

A. The clinician must address three fundamental questions about the **etiology** of anxiety:

1. Is it **situational?**
2. Is it due to a **primary anxiety disorder?**
3. Is it **secondary** to another disorder?

B. The answers to these questions will influence **treatment** selection. Some acutely anxious patients may benefit temporarily from reassurance and the opportunity to verbalize their feelings and concerns. Others require a treatment program that includes psychotherapeutic, psychopharmacologic, and/or behavioral modalities.

C. Moderate to severe anxiety is painful and potentially disabling for the patient and should not be dismissed because a cause is not found in the medical workup. The patient may indeed be relieved to discover that there is no evidence of serious medical illness. However, recurrent panic attacks generally kindle renewed patient fear and concern, leading to repeated requests for medical attention. "Don't worry—it's only your nerves . . ." should not be considered an adequate intervention for the majority of anxious patients.

II. Terminology

A. Experientially, anxiety is similar to **fear.** However, unlike fear, the object (or source) of anxiety is unknown or uncertain.

B. Anxiety is multidimensional and manifests in one or more of the following spheres:

1. **Cognitive.** Worry, obsession, self-consciousness.
2. **Affective.** Uneasiness, dysphoria.
3. **Behavioral.** Avoidance, flight, compulsive repetition.
4. **Physical.** (Table 18-1).

Symptoms may cluster in a single dimension (e.g., physical). The patient whose predominant experience of anxiety is somatic generally presents initially to nonpsychiatric physicians.

C. Anxiety can be regarded as universal and therefore normal response to challenge or uncertainty. **Abnormal or pathologic anxiety** is distinguished by one or more of the following features:

1. **Autonomy.** Spontaneous occurrence unrelated to an external cause.
2. **Intensity.** The degree of suffering exceeds the individual's capacity to bear or cope with the distress.

Table 18-1. Physical signs and symptoms of anxiety

Anorexia	Muscle tension
"Butterflies" in stomach	Nausea
Chest pain or tightness	Pallor
Diaphoresis	Palpitations
Diarrhea	Paresthesias
Dizziness	Sexual dysfunction
Dyspnea	Shortness of breath
Dry mouth	Stomach pain
Faintness	Tachycardia
Flushing	Tremulousness
Headache	Urinary frequency
Hyperventilation	Vomiting
Lightheadedness	

Source: J. F. Rosenbaum. The drug treatment of anxiety. *N. Engl. J. Med.* 306:401, 1982. Reprinted by permission of the *New England Journal of Medicine.*

3. **Duration.** Symptoms persist or recur over time.
4. **Behavior.** The individual develops disabling behavioral strategies (e.g., avoidance, ritualistic or compulsive behavior).

D. A **panic attack** is intense anxiety of sudden onset that is classically associated with a fear of impending doom or loss of control, with a need to flee the circumstances in which the panic attack occurred, and with symptoms of autonomic arousal (Table 18-2). It should be distinguished from **generalized anxiety,** which is characterized by more constant, lower-grade symptoms of uneasiness, worry, and arousal.

E. A **phobia** is an exaggerated and inappropriate fear of and need to avoid a particular stimulus or circumstance.

Table 18-2. DSM-IV draft criteria for panic attack

A discrete period of intense fear or discomfort, in which at least four of the following symptoms developed abruptly and reached a peak within 10 minutes:

1. Palpitations, pounding heart, or accelerated heart rate.
2. Sweating.
3. Trembling or shaking.
4. Sensations of shortness of breath or smothering.
5. Feeling of choking.
6. Chest pain or discomfort.
7. Nausea or abdominal distress.
8. Feeling dizzy, unsteady, lightheaded, or faint.
9. Derealization (feelings of unreality) or depersonalization (being detached from oneself).
10. Fear of losing control or going crazy.
11. Fear of dying.
12. Paresthesias (numbness or tingling sensations).
13. Chills or hot flashes.

Source: Reprinted with permission from the *Diagnostic and Statistical Manual of Mental Disorders, Fourth Edition, Draft Criteria:* 3/1/93. Copyright 1993 American Psychiatric Association.

F. **Obsessions** are unwanted and senseless thoughts that are distressing and intrusive and cannot be suppressed. The thoughts are typically aggressive, sexual, or religious and are repulsive to the patient. Obsessions that are intense or bizarre may be difficult to distinguish from delusions.

G. **Compulsions** are rituals or other behaviors practiced in a repetitious, stereotypic fashion to avoid distress or anxiety. Checking and cleaning rituals are the most common types of clinically significant compulsive behavior.

III. Epidemiology

A. **Anxiety disorders** are the most prevalent form of psychiatric disorder in the general population, with phobic disorders representing the bulk of anxiety disorders (Barlow and Shear, 1988).

1. The lifetime prevalence of **anxiety and phobic disorders** is 17.5%.
2. It has been estimated that at least 10% of the general population have had one or more **panic attacks,** whereas 3–6% have **panic disorder and/or agoraphobia** (see sec. **V.C**).
3. The lifetime prevalence of **obsessive-compulsive disorder** is 2–3% (Jenike, et al. 1990).
4. A **familial pattern of transmission** is common with certain anxiety disorders.
   a. **Panic disorder** occurs in 20–25% of the first-degree relatives of probands with panic disorder. The basis for this familial pattern appears to be genetic, according to twin studies. There is five times greater concordance for panic attacks in monozygotic compared to dizygotic twin pairs.
   b. Up to 35% of first-degree relatives of probands with **obsessive-compulsive disorder** have either obsessive-compulsive disorder (20%) or subclinical obsessive-compulsive disorder (15%).
   c. There is no evidence for a familial pattern in **generalized anxiety disorder.**

B. **Anxiety symptoms** are common in general medical patients.

1. Ten to 27 percent of all primary care patients have anxiety-derived complaints, and approximately half of these are due to an anxiety disorder (e.g., panic disorder, obsessive-compulsive disorder, generalized anxiety disorder) (Barrett et al., 1988).
2. Approximately 10% of North Americans had used a benzodiazepine or related anxiolytic in the year prior to survey (Shurman et al., 1985).

IV. Evaluation

A. General approach

1. The evaluation of anxiety should include a determination of
   a. The anxiety symptoms.
   b. The onset and course of anxiety.
   c. The past history of anxiety, other psychiatric symptoms, and their treatment.
   d. The family history of anxiety and other psychiatric disorders.
   e. Medications used, including over-the-counter medications.
   f. Whether there is a history of substance abuse or medical illness.
2. Acutely anxious individuals may exhibit circumstantial speech and impaired concentration, which can interfere with obtaining the history. It is

best to acknowledge or inquire about the patient's overt discomfort first ("You look nervous and tense. Are you?" or "Are you aware that you jump anxiously from one topic to another and have difficulty answering my questions?") before proceeding with the interview. A calm, measured approach coupled with one's acknowledgment of the patient's distress and impairment can help diffuse anxiety, resulting in improved cognitive performance.

3. If these measures are unsuccessful and anxiety is unusually intense or persistent, it may be necessary to treat the patient with anxiolytic medication (see sec. **VII.A**).

B. History

1. The **chief complaint** of the anxious patient depends generally on the predominant dimension of anxiety experienced—that is, affective, cognitive, physical, or behavioral.

   a. Distressing **somatic symptoms** often prompt the anxious patient to seek emergency medical evaluation. Chest pain, gastrointestinal symptoms, shortness of breath, and light-headedness are common complaints. The physical symptoms are generally atypical, and the patient's report is often intense and dramatic. Certain patients will deny being afraid or anxious. It has been estimated that **nonfearful panic attacks** account for 30–40% of office visits in which there is no identifiable organic basis for the patient's somatic complaint (Beitman et al., 1990).

   b. Presentation to or referral to a psychiatric practitioner or a psychiatric emergency service is more likely when the predominant experience of anxiety is **affective, cognitive,** or **behavioral.** Typical complaints include an irrational sense of impending doom or loss of control, uncontrolled worrying, or limited mobility due to avoidance.

      (1) Fear of "going crazy," dying, or being embarrassed is commonly expressed.

      (2) **Obsessive thoughts,** in particular homicidal or suicidal fantasies, may be the source of concern. Rather than wishing or intending to carry out these acts, the anxious patient fears reacting to unwanted and intrusive fantasies. For example, looking at a knife may trigger frightening, repetitious thoughts of using it to hurt oneself or someone else. Further examination may reveal that the patient harbors unconscious and unresolved resentment toward a boss, a family member, or another significant individual. However, in the patient's life experience there may be no obvious basis for the obsessive thoughts.

      (3) **Fear and avoidance** of travel, of social exposure, or of circumstances that trigger flashbacks or intrusive recollections of past trauma suggest corresponding diagnoses of agoraphobia, social phobia, and post-traumatic stress disorder, respectively (see sec. **V.C**).

   c. Direct requests for sedatives or benzodiazepines made on a crisis or emergency basis should always prompt a careful evaluation for **substance abuse.** The anxious patient who is currently or has previously been in treatment may come to the emergency department expressing a legitimate need for anxiolytic medication. However, when the patient is already in treatment, the instances warranting emergency prescription of benzodiazepines are few, namely, when neither the prescribing nor the covering physician is available to authorize a prescription refill and when face-to-face evaluation of the patient has been recommended. **All other requests are suspect, particularly if the patient is demanding or insistent.** It should be noted that patients with legitimate anxiety disorders rarely overuse these medications and are often reluctant to take an adequate dose.

2. The **onset of symptoms** helps to distinguish different types of anxiety.
   - a. Although anxiety disorders typically present in the late teens and twenties, onset can occur at any time during the life span.
   - b. Since onset after age 40 is more likely to be due to an organic cause, the clinician should delve with special care into the medical history of the older patient. Careful medical evaluation focusing on the presenting symptoms is indicated.
   - c. Symptoms may begin spontaneously or following a discrete and identifiable stresssor.
   - d. Patients with panic disorder seldom forget their first panic attack (**herald attack**). In our experience, those who report a history of panic disorder but cannot remember their first panic attack are likely to have a primary diagnosis other than panic disorder.
3. **Duration and course**
   - a. **Anxiety disorders** are generally either intermittent or persistent.
   - b. **Situational anxiety** is generally self-limited and due to one or more stressors of which the patient may have full, partial, or no awareness. For example, the patient may be aware of heightened stress but may not be fully aware that it is due to anger at his or her spouse. Anxiety is likely to persist until the anger is verbalized and resolved.
4. Given the chronic course of most anxiety disorders, the patient with an anxiety disorder is likely to have a **past psychiatric history** of either prior anxiety episodes, other psychiatric symptoms, or prior psychiatric treatment.
   - a. Fearing stigmatization, many individuals with anxiety disorders tolerate symptoms for years before seeking help. Phobic avoidance, an important cause of delayed evaluation and treatment, can be so severe that individuals remain confined to their homes, sometimes for years. Others may have always attributed their distress to another medical condition.
   - b. If there is a history of treatment, the practitioner should inquire about the nature of treatment received and whether it was psychotherapeutic, behavioral, or pharmacologic.
5. The **family psychiatric history** of the patient with an anxiety disorder is often positive for either anxiety, depression, or alcoholism.
6. The **history of substance use** should be obtained in every anxious patient.
   - a. **Panic disorder** may be triggered by use of **marijuana** or **stimulants** such as cocaine. Anxious patients often consume excessive caffeine and must be told to curtail such use.
   - b. Some individuals use **alcohol** in a misguided attempt to self-medicate an underlying anxiety disorder. Although alcohol may be initially calming, as blood levels fall, the anxiety is likely to become increasingly worse. In these instances, adequate anxiolytic treatment should result in cessation of maladaptive alcohol use.
   - c. The anxious patient who abuses substances is more likely to have a **primary substance abuse disorder** than a primary anxiety disorder. Such patients often distinguish themselves by being insistent, demanding, and manipulative. They seldom derive adequate relief from the prescribed medication, use more than the recommended amount, and commonly report that the medication has been lost or stolen.

Table 18-3. Physical causes of anxiety-like symptoms

Type of cause	Specific cause
Cardiovascular	Angina pectoris, arrhythmias, congestive heart failure, hypertension, hypovolemia, myocardial infarction, syncope (of multiple causes), valvular disease, vascular collapse (shock)
Dietary	Caffeine, monosodium glutamate (Chinese restaurant syndrome), vitamin-deficiency diseases
Drug-related	Akathisia (secondary to antipsychotic drugs), alcohol (or alcohol withdrawal), anticholinergic toxicity, bronchodilators (theophylline, sympathomimetics), decongestants, digitalis toxicity, hallucinogens, hypotensive agents, marijuana, over-the-counter diet pills, stimulants (amphetamines, cocaine, and related drugs)
Hematologic	Anemias
Immunologic	Anaphylaxis, systemic lupus erythematosus
Metabolic	Hyperadrenalism (Cushing's disease), hyperkalemia, hyperthermia, hyperthyroidism, hypocalcemia, hypoglycemia, hyponatremia, hypothyroidism, menopause, porphyria (acute intermittent)
Neurologic	Encephalopathies (infectious, metabolic, and toxic), essential tremor, intracranial mass lesions, postconcussive syndrome, seizure disorders (especially of the temporal lobe), vertigo
Respiratory	Asthma, chronic obstructive pulmonary disease, pneumonia, pneumothorax, pulmonary edema, pulmonary embolism
Secreting tumors	Carcinoid, insulinoma, pheochromocytoma

Source: Adapted from J. F. Rosenbaum. The drug treatment of anxiety. *N. Engl. J. Med.* 306:401, 1982.

d. **Benzodiazepine abuse** is uncommon except in the context of polysubstance abuse. Narcotics abusers in particular are partial to benzodiazepines and may use large amounts to augment a narcotic-induced high. Approximately 10–20% of alcoholics for whom benzodiazepines are prescribed abuse them (Ciraulo et al., 1988).

7. It is important to focus on the patient's **medical history,** particularly when anxiety symptoms are new or atypical. The clinician should
   a. Focus on any medical illness the patient is known to have, including its symptoms, complications, and treatments.
   b. Direct the evaluation toward the somatic system most prominently complained of by the patient (e.g., cardiac, gastrointestinal).
   c. Consider medical illnesses that can fully mimic anxiety (e.g., angina, cardiac arrhythmia, hyperthyroidism, pheochromocytoma). When examined closely, the quality of the anxiety symptoms reported with such illnesses usually differs from those of primary anxiety disorders.
   d. Medical disorders that may present with anxiety-like symptoms are listed in Table 18-3.

e. Assess the patient's use of medications, over-the-counter drugs, illicit drugs, alcohol, and caffeine (including all sources, such as cola drinks or combination analgesics, e.g., Fiorinal). Drugs that have been reported to produce anxiety-like symptoms are listed in Table 18-3.

C. Examination

1. The **mental status examination** of the anxious patient is generally either unremarkable or nonspecific. Speech can be rapid and pressured, mimicking hypomania, or sparse and occasionally mumbled. The range of affect may be constricted and the mood either anxious or depressed. The presence of a thought disorder suggests a diagnosis other than anxiety disorder, although some patients with bizarre or unusual obsessions can appear to be psychotic. Anxiety affects cognition by interfering with attention.

2. The **physical examination** of the anxious patient is also unremarkable or nonspecific unless the cause of anxiety is organic (see Table 18-3).

3. **Laboratory data** can be used either to substantiate or to exclude suspected disorders (e.g., hyperthyroidism, coronary artery disease, substance abuse). Urine and/or serum toxicologic screening should be ordered if ongoing substance abuse is suspected. Electroencephalographic study can be ordered to document a suspicion of complex partial seizures (Weilburg et al., 1987).

V. Diagnosis

A. Phase of life problem or other life circumstance problem. Acute, disabling anxiety can occur following overwhelming stress in an otherwise healthy individual who has no past history of similar reactions or of anxiety disorder. Examples of triggering circumstances include anxiety associated with changes in job, retirement, entering school, marriage, divorce, or birth of a child. The *Diagnostic and Statistical Manual of Mental Disorders, Fourth Edition, Draft Criteria* (DSM-IV) does not provide an Axis I condition that satisfactorily addresses this category of problem but does permit coding of conditions that may be a focus of clinical attention without being due to a mental disorder.

B. Adjustment disorder with anxious mood. This diagnosis is made when either nervousness, worry, or jitteriness occurs within 3 months of an identifiable stressor and persists for no longer than 6 months. The pattern of anxiety is maladaptive, it is excessive or inappropriate to the interpersonal, occupational, or other upheaval that caused it, and it does not constitute merely one instance of overreaction to stress.

C. Anxiety disorders. As defined in DSM-IV, these disorders are characterized by specific patterns of anxiety that are either recurrent or persistent and disabling.

1. **Panic disorder.** Of all individuals suffering from anxiety disorders, those with panic attacks are most likely to come to an emergency department. Patients meeting criteria for this disorder have either experienced at least four panic attacks in a 4-week period or one attack followed by at least a month of sustained fear of having a subsequent attack (see Table 18-2). Panic disorder patients may also suffer mild, moderate, or severe agoraphobia (**panic disorder with agoraphobia**).

   a. **Recurrent panic attacks** typically have their onset in early adult life following a major life event such as a loss, threat of loss, or some physiologic stressor or chemical provocation. The majority of patients will be able to identify some disruption of an attachment bond in the weeks prior to their initial panic attack or recognize unusual life stressors such as relocation, job change, or illness in a loved one. Other patients experience their first panic attack in the context of a medical illness such as hyperthyroidism, but the anxiety disorder may continue beyond the time when the triggering medical condition is controlled. A number of patients describe their initial panic attack as having been provoked by a drug, such as marijuana or cocaine or following a period of excessive caffeine intake.

b. A patient's first panic attack may be considered a **herald attack,** a premonition of more attacks and complications to follow. As many as one-third of the population, however, have experienced one isolated panic attack without recurrence. Panic attacks may be single, intermittent events or erupt in clusters or volleys of attacks.

c. The course of panic attacks is highly variable. Some patients experience **spontaneous** attacks, occurring "out of the blue," in settings where an attack had not been anticipated. Other attacks are deemed **situational,** typically occurring in settings where patients have previously suffered them; these are preceded by anticipatory anxiety. In the typical case of panic disorder with agoraphobia, the patient experiences premonitory anxiety approaching a situation, such as a supermarket or restaurant, where an attack is feared; the anxiety symptoms then crescendo into a panic attack.

d. Another form of panic attack is called the **limited symptom attack.** These spells consist of one or two symptoms only (e.g., dizziness, tachycardia, or respiratory distress) and are particularly difficult for the evaluating physician to differentiate from symptoms of other medical illnesses. Limited symptom attacks may occur early in the course of the disorder before full-blown panic attacks begin, may occur mixed with major panic attacks, or may be residual symptoms in a patient whose disorder has subsided.

e. Adults with panic disorder and agoraphobia frequently describe themselves as having been shy as children or give a history of childhood separation anxiety, such as school phobia.

f. Panic disorder runs in families, and most patients identify other family members with anxiety attacks, histories of phobic avoidance, or depression.

2. **Agoraphobia without history of panic disorder.** Agoraphobia is the fear of settings or places from which escape to what the patient considers a safer place might not be available.

a. Typical agoraphobic situations (i.e., anxiety-provoking circumstances perceived as unsafe) include crowds, restaurants, stores, automobiles, bridges, tunnels, or public transportation.

b. The avoidance of all unsafe circumstances may result in being confined to one's home.

c. Controversy surrounds the role of panic attacks in agoraphobia. Although some experts argue that panic attacks are a necessary precondition of agoraphobia, epidemiologic data indicate that a significant number of individuals suffer from agoraphobia without a history of panic attacks.

3. **Social phobia** reflects anxious distress in situations where the patient is the focus of scrutiny by others and fears humiliation or embarrassment.

a. Common social phobias are stage fright and fear of public speaking. Examples of other variants are the inability to sign one's name in public or to use public lavatories.

b. Social phobic anxiety may be of the lower-grade, generalized variety or may be experienced with the intensity of a panic attack.

c. Social phobia is distinguished from normal anxiety, in part, by the extent of avoidance or social and occupational limitations that occur.

4. **Simple phobia** is the fear of and need to avoid specific stimuli such as particular objects (e.g., snakes, dogs) or situations (e.g., airplanes, heights). If the object or situation is encountered, the individual suffers intense anxiety, which may achieve the level of panic.

5. **Generalized anxiety disorder** is diagnosed if the patient has suffered from unrealistic anxiety and worry (not related to having a panic attack) for a period of 6 months or more, during which time the person has been bothered more days than not by these concerns. Symptoms include motor tension, autonomic hyperactivity, vigilance, and scanning. The symptoms cannot be due to any specific medical or organic cause.

6. **Obsessive-compulsive disorder.** Patients suffer from

   a. Recurrent unwanted and senseless thoughts that are distressing and intrusive but that cannot be suppressed (obsessions), or

   b. The need to repeat certain rituals or other behaviors in a stereotyped fashion or else suffer intense distress or anxiety (compulsions).

7. **Patients with posttraumatic stress disorder** often manifest symptoms resembling the acute symptoms and secondary complications of panic disorder but with onset related to experiencing or witnessing a serious, life-threatening, or violent event. Subsequently the patient re-experiences the event or suffers recurrent dreams and other experiences (e.g., flashbacks) that recall the traumatic event. Anxiety symptoms, the tendency to startle easily, sleep dysfunction, and the need to avoid stimuli reminiscent of the original event characterize this syndrome.

D. **Comorbid disorders.** Studies suggest that diagnostic comorbidity (i.e., cases in which diagnoses of an anxiety disorder and another disorder are made simultaneously) is the rule rather than the exception in clinical populations. In general, comorbidity predicts more severely impaired psychosocial functioning, more intense symptomatology, lower remission rates, and a poorer response to treatment than either diagnosis alone. These characteristics increase the likelihood that patients with diagnostic comorbidity will seek out and require emergency services. The disorders that are commonly comorbid with anxiety disorders include

1. **Depression**

   a. Up to 80% of patients with panic disorder have had a major depressive episode (Breier et al., 1984). In the majority, the depression follows the onset of panic disorder.

   b. In social phobia, 35–70% of patients have a lifetime history of a major depressive episode.

   c. The relationship between generalized anxiety disorder and depression is less distinct.

2. **Other anxiety disorders.** Features of different anxiety disorders commonly overlap. Patients with panic disorder may also suffer from fear of social exposure, obsessions, or compulsions, and those with other anxiety disorders often have panic attacks as well.

3. **Substance abuse disorders.** Some reports suggest that as many as 25% of adult male alcoholics began their substance abuse in an attempt to self-medicate for panic disorder.

4. **Personality disorders.** Dependent and avoidant personality disorders appear to be more common in individuals with panic disorder. It is uncertain whether these personality disorders are a complication of panic disorder or

whether panic disorder is more likely to occur in individuals with these personality traits.

5. **Medical disorders.** The symptoms of some medical disorders (e.g., hyperthyroidism, mitral valve prolapse [MVP], asthma, audiovestibular disorders) not only may mimic anxiety but also may have a higher incidence in patients with anxiety disorders than in the general population. Although auscultatory and echocardiographic criteria for MVP have been reported in up to 50% of panic disorder patients, true or classic MVP due to thickened, redundant mitral valve leaflets probably does not occur more frequently in individuals with panic disorder than in the general population (Katon, 1991).

VI. Differential diagnosis

A. Virtually all psychiatric disorders manifest some degree of anxiety as the sole or predominant symptom at some time during their course. Making the correct diagnosis may require serial observation as the primary disorder (e.g., schizophrenia, depression) evolves.

1. Anxiety may be a heralding sign of **major depression,** particularly the atypical variety. Atypical depression (in the past also referred to as hysteroid dysphoria) is characterized by intense sensitivity to rejection, criticism, or loss. Individuals with this disorder respond to rejection or criticism by becoming immobilized by extreme fatigue; they develop panic attacks, social withdrawal, and a tendency to hibernate and consume excess carbohydrates. Symptoms typically recede in less than 1 week but are recurrent and disabling. Monoamine oxidase inhibitors and serotonin-specific reuptake inhibitors (e.g., fluoxetine) appear to have particular efficacy for this type of depression.

2. **Psychotic symptoms** can both precipitate and be confused with anxiety. The flat affect of the negative-symptom schizophrenic should be distinguished from the constricted affect of an intensely anxious patient. A formal thought disorder characterized by loosening of associations and tangential thinking must be distinguished from anxiety-driven circumstantial speech. Paranoia can be confused with the avoidant style of the social phobic and the agoraphobic.

3. Certain **personality disorders** can manifest intense anxiety. Among the most difficult problems in differential diagnosis is the distinction of panic from the stress-induced fragmentation of identity that occurs in patients with **borderline personality disorder.**

4. Somatization, a tendency to focus on and amplify somatic symptoms, is a common feature of anxiety disorders, particularly panic disorder (Katon, 1991). A diagnosis of **somatization disorder** should be considered when the patient presents with multiple, chronic, and persistent somatic symptoms. At least 13 symptom complaints are necessary for diagnosis, and there must be no identifiable organic pathology for a period of at least 6 months. These symptoms occur at times other than during a panic attack, their pattern and description tend to vary over time, they are grossly in excess of expectation, and they have caused the person to take medicine, to see a doctor, or to alter life-style. Patients with primary somatization disorder generally respond minimally to anxiolytic and antidepressant medication.

5. Anxiety is a prominent feature of alcohol use or withdrawal from alcohol, sedative-hypnotic agents, and opioids and can be difficult to differentiate from the symptoms of a primary anxiety disorder. Studies suggest that **substance abuse tends to be underdiagnosed in walk-in and emergency psychiatric clinics** (Szuster et al., 1990).

B. Medical disorders and **drugs** that produce anxiety-like symptoms are listed in Table 18-3.

VII. Treatment of anxiety

A. Acute anxiety

1. A calm, reassuring manner and use of simple relaxation techniques (e.g., deep breathing using diaphragmatic rather than intercostal muscles) can prove effective as an initial intervention.

2. If acute pharmacologic intervention is indicated as a consequence of the intensity or duration of patient discomfort, **benzodiazepines** are the emergency treatment of choice. Safe and reliable, their acute use, unlike chronic use, does not risk dependency, rebound symptoms, or withdrawal. Several important caveats are worthy of consideration when preparing to treat the acutely anxious patient:

   a. **Withdrawal from alcohol or a sedative-hypnotic agent** must always be considered a cause of acute anxiety. Administration of the responsible substance or of a cross-reactive agent, such as a benzodiazepine, is the appropriate treatment. The dose of medication required to treat symptoms may be higher than the patient's usual daily dose (see Chaps. 29 and 30).

   b. Diagnosis and treatment of sedative-hypnotic withdrawal are best accomplished with the **pentobarbital tolerance test** followed by a **program of phenobarbital withdrawal** (see Chap. 30).

   c. The anxiety and autonomic arousal associated with the **opioid withdrawal syndrome** (see Chap. 30) can be treated with either an increased dosage of opiate, with a benzodiazepine, or with clonidine, the selection of treatment being determined in part by the setting and the likelihood of ongoing substance abuse.

   d. A **neuroleptic agent,** alone or in combination with a benzodiazepine, should be considered for patients whose anxiety is due to psychosis.

3. A benzodiazepine with a rapid onset of effect is most helpful in the setting of acute anxiety. Diazepam, 2–10 mg, or lorazepam, 1–2 mg, is usually adequate.

4. The **route of administration** depends on the circumstances and the intensity of anxiety.

   a. Some emergency physicians favor sublingual lorazepam as a rapidly acting agent. However, a well-designed study comparing the sublingual and oral administration of lorazepam found no differences in the rate of onset or of the achievement of peak blood levels (Spenard et al., 1988).

   b. While intravenous benzodiazepines (e.g., lorazepam, diazepam, and midazolam) are especially potent and rapidly acting, their use must be reserved for unusually severe cases or when medical conditions (e.g., coronary artery disease) create a life-threatening situation. Intravenous benzodiazepines must always be given slowly, never by rapid bolus, and always with immediate access to respiratory equipment and personnel skilled in cardiopulmonary resuscitation.

B. Adjustment disorder

1. A **counseling or psychotherapy referral** is particularly pertinent if a recent psychosocial disruption is apparent, as with the breakup of a relationship or marital turmoil, or if the anxiety is part of a pattern of disturbed interpersonal relationships.

2. The short-term use of a **benzodiazepine** may be helpful as well. The pharmacokinetic differences between benzodiazepines and their individual abuse liability should be taken into consideration when selecting an agent (see Appendix III). For example, lorazepam, 1 mg PO bid–tid, is generally

effective and well tolerated. The patient can be given a short-term supply and asked to return for follow-up evaluation within a week to determine the appropriateness of use and the need for further anxiolytic treatment.

C. Anxiety disorders

1. Optimal treatment of **panic disorder** often requires a combination of pharmacologic and cognitive-behavioral approaches. **Cognitive-behavioral therapy** should be recommended to all panic disorder patients, particularly those suffering from phobic avoidance (Barlow, 1990). However, presentation to an emergency department usually carries with it an implicit request for rapid symptom control. If panic disorder is diagnosed, **an evaluation for pharmacotherapy maintenance is indicated.** A spectrum of psychotropics have anti-panic efficacy: tricyclic antidepressants (TCAs), monoamine oxidase inhibitors (MAOIs), benzodiazepines, and possibly serotonin-specific reuptake inhibitors (SSRIs).

   a. **TCAs** and **MAOIs** are effective for panic disorder (with or without depression) and for depression (with or without anxiety).

      (1) In addition to the SSRIs (see sec. **C**), TCAs and MAOIs are important treatment alternatives for panic disorder patients with comorbid substance abuse, a relative contraindication to use of benzodiazepines.

      (2) The efficacy of TCAs and MAOIs is balanced by side effects that are often not well tolerated by anxious patients, and many anxious patients given TCAs experience transient worsening of symptoms at initiation of treatment.

      (3) For anxiety patients administration of a TCA should be initiated at a low dose (e.g., 10 mg of either imipramine, desipramine, or nortriptyline) and increased gradually to minimize arousal and worsening of baseline symptoms.

      (4) MAOIs (e.g., phenelzine, tranylcypromine) are not first-line treatments for panic disorder but are nevertheless remarkably effective and should be prescribed with the usual precautionary advice to avoid tyramine-containing foods, sympathomimetic agents, and meperidine.

   b. The **benzodiazepines** are effective and well tolerated anti-panic agents. Given in sufficient dosage, a number of benzodiazepines have demonstrated anti-panic efficacy, although the dosage of lower-potency agents (e.g., diazepam, clorazepate, and chlordiazepoxide) necessary to achieve an anti-panic effect may produce unacceptable sedation and ataxia. For these and other reasons, high-potency benzodiazepines, such as alprazolam and clonazepam, have been advocated as the benzodiazepines of choice for panic disorder.

      (1) **Alprazolam,** studied extensively, is the only benzodiazepine approved by the Food and Drug Administration for the treatment of panic disorder. Treatment can be initiated with 0.5 mg tid. Alprazolam's significant abuse potential, however, limits its utility in crisis or emergency patients.

      (2) **Clonazepam,** a high-potency benzodiazepine that is longer lasting than alprazolam and has a slower rate of onset (see Appendix III), also has been shown to be an effective anti-panic agent. Selected patients with alprazolam-associated interdose recurrence of anxiety may be switched successfully to clonazepam (Herman et al., 1987). A starting dose of 0.5 mg, one-half to one tablet bid is recommended. Clonazepam's pharmacokinetic properties theoretically reduce its abuse potential and make it a desirable alternative to alprazolam

for patients who are neither familiar to the clinician nor involved in regular treatment.

c. A relatively new class of agents, the SSRIs—fluoxetine (Prozac), sertraline (Zoloft), and paroxetine (Paxil)—may also be effective for panic disorder and circumvent the side effects associated with TCAs and MAOIs. Again, treatment should begin with lowest possible doses. The SSRIs may also offer preferential efficacy for atypical depression.

2. For **generalized anxiety disorder,** if pharmacologic treatment is indicated, any benzodiazepine (see Appendix III) can be used. Beta-adrenergic blockers, such as propranolol or atenolol, can be used to decrease peripheral autonomic symptoms but are most useful in treating such social phobic symptoms as performance anxiety.

3. If **obsessive-compulsive disorder** is suspected, a benzodiazepine may help to alleviate acute distress, but maintenance treatment should include either clomipramine (not to exceed 250 mg daily) or fluoxetine (up to 80 mg daily) alone or in combination with behavioral therapy. The clinician should be careful to distinguish bizarre or unusual obsessions from delusions to avoid inappropriate prescription of a neuroleptic agent to the patient with obsessive-compulsive disorder.

D. Comorbidity

1. **Depression.** The effective treatment of comorbid anxiety and depression and of atypical depression often requires administration of both an antidepressant and an anxiolytic agent. In this population, the use of benzodiazepines alone often produces some, but transient and suboptimal, symptom reduction. Expecting further improvement, the patient may continue to increase benzodiazepine dosage with limited improvement, possibly fostering an impression of drug abuse. Addition of an antidepressant such as a SSRI, TCA, or MAOI is indicated.

2. **Substance abuse.** Although nearly 40% of alcoholics receive prescription benzodiazepines, the use of benzodiazepines in emergency patients suspected of ongoing substance abuse is to be avoided. Benzodiazepine treatment of selected patients with a history of substance abuse should be guided by the following principles:

   a. Create appropriate expectations by establishing the rules and limits of treatment.

   b. Patients should be forewarned that under no circumstances will extra medication be prescribed between visits unless the physician has recommended a dosage increase. **Such instructions should be documented in the patient's hospital record to alert other clinicians who may see the patient.**

   c. The patient should be advised to consult the physician before adjusting medication. Evidence that medication has been increased without physician involvement is worrisome, and further prescribing should be contingent on modification of such noncollaborative behavior.

Selected Readings

American Psychiatric Association Task Force on DSM-IV. *Diagnostic and Statistical Manual, Fourth Edition, Draft Criteria:* 3/1/93. Washington, D.C.: American Psychiatric Association.

American Psychiatric Association Task Force. *Benzodiazepine Dependence, Toxicity, and Abuse.* Washington, D.C.: American Psychiatric Press, 1990.

Barlow, D. H. Long-term outcome for patients with panic disorder treated with cognitive-behavioral therapy. *J. Clin. Psychiatry* 51(Suppl. A):17, 1990.

Barlow, D. H., and Shear, M. K. (eds.). Panic Disorder. In A. J. Frances and R. E. Hales (eds.), *Review of Psychiatry,* Vol. 7. Washington, D.C.: American Psychiatric Press, 1988. Pp. 5–138.

Barrett, J. E., et al. The prevalence of psychiatric disorders in a primary care practice. *Arch. Gen. Psychiatry* 45:1100, 1988.

Beitman, B. D., et al. Panic disorder without fear in patients with angiographically normal coronary arteries. *J. Nerv. Ment. Dis.* 178:307, 1990.

Breier, A., Charney, D. S., and Heninger, G. B. Major depression in patients with agoraphobia and panic disorder. *Arch. Gen. Psychiatry* 41:1129, 1984.

Cameron, O. G. The differential diagnosis of anxiety: Psychiatric and medical disorders. *Psychiatr. Clin. North Am.* 8:3, 1981.

Ciraulo, D. A., Sands, B. F., and Shader, R. I. Critical review of liability for benzodiazepine abuse among alcoholics. *Am. J. Psychiatry* 10:237, 1988.

Herman, J. B., Rosenbaum, J. F., and Brotman, A. W. The alprazolam to clonazepam switch for the treatment of panic disorder. *J. Clin. Psychopharmacol.* 7:175, 1987.

Jenike, M. A., Baer, L., and Minichiello, W. E., (eds.). *Obsessive-Compulsive Disorder: Theory and Management* (2nd ed.). Chicago: Year Book, 1990.

Katon, W. J. *Panic Disorder in the Medical Setting.* Washington, D.C.: American Psychiatric Press, 1991.

Rosenbaum, J. F. The drug treatment of anxiety. *N. Engl. J. Med.* 306:401, 1982.

Shurman, R. A., Kramer, P. D., and Mitchell, J. B. The hidden mental health network: Treatment of mental illness by nonpsychiatrist physicians. *Arch. Gen. Psychiatry* 42:89, 1985.

Spenard, J., et al. Placebo-controlled comparative study of the anxiolytic activity and of the pharmacokinetics of oral and sublingual lorazepam in generalized anxiety. *Biopharm. Drug Dispos.* 9:457, 1988.

Szuster, R. R., et al. Underdiagnosis of substance-induced organic mental disorders in emergency psychiatry. *Am. J. Alcohol Abuse* 16:319, 1990.

Tesar, G. E., et al. Double-blind, placebo-controlled comparison of clonazepam and alprazolam for panic disorder. *J. Clin. Psychiatry* 52:69, 1991.

Weilburg, J. B., Bear, D. M., and Sachs, G. Three patients with concomitant panic attacks and seizure disorder. *Am. J. Psychiatry* 144:1053, 1987.

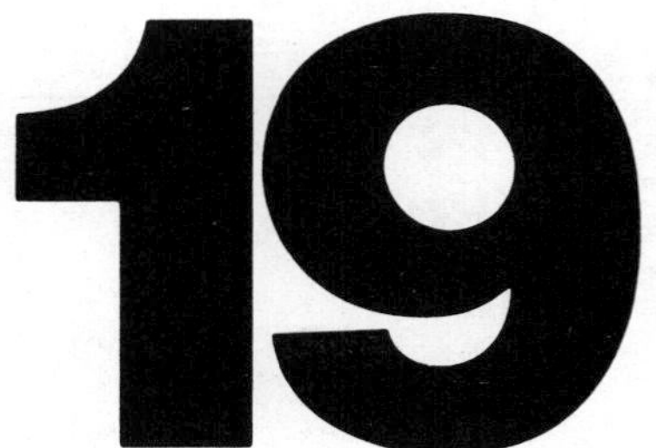

Acute Psychoses and Catatonia

Steven E. Hyman

I. **Acute psychosis** and **catatonia** are not psychiatric diagnoses but clinical syndromes. Possible etiologies of acute psychoses are given in Table 19-1 and of catatonia in Table 19-2. This chapter describes the method of evaluating acutely psychotic and catatonic patients so that the differential diagnosis can be approached systematically and the early steps in psychologic and psychopharmacologic management taken. It is important to recall that the etiology of either an acute psychosis or catatonia cannot be determined from the mental status alone. As is always the case in making a psychiatric diagnosis, the history, including the longitudinal course, must be taken into account. Medical history, physical examination, and relevant laboratory tests are needed to rule out the possibility of a medical illness or drug effect. Prior treatment response and family history of psychiatric or neurologic disorders can provide helpful diagnostic information if used carefully—that is, it must be recalled that many therapeutic agents, such as neuroleptics, are quite nonspecific in their actions; thus their prior effectiveness is not informative as to a specific diagnosis. Family histories may be inaccurate because of attempts to deny mental illness or because relatives were improperly diagnosed in the past.

II. **Acute psychosis**

A. **Evaluation and clinical features.** The acutely psychotic patient is difficult to evaluate and treat because he or she is often excited and disruptive; thus there is often pressure on the physician from emergency department staff to sedate such patients and rapidly transfer them to a psychiatric facility. This sort of pressure combined with the likelihood that the patient will be a poor historian and not compliant with examination makes it a great challenge to perform a careful workup. Obviously if an organic disorder goes undetected there is medical risk to the patient, but even if the problem is a primary psychiatric disorder, early misdiagnosis may lead to a delay or failure to institute proper treatments (such as failure to treat mania with lithium). **Signs and symptoms** of acute psychosis develop rapidly, over a period of days or weeks. The syndrome includes psychotic symptoms—for example, delusions, hallucinations, ideas of reference, or incoherent thought. Other symptoms may include insomnia, anxiety, psychomotor agitation, hyperactivity, or affective derangements (e.g., elation, dysphoria, emotional lability, or blunted affect). The patient usually has severe impairments of thought and judgment. Combined with agitation or hyperactivity, these impairments may result in violence, inadvertent self-injury, or suicide. In addition, judgment may be so poor that the patient may break laws and threaten his or her job, financial well-being, and relationships with family and friends.

B. **Approach to the patient**

1. The more severely psychotic or excited the patient is, the more critical it is that the physician keep questions and requests clear, simple, and direct. This is not the time to delve extensively into the patient's developmental history. Overstimulation of the patient is to be avoided. Limits must be set, but without anger; the need for medication or other interventions should be explained clearly to the patient, but long arguments or discussions are to be avoided.

Table 19-1. Causes of acute psychosis

- Psychiatric causes
  - Mania (including typical and dysphoric mania)
  - Depression
  - Atypical affective disorders (mixed bipolar; schizoaffective)
  - Schizophrenia (first presentation or exacerbation)
  - Schizophreniform illnesses
  - Brief psychotic disorder
  - Factitious psychosis
- Drug abuse
  - Phencyclidine (PCP) and hallucinogens; acute intoxication and "flashbacks"
  - Cocaine (especially freebase or crack)
  - Amphetamine
  - Marijuana use, with panic reaction
  - Alcohol withdrawal, with hallucinosis
  - Sedative-hypnotic withdrawal
- Toxic reactions to medications
  - Alprazolam (Xanax), both intoxication and withdrawal
  - Anticholinergics, including cyclic antidepressants, thioridazine (Mellaril), antihistamines, many antiparkinsonian agents, agents for motion sickness, over-the-counter sleeping pills, drugs, and some plants
  - Cardiac drugs: digitalis toxicity, procainamide, prazosin, captopril (Capoten)
  - Dopamine agonists: levodopa, amantadine, bromocriptine, pergolide, lisuride
  - Glucocorticoids and adrenocorticotropic hormone (ACTH)
  - Monoamine oxidase inhibitors (abrupt discontinuation)
  - Nonsteroidal anti-inflammatory drugs including sulindac, indomethacin
  - Isoniazid
  - Stimulants, including over-the-counter decongestants, diet pills, and pep pills containing sympathomimetics
- Industrial exposures
  - Heavy metals
  - Carbon disulfide
- Metabolic disorders
  - Hypoglycemia
  - Acute intermittent porphyria
  - Cushing's syndrome and, rarely, Addison's disease
  - Hypo- and hypercalcemia
  - Hypo- and hyperthyroidism
- Nutritional deficiencies
  - Korsakoff's psychosis (due to thiamine deficiency)
  - Pellagra (due to niacin deficiency)
  - Vitamin B_{12} deficiency
- Neurologic disorders
  - Encephalitis, meningitis, and brain abscess
  - Neurosyphilis
  - Acquired immunodeficiency syndrome (AIDS) encephalopathy
  - Lupus cerebritis
  - Wilson's disease
  - Huntington's disease
  - Complex partial seizure disorder
  - Stroke
  - Central nervous system neoplasm or paraneoplastic syndrome
  - Early Alzheimer's disease
  - Hypoxic encephalopathy
- Other causes
  - Early hepatic encephalopathy
  - Acute pancreatitis (rarely)

Table 19-2. Causes of catatonia and catatonic-like symptoms

Psychiatric causes
Mania
Depression
Atypical affective disorders (mixed bipolar; schizoaffective)
Schizophrenia (first presentation or exacerbation)
Schizophreniform illnesses
Conversion disorder, dissociative states
Factitious unresponsiveness
Drugs and toxic agents
Neuroleptics
Anticholinergics
Phencyclidine (PCP)
Hallucinogens
Corticosteroids, adrenocorticotropic hormone (ACTH)
Organic fluorides
"Designer drugs"
Neurologic disorders
Parkinsonism
Basal ganglia lesions
Encephalitis
Frontal or temporal lesions
Petit mal or complex partial status epilepticus
Postictal states
Metabolic disorders
Hypercalcemia
Hepatic encephalopathy
Acute intermittent porphyria
Pellagra
Diabetic ketoacidosis

2. If the patient is **too agitated to examine,** the smallest effective dose of a sedative drug should be used; more definitive treatments should be withheld until the diagnosis becomes clear. In practice, lorazepam, 1–2 mg PO or IM, or diazepam, 5–10 mg PO, is usually effective, indeed more reliably sedating than high-potency neuroleptics. Depending on the degree of agitation, more may be needed, but oversedation is best avoided in order not to cloud the diagnostic picture. It is best to withhold neuroleptic drugs until adequate diagnostic data are obtained. This is particularly true if the patient may have previously been medicated and has symptoms that could represent neuroleptic toxicity, such as akathisia, or symptoms of movement disorder, or catatonic-like symptoms. Premature administration of neuroleptics to such patients could severely hamper subsequent efforts at workup. In addition, low-potency neuroleptics can exacerbate the symptoms of certain ingestions (e.g., phencyclidine (PCP) or anticholinergic compounds). In many cases it may be optimal to observe diagnostically puzzling patients drug-free for several days or, if sedation is needed, to use the lowest effective doses of benzodiazepines alone. The early management problems created by this approach are usually amply compensated by diagnostic clarity in the long run. If the patient is extremely agitated or violent, restraints may be needed in addition to sedatives.

C. Workup

1. **Vital signs** should be obtained immediately. If the patient is febrile or has marked abnormalities of blood pressure, respiration, or heart rate, rapid

medical assessment will be needed. It should be recalled that agitated patients may have some degree of hypertension, tachycardia, and tachypnea due to sympathetic arousal.

2. **History.** The history may be impossible to obtain from the patient. Therefore friends and family members will be important sources of information. The order in which the history is obtained will depend on the clinical situation. Thus, for example, if the patient has a fever, early history taking should center on the possibility of infection or possible toxic reactions to neuroleptic, cocaine, or anticholinergic compounds. If, on the other hand, the patient appears medically stable, a more detailed psychiatric history should be the early focus of the examination. Information pertinent to differential diagnosis must be obtained.

   a. **Premorbid history**

      (1) Has the patient had any similar episodes previously?

      (2) Did the patient seem well psychiatrically prior to the episode or, for example, chronically maladjusted or bizarre?

      (3) Is there a history of significant drug abuse or dependence?

   b. **The course and nature of the illness**

      (1) How rapidly did symptoms develop, and what is their total duration?

      (2) Has the patient exhibited any neurovegetative signs?

         (a) What is the patient's pattern of sleep? Of eating?

         (b) Has the patient been hyperactive or had periods of akinesia and mutism?

      (3) What are the patient's mental symptoms?

         (a) Are delusions or hallucinations present? It is important to determine whether the patient is experiencing hallucinations commanding dangerous actions and whether the patient has delusions that could lead to harm of self or others or interfere with treatment. Content or degree of bizarreness is not diagnostic of any particular illness. In particular, acute mania in adolescents may present with bizarre delusions indistinguishable from symptoms of schizophrenia.

         (b) Does the patient feel frightened, suspicious, or irritable? It is important to know this, both in order to be empathic and to manage the patient successfully.

         (c) Does the patient have any suicidal or violent ideas, plans, or intentions?

   c. **Medical history,** including all prescription and over-the-counter drug use, must be obtained. (Most over-the-counter sleeping pills are strongly anticholinergic; decongestants, diet pills, and pep pills may include stimulants such as phenylephrine and caffeine.)

   d. Has the patient used **illicit drugs** in the period during which symptoms developed? It is particularly important to ask about use of cocaine, amphetamines, phencyclidine (PCP, "angel dust"), and hallucinogens.

   e. **Family history**

      (1) A history of affective disorders in biologic relatives, including manic-depressive illness and major depressions makes a diagnosis of mania, depression, or atypical affective disorder more likely.

      (2) A family history of schizophrenia may be difficult to interpret be-

cause this disorder was overdiagnosed in the past; however, it makes schizophrenia the more likely diagnosis in the patient.

(3) A family history of neurologic diseases, such as Huntington's disease, Wilson's disease, or porphyria, would be helpful in focusing the investigation.

3. Mental status examination. All psychiatric patients deserve a full mental status examination, especially those whose symptoms appear acutely without prior psychiatric illness (see Chap. 1).

a. Fluctuating levels of alertness strongly suggest drug use or delirium.

b. Inattention may be produced by either delirium or psychoses—for example, manic patients may be extremely distractable; patients may be attending to their hallucinations.

c. Confusion (disorientation to time and place) is common in acute psychoses (especially acute mania) as well as in delirium or dementia (see Chap. 1).

d. In addition to typical psychotic symptoms, such as delusions, auditory hallucinations, or ideas of reference, is the patient experiencing visual, tactile, or olfactory hallucinations? These are more common with organic, rather than primary psychiatric disorders.

e. Is the patient experiencing visual distortions? These are most common with hallucinogenic drugs and organic deliria, although they may occur with primary psychiatric disorders.

f. Apparent manipulativeness or wildly histrionic presentation of psychotic symptoms suggests factitious psychosis or brief reactive psychosis (see sec. **II.D.1.d**).

g. It is important to be satisfied that the apparent psychosis is not simply a fluent aphasia (see Chap. 1).

4. Laboratory screening requires clinical judgment of likely diagnostic possibilities, but as discussed in Chap. 25, all patients presenting with acute psychiatric symptoms should have at least the following analyses done:

a. Electrolytes.

b. Blood urea nitrogen (BUN), creatinine.

c. Blood glucose.

d. Calcium.

e. Serum glutamic-oxaloacetic transaminase (SGOT), bilirubin, and alkaline phosphatase.

f. Free thyroxine (T_4) and thyroid stimulating hormone (TSH).

g. Complete blood count including a differential and mean corpuscular volume (MCV).

h. Urinalysis.

i. Urine drug screen.

D. Differential diagnosis (see Table 19-1)

1. Psychiatric disorders

a. Mood disorders

(1) Mania (see Chap. 20) commonly presents as an acute psychosis. Although the diagnosis of classic mania may be straightforward, the presentation of mania can vary remarkably. Some patients exhibit little or no euphoria or are euphoric only early in the manic episode; such patients may be predominantly irritable, paranoid, and dysphoric. It is not uncommon for clinicians to misclassify such patients as depressed. The diagnosis of dysphoric mania is based on a known history of bipolar disorder, the progression of the current episode, and the presence of other components of the manic syndrome (e.g., increased energy, decreased need for sleep). Psychotic symptoms are common during manic episodes. Although these are most often congruent with the elevated mood (e.g., grandiose delusions), some patients, especially adolescents, may have florid psychotic symptoms including bizarre delusions, once thought to be pathognomonic for schizophrenia. The correct diagnosis is based on the course of illness (acute onset and episodic course in mania versus insidious onset and chronic course in schizophrenia) and the presence of neurovegetative symptoms. A history of prior manic or depressed episodes (with or without psychosis) and a family history of affective disorder are also helpful in diagnosing mania.

(2) Depression may be a relatively common cause of catatonia but less commonly can manifest itself as an acute agitated psychosis. Depressed patients may primarily be paranoid or irritable or may even have blunted rather than sad affect. A neurovegetative syndrome consistent with depression, prior history of affective disorder, family history of affective disorder, and onset from a relatively normal baseline help make the diagnosis of depression (see Chap. 17).

(3) Atypical affective disorders are a diagnostically difficult area.

(a) Some patients have concurrent manic and depressed symptoms, called **mixed bipolar disorder.** These patients may be extremely agitated or, alternatively, may have intermittent or more protracted catatonic symptoms.

(b) Other patients have a past history of clear manias or depressions but presently have prominent psychotic symptoms despite relative remission of the affective symptoms. These patients are described by the *Diagnostic and Statistical Manual of Mental Disorders, Fourth Edition, Draft Criteria* (DSM-IV) as having **schizoaffective disorder** (see Table 21-2). It is important to determine whether acute decompensations represent a relapse of affective symptoms, which might respond to treatment with antidepressants, lithium, or electroconvulsive therapy (ECT), or whether the affective symptoms are in the background during the acute episode; focus on the antipsychotic medication might be the critical first step in diagnosis (see Chap. 21).

b. Schizophrenia may present as an acute psychosis either as the initial psychiatric contact or as an exacerbation of previously stabilized illness. In either case, schizophrenia is now understood as a chronic illness; DSM-IV requires at least 6 months of illness for diagnosis (see Table 21-1). Acute psychotic exacerbations of schizophrenia may be caused by noncompliance with medication, toxic effects of medication, superimposed drug abuse, or relapse despite apparently adequate treatment (see Chap. 21).

c. Schizophreniform disorder is diagnosed in patients who have symptoms of schizophrenia but whose illness has lasted less than 6 months (Table 19-3). These patients can present with the gamut of psychotic symptoms ranging from an acute, agitated psychosis to catatonia. This DSM-IV diagnosis is unlikely to represent a valid disease entity. Patients with good prognostic signs (Table 19-3) or a family history of affective disorder are likely to represent atypical presentations of mania, depression,

Table 19-3. DSM-IV draft criteria for schizophreniform disorder

A. Meets criteria A, D, and E of schizophrenia (see Table 21-1).
B. An episode of the disorder (including prodromal, active, and residual phases) lasts at least 1 month but less than 6 months. (When the diagnosis must be made without waiting for recovery, it should be qualified as "provisional.")

Specify if:

Without good prognostic features, *or*
With good prognostic features as evidenced by at least two of the following:

1. Onset of prominent psychotic symptoms within 4 weeks of the first noticeable change in usual behavior or functioning.
2. Confusion or perplexity at the height of the psychotic episode.
3. Good premorbid social and occupational functioning.
4. Absence of blunted or flat affect.

Source: Reprinted with permission from the *Diagnostic and Statistical Manual of Mental Disorders, Fourth Edition, Draft Criteria:* 3/1/93.

or mixed bipolar disorder and to have an indistinguishable prognosis. The remainder of patients probably represent a mixed diagnostic group including early schizophrenia. The critical point is that a diagnosis of schizophreniform disorder should not exclude patients from trials of lithium, valproic acid (Depakene), carbamazepine (Tegretol), and other drugs for mood disorders.

d. **Brief psychotic disorder** (Table 19-4) is the DSM-IV diagnosis used when psychotic symptoms develop acutely and last for a period of no longer than 1 month. This syndrome is most likely to occur in patients who have severe personality disorders at baseline, following an acute stressor. Behavior during the psychotic episode is often bizarre and histrionic. The validity of this diagnostic category is unsettled. It is possible that a significant proportion of patients who receive this diagnosis either have an affective disorder or display factitious psychotic symptoms in response to stress. Further research is needed.

Table 19-4. DSM-IV draft criteria for brief psychotic disorder

A. Presence of at least one of the following symptoms*:
   1. Delusions.
   2. Hallucinations.
   3. Disorganized speech (e.g., frequent derailment or incoherence).
   4. Grossly disorganized or catatonic behavior.
B. Duration of an episode of the disturbance is at least 1 day and no more than 1 month, with eventual full return to premorbid level of functioning. (When the diagnosis must be made without waiting for recovery, it should be qualified as "provisional.")
C. Not better accounted for by a mood disorder (i.e., no full mood syndrome is present) or schizophrenia, and not due to the direct effects of a substance or a general medical condition.

*Do not include a symptom if it is a culturally sanctioned response pattern.
Source: Reprinted with permission from the *Diagnostic and Statistical Manual of Mental Disorders, Fourth Edition, Draft Criteria:* 3/1/93.

e. **Factitious psychoses and malingering** occur most commonly in patients with underlying personality disorders or somatiform disorders (see Chap. 28). The psychotic symptoms are often atypical in onset and offset, are histrionic in nature, and often have a manipulative quality (e.g., occurring in such a way as to gain care or attention). The diagnosis requires the identification of some secondary gain and, preferably, the admission of voluntary control. This is an important diagnosis to make because the treatment is clearly different from that of the major psychoses. Neuroleptics are of no proven benefit in this disorder. Psychologic interventions are the therapies of choice.

2. **Drug-induced psychoses.** Drug-induced psychoses may be caused by acute or chronic abuse or by withdrawal. A history of drug use by the patient must raise the physician's suspicion. The patients themselves are often unreliable reporters, making data obtained from objective tests, such as a toxic screen, and from friends and family invaluable. It is important to note that patients with major psychoses such as schizophrenia often abuse drugs, which can produce a very clinically confusing picture. At times the components of such mixed states can only be sorted out in a drug-free inpatient environment. Drug abuse emergencies are fully reviewed in Chap. 30. Differential diagnostic points concerning drug-induced psychoses are covered briefly here:

a. **Phencyclidine (PCP,** or **"angel dust")** psychosis may result from a small or moderate dose, often in an inexperienced user. High doses of PCP may initially produce coma with behavioral excitation emerging as levels fall.

(1) The psychosis may include delusions, hallucinations, bizarre behavior, agitation, anxiety, panic, and aggressiveness or assaultiveness; it may mimic manic or schizophrenia-like symptoms.

(2) On examination, there is often a blank stare. Tachycardia and hypertension are the rule; there may be mydriasis, horizontal and vertical nystagmus, salivation and vomiting, ataxia, and muscular rigidity. In addition, there may be analgesia, which can be tested with a pin.

b. **Hallucinogens** include LSD, psilocybin, mescaline, and MDMA (3, 4-methylenedioxyethamphetamine, "ecstasy").

(1) The symptoms may include visual hallucinations, distortions of all senses, hyperesthesia, and euphoria.

(2) Mescaline produces tachycardia, hypertension, mydriasis, sweating, tremor, and motor restlessness and may also produce severe vomiting. The physical examination may be normal if LSD, psilocybin, or MDMA has been ingested.

c. **Cocaine and amphetamines**

(1) **Acute, high-dose use,** as may especially occur with use of intravenous cocaine or amphetamine, freebased cocaine or crack, or smoked amphetamine ("ice") may lead to paranoid states and violence (see Chap. 30).

(2) **Chronic use** or high doses of cocaine or amphetamines may produce a psychotic syndrome with paranoia, irritability, restlessness, emotional lability, formication, and stereotypy such as skin-picking, lip-biting, bruxism, or pacing. Examination reveals sympathetic excess (see Chap. 30).

d. **Withdrawal from alcohol or sedative hypnotics** may produce a state with visual hallucinations, agitation, delirium, and seizures. This state is usually readily distinguished from acute psychosis and is a medical emergency (see Chaps. 30 and 31).

3. **Medical and neurologic disorders** may present with a variety of psychiatric symptoms and signs including acute psychoses (see Table 19-1). The medical and neurologic disorders are reviewed in Chaps. 25 and 26.

E. **Management of acute psychoses** depends on the etiology. If the acute psychosis is due to one of the major psychiatric disorders, the initial symptomatic management is similar, even though definitive treatments differ. The cardinal points in emergency management are a safe environment, low stimulation, and antipsychotic medication with additional sedation if necessary. If an organic cause is suspected, the specific treatment of that disorder is the cornerstone of management. However, unless there are contraindications or a real need to observe the patient unmedicated, judicious use of a short-acting benzodiazepine or low doses of a high-potency antipsychotic agent may be extremely helpful in the early stages of management.

1. Patients who are acutely psychotic often refuse treatment, raising important **legal issues** (see Chap. 10). In emergency situations in which serious harm to the patients or others is likely, the physician must treat the patient. The nature of the emergency should be clearly documented in the record. If, on the other hand, there is no true emergency, a psychotic patient is allowed to refuse treatment pending a judicial ruling on his or her competency and need for treatment. It is worth consulting with hospital attorneys if the situation is unclear.

2. **Emergency behavioral management**

   a. As note above, the physician's first task is to ensure the **safety** of the patient and the staff. If the patient is violent or threatening violence, or is wildly psychotic and agitated, he or she should be put into four-point leather restraints (see Table 5-1). Even if violence is not an immediate problem, it is important to remove all potentially dangerous objects from the patient's possession, such as sharp objects, sources of flame, or belts. The need to do this should be explained in a firm way, but with respect for the patient's dignity. For example, the physician might say, "The symptoms of your illness are unpredictable, so it is important that you have nothing that you could hurt yourself with. We will return these to you as soon as we can."

   b. Patients benefit from a **low stimulation environment.** A specially designated "quiet room" is optimal if available. If not, the patient should be placed in a room that is free of any potentially dangerous objects (including extra furniture), that is out of the way of loud emergency department traffic but is not out of the way of observation.

   c. The patient should be **observed closely.** A staff member should look in at least every 5 minutes; some patients will require constant attendance.

   d. **Limits** should be clearly and simply set. Long discussions should be avoided. Explanations should be given for everything done, clearly and simply.

3. **Emergency pharmacologic management**

   a. **Pharmacologic management of the quiet and compliant patient** is an adequate dose of an antipsychotic drug, such as haloperidol 5 mg as part of a 5 mg bid regimen, or its equivalent. Liquid concentrates are preferable to pills because of more rapid absorption and because compliance with the dose is easier to monitor. The clinician should add a prophylactic antiparkinsonian, e.g., benztropine mesylate (Cogentin) 2 mg PO bid, especially if there is a history of prior dystonias or if the patient is at high risk of dystonia, i.e., a young male.

   b. Optimal pharmacologic management of **agitated, more severely disturbed patients** requires the administration of an antipsychotic agent and additional sedatives as needed.

(1) An effective regimen is haloperidol 5 mg of liquid concentrate PO or 5 mg IM as part of a 5 mg bid regimen (or an equipotent dose of another high-potency antipsychotic), with a prn benzodiazepine titrated to avoid the extremes of agitation and oversedation. Lorazepam 1–2 mg PO or IM every 30–60 minutes is a good choice. For severely agitated patients, lorazepam can be given slightly more frequently or by the IV route (1–2 mg given slowly to avoid respiratory depression), but vital signs must then be monitored very closely and the patient kept under constant observation. Intravenous benzodiazepines should only be used when personnel skilled in resuscitation are present. The combination of a high-potency antipsychotic and a benzodiazepine appears to produce fewer side effects than very high doses of either agent alone; the benzodiazepine may, in fact, exert a protective effect against akathisia and other neuroleptic-induced side effects. Use of a benzodiazepine in this situation poses little or no risk of tolerance or addiction because it is short-term. Addition of a prophylactic antiparkinsonian, e.g., benztropine 2 mg PO bid, is recommended.

(2) Although rapid high-dose neuroleptic administration ("rapid neuroleptization") was used by some clinicians in recent years, on closer examination this approach had more liabilities than advantages. Short-acting benzodiazepines are more reliably sedating than high-potency neuroleptics and have far fewer side effects. More sedating low-potency neuroleptics, such as chlorpromazine (Thorazine), should not be used in emergency situations because of the risk of hypotension and the risk of exacerbating the symptoms of certain ingestions, such as PCP and anticholinergics. The argument that rapid neuroleptization protocols produce faster improvement in psychotic symptoms than standard doses was not borne out; early improvement in psychotic symptoms with high-dose neuroleptic regimens probably represented no more than nonspecific sedation. The major problems with high-dose neuroleptic regimens are side effects, especially akathisia and parkinsonism. The former is uncomfortable, is difficult to treat, and may produce clinical worsening (e.g., agitation). Less common but more serious is the risk of severe extrapyramidal effects. Even when rapid neuroleptization appeared to be successful in the emergency department, over the ensuing 24–72 hours parkinsonian symptoms including catatonic-like symptoms of akinetic mutism appeared all too often. The clinician was then faced with the dilemma of determining which symptoms were due to the illness and which to medication.

III. Catatonia

A. Definition. Catatonia is a syndrome, not a specific disease or subtype of schizophrenia. Although the term is usually applied to patients with a primary psychiatric disorder, indistinguishable symptoms may be caused by a variety of organic causes, including neuroleptic drug toxicity (see Table 19-2). Since the emergency physician is faced with sorting out the etiology and beginning treatment, the full range of causes of catatonic-like symptoms are considered in this section.

1. Clinical features. The catatonic syndrome is characterized by some or all of the following:

a. Mutism (paucity or absence of spontaneous speech; lack of response to questioning).

b. Negativism (apparently motiveless resistance to all instructions or attempts to be moved; if active, the patient may do the opposite of what is asked).

c. Grimacing and posturing (assumption of bizarre facial expressions or postures, which may be transient or held for prolonged periods of time).

d. Catalepsy or waxy flexibility (a steady, slight resistance to movement that makes the limb feel like pliable wax); whether or not this abnormal resistance is present, the limb will often remain in the position in which it was left by the examiner.

e. Apparent stupor (little or no spontaneous movement and a marked decrease in reactivity to the environment despite being physiologically awake by electroencephalographic criteria).

2. The catatonic patient is at risk for dehydration and inanition. If the syndrome is due to a medical disorder, there is the additional risk from the underlying illness.

B. **Diagnostic workup.** Because this syndrome may result from the wide variety of causes listed in Table 19-2, the approach to diagnosis must be open-minded and systematic. Even in patients with an established major psychiatric diagnosis, difficulties remain. Catatonia may be the result of the underlying disorder, the result of the neuroleptic drugs given to treat the disorder, or the result of superimposed drug abuse or neurologic illness. On the basis of examination alone, it is often impossible to distinguish different causes of the syndrome.

1. **History** will have to be obtained from family and friends but should include a history of any psychiatric illness, recent medical symptoms, all prescribed medications, drug abuse, exposures to toxic substances, and family history of psychiatric disorders.

2. **Physical examination** should be thorough. It is important not to be blinded by prior psychiatric diagnoses but to be satisfied that the patient has the catatonic syndrome and is not stuporous or delirious on a medical basis. On examination the patient with catatonia may lie or stand with eyes open but apparently be unresponsive to visual stimuli. There are usually few or absent spontaneous movements. The patients are usually mildly tachycardic; slight elevations of blood pressure and temperature also occur. The pupils are normally reactive; oculocephalic (doll's head) responses are absent. Ice water calorics are rarely needed to rule out other diagnoses but produce normal rapid-phase nystagmus away from the irrigated ear. Other findings are as described in the definition of catatonia (see sec. **III.A**).

3. **Diagnostic tests**

a. **Laboratory tests** for all patients should include electrolytes, calcium, renal and liver function, glucose, a complete blood count, and a toxic screen.

b. **Electroencephalogram (EEG).** If the physician is unsure from the history and physical examination whether the patient has an organic delirium or catatonia on a psychiatric basis, the EEG is the most helpful additional test. Toxic deliria due to alcohol, sedative-hypnotic drugs, encephalitis, or early hepatic encephalopathy will result in abnormal slow activity on the EEG. Deliria due to withdrawal from alcohol or sedative-hypnotics will produce low-voltage fast activity. Petit mal, or complex partial status epilepticus, will also be apparent on the EEG.

c. **A lumbar puncture** should be performed if there is fever, and especially if there is a concomitant leukocytosis.

d. **An amobarbital (Amytal) interview** is advocated by some authorities as a way of distinguishing organic, psychotic, and hysterical causes of a catatonic appearance. Amobarbital sodium is given IV, at a rate no faster than 50 mg/minute, up to a total of 500–750 mg (the lower dose for small or elderly patients). The drug should be given through a secure, freely flowing IV line, in case respiratory arrest or another emergency requiring venous access should ensue. The dose is titrated to the degree of sedation desired. Usually the interview should begin with light sedation, a state in which patients will have lateral nystagmus. Deeper sedation will usually produce some degree of dysarthria. While the amobarbital is being given the physician should interview the patient in a nonjudgmental fashion and perform repeated neurologic examinations. Patients who are catatonic on an organic basis should worsen rapidly, whereas those with psychotic or hysterical disorders will tolerate higher doses and begin to improve. If the patient has a nonorganic cause of catatonia, further diagnostic information can be obtained by a skillful interview in which the patient is asked about symptoms and precipitants. The amobarbital interview is not a substitute for a careful diagnostic workup. A substitute for amobarbital is lorazepam, 1–2 mg, given slowly IV.

C. **Specific causes of catatonic symptoms** (see Table 19-2)

1. **Psychiatric causes**

a. **Major affective disorders** are probably the most common psychiatric causes of acute catatonia. In a series reported by Abrams and Taylor (1976) 39 (71%) of 55 patients with catatonic symptoms had affective disorders. A prior history of a manic or depressed episode or a family history of affective disorder will obviously help the physician in making the diagnosis. In the absence of such a history, acute onset of symptoms from a relatively normal baseline of functioning favors an affective diagnosis (or an organic cause); patients with acute onsets have the best prognoses.

b. **Schizophrenia** is probably a less common cause of acute catatonia. In the series of Abrams and Taylor, only 4 (7%) of 55 patients with catatonic symptoms met criteria for schizophrenia.

c. **Causes of psychogenic unresponsiveness** mimicking catatonia include conversion disorder, dissociated states, factitious disorders, and malingering. It may be difficult to differentiate unresponsiveness on the basis of these disorders from catatonia caused by a psychotic disorder. It is important to make a diagnosis, however, since the treatments are markedly different. In patients with hysterical and factitious disorders, neuroleptics are of no proven value; psychologic interventions are the treatments of choice.

(1) The major clues to the diagnosis are an atypical presentation and often, prior evidence of a personality disorder. The typical patient with **factitious stupor or coma** lies quietly with the eyes closed. He or she is usually unresponsive to stimuli or questions. If the patient is accompanied or if a prior hospital record is available, a history of similar episodes should be sought. The differential diagnosis of stupor and coma is complex, but medical causes obviously must be ruled out.

(2) The **neurologic examination** reveals the patient to be physiologically awake. The pupils are equal and reactive to light. The eyelids sre often held tightly closed and, if opened, usually close rapidly. It is virtually impossible to mimic the slow steady closure of the lids often seen in coma. Oculocephalic responses may or may not be present. Muscle tone is usually normal, as patients rarely resist passive movement of their limbs. True waxy flexibility is hard to mimic but is also absent in many genuinely catatonic patients. Deep tendon reflexes may be voluntarily suppressed, but if present, they are symmetric.

(3) Useful **diagnostic maneuvers** include the following:

(a) Although patients may not respond to noxious stimuli, they usually avoid self-injury. Thus if the patient's hand is released over his or her face, the hand will usually fall so as to miss the face.

(b) **Ice water calorics** always reveal quick-phase nystagmus away from the irrigated side. Lack of response or tonic deviation suggests a focal neurologic lesion.

(c) **The EEG** reveals the patient to be awake. Usually there is alpha rhythm inhibited by opening the patient's eyes.

2. Toxic states

a. A catatonic-like state can be produced by **neuroleptic drugs.** Although typically patients will have received high doses of neuroleptics, there are reports of a catatonic-like picture developing after only a single dose of medication. These patients may have all of the classic catatonic symptoms. Not all patients who develop catatonia in response to neuroleptics have an underlying psychiatric disorder; the syndrome also occurs in patients given neuroleptics for organic deliria. Neuroleptic-induced catatonia must be ruled out in any patient who develops catatonic symptoms after receiving neuroleptic drugs. Antiparkinsonian agents or benzodiazepines can be administered as a diagnostic maneuver, but in such cases they may work very slowly, and adequate doses must be given before iatrogenic catatonia is considered ruled out. Benztropine (Cogentin) can be given IV or IM in 2-mg doses. It has the advantage over diphenhydramine (Benadryl) of producing less sedation and therefore not clouding the diagnostic picture. If there is no improvement, the dosage should be repeated at least once after 20–30 minutes unless anticholinergic symptoms develop. Alternatively, lorazepam 1 mg can be given IM and repeated in 30 minutes if there is no response. Anticholinergic and benzodiazepine drugs can also be given serially. If neuroleptic-induced catatonia is diagnosed, the neuroleptic should be temporarily discontinued and resumed only after symptoms have cleared, obviously at a lower dosage. During the interim, treatment with an anticholinergic alone may be warranted.

b. **PCP and hallucinogens** can cause a catatonic syndrome with either excited or retarded features. PCP is the drug of abuse that is most likely to cause a catatonic syndrome and is unfortunately an adulterant in much of what is sold as LSD, mescaline, or tetrahydrocannabinol (THC). A history of drug ingestion and a positive toxic screen are the fundamental diagnostic clues. During the phase of stupor the only recommended treatment is supportive. As levels of PCP fall other symptoms may emerge; their management is described in Chap. 30, sec. **V.** Catatonia due to LSD and other hallucinogens often responds to low doses of high-potency neuroleptics such as haloperidol 5 mg.

c. **Other toxic substances.** The history of exposure is the crucial point in making the diagnosis. Catatonic states due to adrenocorticotropic hormone (ACTH) or glucocorticoids may respond to neuroleptic treatment.

3. Neurologic disorders

a. **Disorders of the basal ganglia.** Catatonic states can be caused by lesions of the basal ganglia. Indeed the basal ganglia are likely to be the site at which neuroleptic drugs cause catatonic symptoms as well. Catatonic-like symptoms have been observed in patients with end-stage parkinsonism and also in patients with bilateral surgical lesions of the globus pallidus made in an attempt to relieve parkinsonism.

b. **Other lesions.** Catatonia has been reported in patients with petit mal or complex partial status epilepticus, postictal syndromes, frontal lobe lesions, temporal lobe lesions, third ventricle tumors, and with the onset of viral encephalitis. The presence of fever or focal abnormalities on the neurologic examination should prompt further neurologic workup.

4. **Metabolic conditions** reported in association with catatonia include hypercalcemia, hepatic encephalopathy, pellagra, acute intermittent porphyria, and diabetic ketoacidosis.

D. Treatment of catatonic patients with psychiatric disorders

1. Once a psychiatric disorder has been diagnosed on the basis of history, physical examination, and any necessary diagnostic tests, appropriate psychiatric treatment can be started. It is critical that no neuroleptics be administered until neuroleptic-induced catatonia has been satisfactorily ruled out. Recent anecdotal reports suggest that lorazepam may be useful in the treatment of catatonia.

2. **Treatment of specific psychiatric causes of catatonia**

   a. **Affective disorders.** The single most effective treatment for catatonia due to mania or depression is electroconvulsive therapy (ECT). The value of ECT lies in its safety and in the rapidity with which it alleviates symptoms. However, because of the "invasive" nature of ECT in the minds of many people, and because court orders must usually be obtained to use it in unresponsive patients, ECT is usually reserved for patients who are medically at risk from the catatonic state and for patients who have not responded to other treatments. The standard first-line treatment, therefore, is to begin with a neuroleptic. Low-potency neuroleptics should be avoided because of the risk of hypotension and, in stuporous patients, worsened sedation. Haloperidol can be started at 5 mg PO or IM bid. As patients improve enough to take oral medication, antidepressants or lithium carbonate can be added depending on whether depression or mania has been diagnosed. Parenteral amitriptyline and imipramine are available in the United States, but for patients whose depression is so severe that they are unable to take oral medication, ECT remains the treatment of choice because of its rapidity of action.

   b. **Schizophrenia** is treated with neuroleptic drugs. As in the case of affective disorders, haloperidol 5 mg bid or the equivalent may be begun. ECT is of no proven value in schizophrenia.

   c. **Conversion reactions, factitious psychosis, and malingering** are difficult to distinguish from one another because the diagnostic differences are based on the degree to which the factitious symptoms are under conscious control. The degree of volition is notoriously hard to sort out unless the patient directly admits to malingering. In most cases of conversion, suggestion or noxious stimuli may be used to help the patient regain alertness. An amobarbital interview may also be helpful both diagnostically and therapeutically in such cases. A psychiatric referral can be offered once the patient resumes alertness, but it is often resisted.

Selected Readings

Abrams, R., and Taylor, M. A. Catatonia: A prospective clinical study. *Arch. Gen. Psychiatry* 33:579, 1976.

American Psychiatric Association Task Force on DSM-IV. *Diagnostic and Statistical Manual of Mental Disorders, Fourth Edition, Draft Criteria:* 3/1/93. Washington, D.C.: American Psychiatric Association.

Arana, G. W., et al. Efficacy of anticholinergic prophylaxis for neuroleptic-induced acute dystonia. *Am. J. Psychiatry* 145:993, 1988.

Ballenger, J. C., Reus, V. I., and Post, R. M. The "atypical" clinical picture of adolescent mania. *Am. J. Psychiatry* 139:602, 1982.

Coryell, W., and Tsuang, M. T. Outcome after 40 years in DSM III schizophreniform disorder. *Arch. Gen. Psychiatry* 43:324, 1986.

Cremona-Barbaro, A. Neuroleptic-induced catatonic symptoms. *Br. J. Psychiatry* 142:98, 1983.

Gelenberg, A. J. The catatonic syndrome. *Lancet* 1:1539, 1976.

Gelenberg, A. J., and Mandel, M. R. Catatonic reactions to high potency neuroleptic drugs. *Arch. Gen. Psychiatry* 34:947, 1977.

McEvoy, J. P., and Lohr, J. B. Diazepam for catatonia. *Am. J. Psychiatry* 141:284, 1984.

Perry, J. C., and Jacobs, D. Overview: Clinical applications of the amytal interview in psychiatric emergency settings. *Am. J. Psychiatry* 139:552, 1982.

Pope, H. G., Jr., and Lipinski, J. F. Diagnosis in schizophrenia and manic-depressive illness. *Arch. Gen. Psychiatry* 35:811, 1978.

Post, R. M., et al. Dysphoric mania: Clinical and biological correlates. *Arch. Gen. Psychiatry* 46:353, 1989.

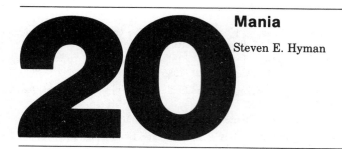

Mania

Steven E. Hyman

I. Manic episodes (Table 20-1) are frequently extremely disruptive to patients' personal lives, families, and jobs; may endanger the patients' safety; and often require emergency treatment.

A. By convention, patients with mania are said to have **bipolar disorder** (the *Diagnostic and Statistical Manual of Mental Disorders, Fourth Edition, Draft Criteria* [DSM-IV] term) or **manic depressive illness** even if they have never had a depressive episode.

B. The emergency evaluation and management of manic patients can be quite difficult.

1. Although classic mania is easy to diagnose, mania can also mimic other psychiatric disorders, such as schizophrenia, or even personality disorders.

2. It is common for individuals with mania to deny that they have a psychiatric illness or that they require treatment. They are often disruptive and argumentative. Effective intervention therefore requires great patience, calm, firmness, and sometimes even a degree of coercion on the part of the physician.

II. Clinical manifestations

A. Symptoms and signs. Manic episodes are subdivided into *hypomania* and *mania.* Hypomanias are less severe forms of mania. Hypomanias are diagnosed when there are unequivocal observable changes in functioning that are uncharacteristic of the person when not symptomatic, but the episode is not severe enough to cause marked impairment. If psychotic symptoms occur, the diagnosis of mania is made. DSM-IV refers to patients who have had at least one full manic episode as having *bipolar I disorder* and to those who have had only hypomanias as having *bipolar II disorder.* Patients who have only had hypomanic or manic episodes as a clearly precipitated result of antidepressant medication, electroconvulsive therapy, or light therapy are classified as *bipolar III* by some clinicians, but this is not a DSM-IV category. The cardinal symptoms of mania are often said to be elevated mood, flight of ideas, and motor overactivity, but presentations can be quite variable with a substantial fraction having atypical presentations. Thus a fuller description of presenting signs and symptoms is given here than is provided in the DSM-IV criteria (Table 20-1):

1. **Mood.** When elevated, mood is usually cheerful, high, and unselectively enthusiastic and has an infectious quality to it—that is, the examiner is often made to smile or laugh. It must be recognized, however, that the cheerfulness may be quite brittle, with patients suddenly becoming irritable, angry, or sad with little provocation. Indeed, it is characteristic of mania that affect can be markedly labile; thus even if the predominant mood is euphoric, the patient may have brief periods of tearfulness or even of feeling depressed and suicidal. The examiner can be fooled about the state of the patient's mood disorder if the patient is seen only once—for example, during a brief depressive swing. Some patients have little or no euphoria

Table 20-1. DSM-IV draft criteria for manic episode

A. A distinct period of abnormally and persistently elevated, expansive, or irritable mood, lasting at least 1 week (or any duration if hospitalization is necessary).

B. During the period of mood disturbance, at least three of the following symptoms have persisted (four if the mood is only irritable) and have been present to a significant degree:
   1. Inflated self-esteem or grandiosity.
   2. Decreased need for sleep (e.g., feels rested after only 3 hours of sleep).
   3. More talkative than usual or pressure to keep talking.
   4. Flight of ideas or subjective experience that thoughts are racing.
   5. Distractibility (i.e., attention too easily drawn to unimportant or irrelevant external stimuli).
   6. Increase in goal-directed activity (either socially, at work or school, or sexually) or psychomotor agitation.
   7. Excessive involvement in pleasurable activities that have a high potential for painful consequences (e.g., person engages in unrestrained buying sprees, sexual indiscretions, or foolish business investments).

C. The mood disturbance is sufficiently severe to cause marked impairment in occupational functioning or in usual social activities or relationships with others, or to necessitate hospitalization to prevent harm to self or others.

D. Not due to the direct effects of a substance or a general medical condition.

Source: Reprinted with permission from the *Diagnostic and Statistical Manual of Mental Disorders, Fourth Edition, Draft Criteria:* 3/1/93. Copyright 1993 American Psychiatric Association.

or are euphoric only during the early stages of the episode; such patients may be predominantly irritable, paranoid, or dysphoric. It is not uncommon for clinicians to mistake such patients as depressed or schizophrenic based on their mental status. Prior history, the **progression of the present episode, and the presence of other components of the manic syndrome** help make the correct diagnosis. Many of the irritable patients are easy to anger, may be quite litigious, and constantly threaten to sue or jail anyone who tries to treat them. Dysphoric manic patients are also at increased risk for suicide or committing acts of violence.

2. **Inflated self-esteem** is often marked; patients are often grandiose or have grandiose delusions, such as the belief that they have special powers.

3. **Hyperactivity** is often observed and may be accompanied by a subjective sense of increased energy. There is often an increase in social interactions and increased planning of and involvement in a variety of goal-directed activities, such as business or religious activities.

4. **Speech** is often loud, rapid, and difficult to interrupt (pressured). The examiner may find that he or she is speaking loudly and rapidly in an attempt to get a point across to the patient. (It is better to get the patient's attention and to make points briefly, slowly, and clearly.)

5. **Flight of ideas** presents itself as a rapid and continuous flow of speech with many changes from topic to topic. The flow is often based on small distractions in the environment. The subjective experience of the patient is of his or her thoughts going very quickly (racing), often so quickly as to be confus-

ing. Even when flight of ideas is not present, the patient's thinking is often **tangential.**

6. **Patients are easily distractible;** subjectively they will complain of an inability to concentrate.

7. Patients often become involved in activities that have a **high potential for bad consequences** that the patient does not recognize, such as going on spending sprees, driving recklessly, or inviting fights.

8. **Hypersexuality** is common; the patient may dress inappropriately and may flirt with the examiner. There may be a history of recent promiscuity that is otherwise uncharacteristic of the patient.

9. **Decreased need for sleep** is nearly universal. This is different from the poor sleep of the depressed patient because the patient will usually not feel tired. In severe mania patients may go for days without sleeping. Patients may also neglect to eat, often because they are preoccupied with other things.

10. **Psychotic symptoms** may occur. Many such symptoms are **mood-congruent** delusions and hallucinations, such as grandiose delusions. However, any kind of psychotic symptom may occur during a manic episode; the content of psychotic symptoms cannot be used to distinguish mania from schizophrenia. Ideas of reference are common in mania; bizarre hallucinations and delusions also occur, more commonly in adolescents. Many predominantly paranoid manic patients have been misdiagnosed in the past as paranoid schizophrenics.

11. **Confusion.** The generalization is often made that patients with organic deliria are likely to be confused, but those with major psychotic disorders have a clear sensorium. That generalization often does not hold for acute mania or other acute psychoses. Patients commonly are not oriented to time or place.

B. Clinical course

1. Classically, bipolar disorder is a remitting and relapsing illness with periods of normal functioning between episodes, but a minority of patients will develop chronic mania or depression that is refractory to treatment or chronic psychotic symptoms even when the affective symptoms are in relative remission. The latter group are called schizoaffective by DSM-IV (see Chap. 21, sec. **II.B**).

2. In general, the onset of a manic episode is relatively acute, occurring over days to weeks. Rarely mania can have a hyperacute onset over a period of hours. If symptoms were present for a long period before onset of the full manic episode, the prodromal symptoms often turn out to be typical manic symptoms in muted form (hypomania) or symptoms of an antecedent depression.

C. Past psychiatric history may reveal prior manic or depressed episodes.

D. Family history is often positive for mood disorder (depression or bipolar disorder), but it is often impossible to elicit such a history in the emergency department. It must be recalled that family members called schizophrenic in the past might now receive a different diagnosis, so it is worth considering how such individuals would be diagnosed currently based on their history rather than by accepting older diagnostic labels.

E. Other clinical considerations

1. All of the currently available antidepressant drugs may:

   a. **Precipitate mania** even if being used concomitantly with lithium. Precipitated mania may occur in already established bipolar patients or may represent the patient's first manic episode. Some patients only develop mania while on antidepressant drugs. In many cases, the manic episode continues even if the antidepressants are withdrawn, but in any case, **antidepressants should be discontinued when mania occurs,** and the overall influence of antidepressants on the course of the patient's illness should be considered.

b. Speed up the patient's rate of cycling, thus increasing the number of manic and depressed episodes suffered per year. In fact, antidepressant administration may induce rapid cycling (more than three cycles per year), a form of bipolar disorder, which is relatively treatment resistant. In general, it is worth minimizing antidepressant use in bipolar patients. Antidepressants should only be used when clearly needed and should be discontinued within a few weeks of resolution of acute depressive symptoms, with continuation therapy and prophylaxis being obtained from lithium alone. (This differs from unipolar depressives who generally benefit from 6 months of continuation therapy with antidepressants after their symptoms resolve.)

2. Postpartum, either depression or mania may occur. Women with a previous history of affective disorders during the puerperium are at increased risk during later pregnancies.

III. Epidemiology

A. The prevalence of bipolar disorder approaches 1% of the population.

B. Unlike unipolar depression, which occurs more commonly among women, the incidence of bipolar disorder appears to be equal between the sexes.

C. The age of risk extends throughout life, but almost all cases appear to begin between the ages of 15 and 60. The mean age of onset is in the early 30s, but one-third of cases begin before the age of 20 years. Estimates of age of onset may have to be revised downward as modern diagnostic tools are applied to children and adolescents.

IV. Differential diagnosis

A. Organic mood disorders (secondary mania). Just as depression can have an organic etiology (e.g., reserpine-induced, or pancreatic cancer), manic symptoms can be caused by physical illness or drug toxicity. The possibility of secondary mania should be considered in all patients. Thus the physician should always obtain a medical history, including a history of all prescription and illicit drug use. A neurologic and general physical examination should also be performed, although this may be extremely difficult if the patient is uncooperative. Causes of secondary mania are listed in Table 20-2.

B. Schizophrenia

1. Differential diagnosis may be difficult if the patient presents with a florid psychosis or predominant paranoia.

2. The presence of the manic syndrome (see Table 20-1) makes the diagnosis of mania despite the presence of even bizarre psychotic symptoms.

3. Unlike bipolar disorder, with its pattern of remissions and relapses, the course of schizophrenia, as defined by DSM-IV is chronic. DSM-IV requires a minimum of 6 months of illness before schizophrenia can be diagnosed. In general, psychoses developing rapidly from a good baseline of functioning are either organic or affective. If no organic cause is found and affective features are absent in a psychosis of less than 6 months duration, schizophreniform disorder should be diagnosed. This diagnosis probably does not represent a true "disorder," but a heterogeneous mix of patients, many of whom have atypical mood disorders (see Chap. 19, sec. **II.D.1.c**) and others of whom will go on to manifest schizophrenia. The important clinical point

Table 20-2. Organic causes of a manic syndrome (secondary mania)*

Drug-induced causes
- Glucocorticoids and adrenocorticotropic hormone (ACTH)
- Levodopa
- Isoniazid
- Psychostimulants
- Cyclobenzaprine (Flexaril)
- Bromides

Related to drug abuse
- Psychostimulant abuse, especially high-dose or chronic cocaine or amphetamine abuse
- Phencyclidine abuse
- Alcohol abuse or withdrawal

Toxic-metabolic causes
- Early hepatic encephalopathy
- Cushing's syndrome
- Hemodialysis
- Addison's disease
- Hyperthyroidism

Neurologic disorders
- Encephalitis
- Multiple sclerosis
- Wilson's disease
- Huntington's disease
- General paresis
- Brain tumors
  - Parasagittal meningiomas
  - Diencephalic gliomas
  - Craniopharyngiomas
- Organic deliria
- Temporal lobe lesions (usually nondominant)

*Manic episodes may be precipitated in bipolar patients by all antidepressant treatments (tricyclics, tetracyclics, trazodone, monoamine oxidase inhibitors, electroconvulsive therapy) and by psychostimulants. This is a different phenomenon from an organic etiology of mania (secondary mania) in that the patient has an underlying bipolar disorder.

is that a diagnosis of schizophreniform disorder should not rule out trials of lithium or other drugs used in the treatment of mood disorders, especially if certain features, such as family history, make the possibility of mood disorder greater.

C. **Cyclothymic disorder** involves cyclic periods of both hypomania and mild depression, but a full manic episode does not develop. Some patients may develop mania after a prior history of cyclothymia, at which time both diagnoses are appropriate. Cyclothymia may respond to lithium, although slowly and often less completely than bipolar disorder.

D. **Drug or alcohol abuse.** Although many drugs and alcohol can produce a picture of disinhibition, expansive mood, irritability, emotional lability, and even psychosis, perhaps those that can most readily mimic acute mania are phencyclidine (PCP) and cocaine or other psychostimulants (see Chap. 30). A drug history and toxic screen are critical parts of the workup for mania in the emergency department.

E. **Personality disorders** with affective instability may produce symptoms similar to hypomania or cyclothymia. It is important to try to make a diagnosis because the treatments are clearly different (e.g., psychotherapy versus a long-term trial of lithium with or without psychotherapy).

F. Complex partial seizure disorders (temporal lobe epilepsy) may produce a psychosis that can mimic mania or schizophrenia.

V. Emergency evaluation and management

A. Evaluation must include the history and mental status examination. The physician must not neglect to ask about suicide or potential violence; manic patients may be suicidal on a delusional basis. **Family history** should be obtained, concentrating on any history of psychiatric disorders, and **social history** bearing on the ability of those in the patient's living environment to care for him or her if discharge is contemplated.

B. Once a diagnosis of mania has been made, the physician must decide whether the patient is so disruptive and potentially dangerous as to require emergency intervention and transfer to an inpatient psychiatric unit. If the patient is less ill, the physician must evaluate the severity and nature of the symptoms and the resources of the home environment in order to determine whether further treatment requires a hospital setting. It must be recalled that the effects of antimanic medications might take as long as 10 days to 2 weeks to become apparent, and full remission might take 4 to 6 weeks. Thus even if the symptoms are mild, treatment beyond the emergency department must be planned.

C. Emergency treatment

1. If the patient is violent, hyperactive, or extremely disruptive in the emergency department, emergency intervention is necessary. Although the long-term treatment of choice for mania is lithium, its onset of action is so slow that it has no use in emergency situations. Even if the patient does not exhibit psychotic symptoms, the drugs of choice for treatment of acute mania are the antipsychotic drugs. In addition, if the patient is violent or uncontainable, the use of adjunctive sedative drugs is indicated, and restraint may be necessary.

2. The emergency regimen for an excited manic patient is identical to that for all acute psychoses discussed in Chap. 19.

   a. The patient should be placed in a low stimulation environment, free of any dangerous objects. (Some emergency departments have a designated quiet room for treating agitated patients.)

   b. The patient must be closely watched, but not stimulated. It is not helpful for the staff to get drawn into long discussions with the patient, especially if the patient's hyperactivity begins to worsen. Limits should be simple and clearly set.

   c. The patient should be told what the physicians believe the problem to be and offered medication. Short, simple explanations should be given.

   d. Medication should include an antipsychotic drug; haloperidol (Haldol) 5 mg as part of a 5 mg bid regimen (or an equipotent dose of another neuroleptic) is generally effective. Most patients will also require additional sedation. This is safely and effectively achieved with the short-acting benzodiazepine, lorazepam (Ativan) 1–2 mg PO or IM every 20–30 minutes as needed. The rationale for this regimen in acute psychoses is discussed in Chap. 19, sec. **II.E.3.b.**

   e. For patients already on lithium who are suffering a **breakthrough episode,** the lithium level should be checked in the emergency department and interpreted in the light of the elapsed time since the last dose. These patients should be continued on lithium and should have an antipsychotic and sedatives added to their regimen at doses identical to those for other manic patients. In addition, the reasons for the failure of lithium prophylaxis should be considered (see sec. **VI**).

   f. Patients who are ill enough to require emergency sedation will need inpatient treatment, preferably on a locked psychiatric unit. Unfortunately, involuntary hospitalization is often necessary.

D. Disposition. The need for hospitalization must be decided based on a variety of factors. In general, hospitalization is indicated if:

1. Symptoms are serious—for example, if the patient is at high risk for self-damaging acts, hurting others, or ruining his or her personal affairs.
2. The patient is at physical risk because he or she is not sleeping or eating or is extremely hyperactive.
3. The patient is psychotic or extremely impulsive.
4. There is a history of poor response to treatment.
5. The family feels unable to supervise outpatient treatment, or if the patient lives in a chaotic environment.

E. If the patient is to be treated as an outpatient:

1. The patient should be given a dose of an antipsychotic drug and a few days' supply to last until the first follow-up appointment. Haloperidol 5 mg bid or perphenazine 16 mg bid or the equivalent would be effective. Alternatively, the patient may have used a different antipsychotic successfully in the past and may want to use it again.
2. The patient should be given an appointment with a physician skilled in the use of lithium. (The use of lithium is discussed in sec. **VII.**) To expedite the subsequent initiation of lithium, the necessary baseline medical workup can be obtained.
   a. Serum creatinine and blood urea nitrogen (BUN).
   b. Thyroid stimulating hormone (TSH), and free thyroxine (T_4).
   c. An electrocardiogram (ECG) if the patient is over 40 years old or has a history of cardiac illness.
3. A member of the family should be asked to monitor the patient's compliance, since many manic patients do not recognize their illness and do not comply with treatment. This person should be instructed to bring the patient back to the emergency department if symptoms worsen or if the patient will not take medication.
4. The family should receive some instruction about manic-depressive illness so that the patient's behaviors (e.g., hypersexuality, intrusiveness) are understood.
5. The patient should be restricted from going to work or managing financial or personal affairs during the acute episode.
6. Psychotherapy should not be attempted while the patient is acutely manic.

VI. Determining the reason for the episode if a relapse. It is useful if the emergency physician considers the possible reasons for relapse because he or she may have the most data available to help optimize long-term management. Relapse may be due to the following:

A. Breakthrough symptoms despite an adequate prophylactic lithium level—that is, 0.8–1.0 mEq/liter. (A level should be drawn in the emergency department; it must be interpreted in the light of time since the last dose.) Lithium is not a perfect prophylaxis; if breakthroughs recur repeatedly, despite good compliance:

1. A higher prophylactic lithium level may be needed, although levels above 1.0 mEq/liter are not recommended because of side effects.
2. The patient may not have been on lithium long enough (a full prophylactic effect occasionally takes months to develop).

3. The patient may need an alternative or adjunctive treatment, such as carbamazepine (Tegretol) or valproic acid (Depakene).

B. Breakthroughs may be caused by **antidepressant** precipitation of mania in which case the antidepressant should be stopped in the emergency department and a note made to the patient's physician to reconsider the pattern of antidepressant use.

C. **Noncompliance** may be difficult to sort out. Many patients begin to become manic and then, because of the ensuing feeling of well-being, stop their medication. Others stop their lithium first with subsequent emergence of manic symptoms.

1. Causes of noncompliance include:

   a. Patient's unwillingness to give up manic "highs" or denial of illness.

   b. Side effects of lithium (see Chap. 24, sec. **VI**).

   c. Personal or cultural biases against somatic treatments not previously expressed to the patient's physician.

   d. A superimposed personality disorder leading to—for example, variable medication-taking, poor rapport with physicians, and threats of suicide with medication.

   e. Family interference—for example, pressuring the patient to deny the illness because of stigma, or providing a chaotic home life.

2. Noncompliance can often be avoided by paying attention to:

   a. Patient education

      (1) Discussion of need for medication, of lag periods prior to onset of efficacy (especially for antidepressants, lithium), and of the way in which the medication helps—that is, antidepressants and lithium are effective only with continuous usage and do not relieve acute symptoms when used prn.

      (2) Discussion of side effects (this should be documented in the record).

      (3) Exploring for misconceptions, possible symbolic meanings of the medication, and family disapproval.

   b. Keeping regimens as simple as possible.

   c. Side effects (see Chap. 24).

D. **Hypothyroidism** may either mimic depressive recurrences or make patients relatively treatment-resistant. Since lithium has pronounced antithyroid effects, emergence of fatigue, listlessness, and other symptoms of hypothyroidism, or an otherwise inexplicable worsening in the course of the manic-depressive illness, should prompt ordering of thyroid function tests including a TSH. Given lithium's antithyroid properties, a TSH should be checked every 6 months in the course of routine follow-up. Since this is the most sensitive test for hypothyroidism, other thyroid indices need only be checked if it is abnormal.

VII. **Lithium** is effective in treating manic episodes and is the drug of choice for prophylaxis against relapse. As noted above, however, it is not useful in emergency departments because of the slow onset of its therapeutic effect.

A. **Using lithium.** Lithium should be started slowly since a rapid rise in serum levels produces side effects. The usual procedure is to draw baseline renal function and thyroid studies and to perform an ECG if indicated. Lithium carbonate can be started at 300 mg PO tid in healthy adults but should be started at half that dose in the elderly or if renal disease is suspected. Although there are algorithms for choosing the maintenance dose from the level produced by a single oral dose, it is safest to increase the dose slowly as serum levels and side effects allow. Levels can be drawn every 4–5 days until a stable dose is achieved. The target serum level for acute manic episodes is 0.8–1.2 mEq/liter. For prophylaxis, levels can be in the range of 0.8–1.2 mEq/liter. Levels should be drawn 12 hours after the last oral dose. For patients with normal renal function, the oral dose that results in therapeutic levels is usually between 1500–2100 mg/day. Mild toxicity often occurs at the beginning of therapy and can usually be managed by temporarily decreasing the dose. Lithium toxicity is fully discussed in Chap. 24, sec. **VI.B.**

B. Indications for use. If a manic episode is mild, lithium may be used alone, provided the patient is closely supervised. For more severe mania, neuroleptic medication is usually begun first, but lithium can be added to the neuroleptic. It is generally preferable to wait for a day or two before adding lithium so that if side effects occur, it will be easier to identify the offending agent. Once the acute episode has resolved, the neuroleptic should be weaned and lithium continued alone as a prophylactic agent. The duration of lithium prophylaxis depends on the frequency and seriousness of recurrences and is a matter to be decided individually for each patient. After resolution of the acute episode the patient should be maintained at the lowest effective prophylactic dose. Once a stable dose is achieved, lithium levels can be monitored every 2–3 months, and renal function and thyroid function tests should be monitored every 6 months. The patient should be instructed about the symptoms of lithium toxicity and should report these promptly. Sodium restriction, volume depletion, and diuretic use will raise lithium levels. Thus lithium doses and levels will have to be carefully monitored during intercurrent illnesses, if diuretics are to be used, or if the patient plans to change his or her dietary habits. (Fuller descriptions of the use of lithium can be found in other sources [e.g., Hyman and Arana, 1987]).

VIII. Other antimanic agents

A. For patients who have repeated relapses despite adequate lithium therapy, the addition or substitution of carbamazepine or valproate in the pharmacologic regimen can be considered. This is a step best considered in conjunction with the physician treating the patient over the long term and should not be undertaken in the emergency department.

B. For manic patients who are uncontrollable in the hospital, despite the use of maximal regimens of neuroleptics, lithium, and/or carbamazepine, and sedatives, or whose hyperactivity threatens inanition despite sedation and restraint, emergency electroconvulsive therapy (ECT) is the treatment of choice.

Selected Readings

DIAGNOSIS

American Psychiatric Association Task Force on DSM-IV. *Diagnostic and Statistical Manual of Mental Disorders, Fourth Edition, Draft Criteria:* 3/1/93. Washington, D.C.: American Psychiatric Association.

SECONDARY MANIA

Cummings, J. L., and Mendez, M. F. Secondary mania with focal cerebrovascular lesions. *Am. J. Psychiatry* 141:1084, 1984.

Goggans, E. C. A case of mania secondary to vitamin B_{12} deficiency. *Am. J. Psychiatry* 141:300, 1984.

Jampala, V. C., and Abrams, R. Mania secondary to left and right hemisphere damage. *Am. J. Psychiatry* 140:1197, 1983.

Krauthammer, C., and Klerman, G. L. Secondary mania. Manic syndromes associated with antecedent physical illness or drugs. *Arch. Gen. Psychiatry* 35:1333, 1978.

RAPID CYCLING

Oppenheim, G. Drug-induced rapid cycling: Possible outcomes and management. *Am. J. Psychiatry* 139:939, 1982.

Roy-Byrne, P. R., et al. Aproaches to the evaluation and treatment of rapid cycling affective illness. *Br. J. Psychiatry* 145:543, 1984.

Wehr, T. A., and Goodwin, F. K. Rapid cycling in manic-depressives induced by tricyclic antidepressants. *Arch. Gen. Psychiatry* 37:555, 1979.

LITHIUM

Hyman, S. E., and Arana, G. W. *Handbook of Psychiatric Drug Therapy*. Boston: Little, Brown, 1987.

Prien, R. F., et al. Drug therapy in the prevention of recurrences in unipolar and bipolar affective disorders. *Arch. Gen. Psychiatry* 36:847, 1984.

BENZODIAZEPINES FOR SEDATION

Modell, J. G., Lenox, R. H., and Weiner, S. Inpatient clinical trial of lorazepam for the management of manic agitation. *J. Clin. Psychopharmacol.* 5:109, 1985.

CARBAMAZEPINE (TEGRETOL)

Ballenger, J. C., and Post, R. M. Carbamazepine in manic-depressive illness: A new treatment. *Am. J. Psychiatry* 137:782, 1980.

Lipinski, J. F., and Pope, H. G. Possible synergistic action between carbamazepine and lithium carbonate in the treatment of three acutely manic patients. *Am. J. Psychiatry* 139:948, 1982.

Post, R. M., et al. Prophylactic efficacy of carbamazepine in manic-depressive illness. *Am. J. Psychiatry* 140:1602, 1983.

ELECTROCONVULSIVE THERAPY FOR MANIA

Thomas, J., and Reddy, B. The treatment of mania. A retrospective evaluation of the effects of ECT, chlorpromazine, and lithium. *J. Affective Disord.* 4:85, 1982.

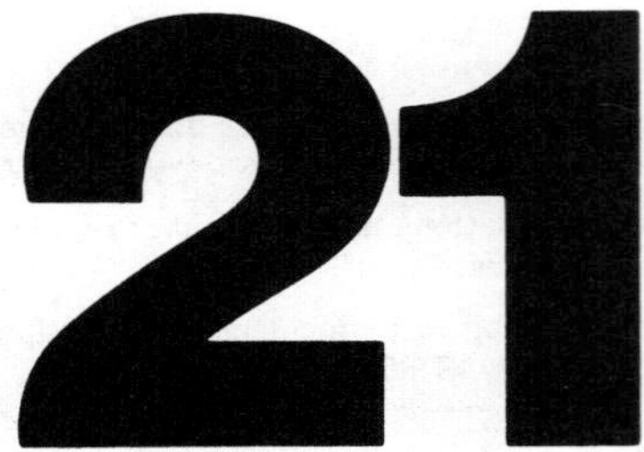

Schizophrenic and Other Chronically Psychotic Patients in Crisis

Steven E. Hyman
Donald C. Goff

I. Schizophrenic and other chronically psychotic patients may be brought for emergency treatment for many reasons, most dramatically when they develop a florid acute psychosis or catatonia superimposed on their chronic course, but also because of particular symptoms such as agitation, worsening in severity or frequency of hallucinations, increasingly bizarre behavior, or increasing withdrawal and apathy. Alternatively, emergency department visits may be precipitated by inadequate shelter, malnutrition, or intercurrent medical illness. The care of chronically psychotic patients represents a serious medical and social problem. Although antipsychotic medications have made it possible to discharge the majority of such individuals from psychiatric hospitals, these drugs generally do not produce a full recovery and may produce a host of neuropsychiatric side effects, some of which (e.g., akathisia or akinesia) may mimic the symptoms of the underlying illness. While antipsychotics are fairly effective in treating or at least dampening psychotic symptoms such as auditory hallucinations, they are less effective in treating the withdrawal, apathy, and idiosyncratic thinking that frequently impair the lives of these patients. Relapses of florid psychosis mark the course of many of these individuals; these relapses may be due to a variety of causes and require careful evaluation. In addition, release from psychiatric hospitals has created a new set of social problems, including homelessness, for many of these patients. Although the preponderance of chronically psychotic patients carry the diagnosis of schizophrenia, many suffer from poor prognosis forms of major affective disorder or organic psychoses—for example, due to head injury or as long-term sequelae of partial complex epilepsy. Although there are specific factors to be considered for each etiology of chronic psychosis, there are many similarities in the management of all such patients, including rational use of antipsychotic drugs and a proper level of social and psychologic support.

II. Specific disorders

A. Schizophrenia probably represents a heterogeneous group of disorders with certain clinical features in common.

1. The core features of schizophrenia, as defined by the *Diagnostic and Statistical Manual of Mental Disorders, Fourth Edition, Draft Criteria* (DSM-IV) are prominent psychotic symptoms and a chronic, downhill course (Table 21-1). The onset is usually insidious. Acute onset from an asymptomatic state or late in life suggests an organic or affective etiology.

   a. If symptoms have persisted for less than 6 months, a diagnosis of schizophrenia cannot be made. Patients with symptoms or schizophrenia for less than 6 months who do not have an affective syndrome or organic disorder are diagnosed as having **schizophreniform disorder** (see Chap. 19, sec. **II.D.1.c**).

   b. From the current state of research, it appears that a substantial proportion of patients with schizophreniform disorder do not go on to develop schizophrenia, with its chronic, downhill course. Indeed, there is evidence to suggest that if symptoms come on acutely, from a good baseline of functioning, or if there is a family history of affective illness, schizo-

Table 21-1 DSM-IV draft criteria for schizophrenia

A. **Characteristic symptoms.** At least two of the following, each present for a significant portion of time during a 1 month period (or less if successfully treated):*
   1. Delusions.
   2. Hallucinations.
   3. Disorganized speech (e.g., frequent derailment or incoherence).
   4. Grossly disorganized or catatonic behavior.
   5. Negative symptoms, i.e., affective flattening, alogia, or avolition.

B. **Social/occupational dysfunction.** For a significant portion of the time since the onset of the disturbance, one or more major areas of functioning such as work, interpersonal relations or self-care is markedly below the level achieved prior to the onset (or when the onset is in childhood or adolescence, failure to achieve expected level of interpersonal, academic, or occupational achievement).

C. **Duration.** Continuous signs of the disturbance persist for at least 6 months. This 6-month period must include at least 1 month of symptoms that meet criterion A (i.e., active phase symptoms), and may include periods of prodromal or residual symptoms. During these prodromal or residual periods, the signs of the disturbance may be manifested by only negative symptoms or two or more symptoms listed in criterion A present in an attenuated form (e.g., odd beliefs, unusual perceptual experiences).

D. **Schizoaffective and mood disorder exclusion.** Schizoaffective disorder and mood disorder with psychotic features have been ruled out because either:
   1. No major depressive or manic episodes have occurred concurrently with the active phase symptoms; *or*
   2. If mood episodes have occurred during active phase symptoms, their total duration has been brief relative to the duration of the active and residual periods.

E. **Substance/general medical condition exclusion.** The disturbance is not due to the direct effects of a substance (e.g., drugs of abuse, medication) or a general medical condition.

*Only one A symptom is required if delusions are bizarre or if hallucinations consist of a voice keeping up a running commentary on the person's behavior or thoughts, or of two or more voices conversing with each other.

Source: Reprinted with permission from the *Diagnostic and Statistical Manual of Mental Disorders, Fourth Edition, Draft Criteria:* 3/1/93. Copyright 1993 American Psychiatric Association.

phreniform disorder may, in fact, represent an atypical presentation of affective disorder. Thus consideration of use of lithium and antidepressants should not be ruled out in these patients.

2. **Prognosis.** For patients who meet criteria for schizophrenia, the prognosis is generally poor. Complete recovery is uncommon and should prompt reconsideration of the diagnosis. Partial recovery with remission of the florid psychotic symptoms is most typical, although about 20% of patients demonstrate little or no response to conventional antipsychotic agents. Unfortunately, the acute psychotic symptoms tend to recur, and even when the disease is quiescent, patients have residual symptoms (see Table 21-1) that may be disabling. The severity of these residual symptoms varies markedly among patients, but poor functioning in major life roles is the rule.

Table 21-2. DSM-IV draft criteria for schizoaffective disorder

A. An uninterrupted period of illness during which, at some time, there is either a major depressive episode or manic episode concurrent with symptoms that meet criterion A for schizophrenia (see Table 21-1).
B. During the same period of illness, there have been delusions or hallucinations for at least 2 weeks in the absence of prominent mood symptoms.
C. Symptoms meeting criteria for a mood episode are present for a substantial portion of the total duration of the active and residual periods of the illness.
D. Not due to the direct effects of a substance (e.g., drugs of abuse, medication) or a general medical condition.

Specify type:

Bipolar type: if manic episode (or both manic and major depressive episodes).

Depressive type: if major depressive episode only.

Source: Reprinted with permission from the *Diagnostic and Statistical Manual of Mental Disorders, Fourth Edition, Draft Criteria:* 3/1/93.

B. Schizoaffective disorder. These patients have had clear affective disorder at certain times but have prominent psychotic symptoms, even when their affective symptoms are in relative remission. Using current nomenclature, these patients are best described by the DSM-IV category of schizoaffective disorder (Table 21-2). A substantial fraction of these patients have chronic psychotic symptoms and a downhill course often indistinguishable from schizophrenia. Acute decompensations may be more disruptive than those of typical schizophrenic patients, however, because they may be accompanied by severe affective symptoms as well as by florid psychotic symptoms. It is important to determine whether acute decompensations include affective symptoms that might respond to treatment with antidepressants, lithium or carbamazepine, or electroconvulsive therapy (ECT), or whether the affective symptoms are in the background during the acute episode and therefore that treatment with an antipsychotic drug alone might be adequate. In schizoaffective patients use of treatments for affective disorder often improves mood and neurovegetative symptoms, but the response of psychotic symptoms is often incomplete and requires the addition of an antipsychotic drug.

C. Chronic organic psychoses may have specific therapies depending on the etiology, but treatment of the psychotic symptoms and behavioral disturbances is often empiric and based on the use of antipsychotic drugs in analogy with their use in primary (nonorganic) psychotic disorders. Thus, for example, if a seizure disorder is present, anticonvulsant treatment will be needed but will often not adequately treat the psychotic symptoms; these symptoms often respond, at least partially, to an antipsychotic drug. (High-potency antipsychotic drugs appear to have little effect on the seizure threshold.) If, in addition, a patient with an organic brain syndrome, e.g., on the basis of head injury or a dementing process, is unpredictably violent, consideration can be given to empiric trials of propranolol, lithium, or carbamazepine (Tegretol) (see Chap. 5).

III. Acute deterioration, whether a major psychotic episode or simply worsening in one or more chronic symptoms, may be due to a variety of causes and does not always reflect a worsening of the underlying process. Thus it is important that the patient not simply be given an extra dose of antipsychotic medication and hospitalized or discharged, but that a careful evaluation be performed, including a full history and mental status and physical examinations.

A. The history should provide information about the current problem, any possible precipitants, and the patient's overall course of illness and level of functioning. In addition, it is important to ask about medication compliance and side effects, demoralization, symptoms of depression, suicidality, drug abuse, family problems, living arrangements, lack of funds, and physical symptoms.

B. The reliability of the patient's answers must be considered with care and will depend, in part, on the severity of his or her pychosis. Often family and friends can supply important information about the patient's overall course, recent behavior, and compliance with treatment.

C. The management of the acute deterioration will depend on what, in particular, has destabilized the patient. **Causes of acute deterioration and their management** are discussed below:

1. Noncompliance with antipsychotic medication is a common cause of relapse. If the result of noncompliance is an acute agitated psychosis or catatonia, a full exploration of the compliance problem will obviously have to wait until the acute symptoms have been treated; otherwise it is worth taking up the problem of suspected noncompliance in the emergency department.

a. Evaluation. It is important to discuss with the patient his or her thoughts about whether the medications are helpful and to explore for any delusional ideas attached to the medication. In addition, it is important to ascertain whether there are any side effects (e.g., akathisia) that have discouraged the patient from taking medication. If a symptom being interpreted as a side effect is actually due to another cause, it may be possible to educate the patient. (For a full discussion of the side effects of antipsychotic drugs, see Chap. 24.) Finally, it should be determined whether the patient is unlikely to comply with an oral medication despite any treatment arrangements that can realistically be made.

b. Management

(1) If an **acute psychosis or catatonia** has emerged, it must be treated before other problems can be addressed. Even if a patient admits to noncompliance, it cannot be assumed that noncompliance is the only problem. Drug abuse or a superimposed organic disorder must still be ruled out. Catatonia, in particular, should not be treated with an antipsychotic drug until the physician is satisfied that the symptoms are not, in fact, due to prior neuroleptic treatment (see Chap. 19). If the physician is satisfied that the acute symptoms represent reemergence of the underlying disorder due to noncompliance or even despite adequate compliance, the treatment consists of an antipsychotic with addition of a sedative as needed (see Chap. 19)—for example, haloperidol 5 mg bid (or the equivalent) and lorazepam 1–2 mg PO or IM q20–30min as needed. Alternatively, use of an antipsychotic drug regimen that has succeeded in the past for this patient is reasonable unless the prior antipsychotic drug dosage appears to have been excessive. Young patients started on high-potency antipsychotic agents should also receive an anticholinergic drug (e.g., benztropine 2 mg bid) for prophylaxis against dystonic reactions during the first 2 weeks of therapy.

(2) If the patient has refused to take a particular medication (the reasons may be delusional) another antipsychotic drug at equipotent dose can be substituted, but compliance will have to be followed closely. Some patients will require long-acting antipsychotic drug therapy (see sec. **IV.A.3**).

(3) If **side effects** are the apparent cause of noncompliance, an attempt should be made to do the following:

(a) After resolution of acute symptoms, use the lowest dose of an antipsychotic that keeps the patient's symptoms under control (see **IV.A.2**). In practice, many chronic patients are probably being overmedicated.

(b) If the side effects of a particular agent are bothersome—for example, sedation or retrograde ejaculation with thioridazine (Mellaril)—an agent with a different side effect profile can be chosen (see Appendix I).

(c) Side effects remaining after medication doses have been decreased to the lowest effective should be treated—for example, akathisia can be treated with a benzodiazepine, propranolol, or an anticholinergic; parkinsonism can be treated with an anticholinergic (see Chap. 24).

2. **Side effects of antipsychotic drugs** may be the direct cause of deterioration in chronic patients.

   a. **Akathisia,** or a subjective need to be in motion (often accompanied by agitation, pacing, and irritability) is frequently misdiagnosed as an exacerbation of the underlying disorder. If this side effect is not recognized, the antipsychotic drug doses might be increased when it is a decrease or other treatment that is indicated. Thus agitated patients should be asked about feeling a need to move or to pace, and patients should be observed for repetitive motor behaviors consistent with akathisia. About half of patients with akathisia also have other extrapyramidal symptoms.

   b. **Akinesia** or a paucity of movement is an extrapyramidal effect of antipsychotic drugs. The patient may appear withdrawn with little expressiveness, symptoms easily misattributed to worsening schizophrenic withdrawal or blunted affect or to depression. Akinesia improves with reduction in drug dosage or addition of an anticholinergic. In its extreme form, neuroleptic-induced akinesia may be indistinguishable from **catatonia.** Depot antipsychotic drugs (fluphenazine and haloperidol are available as depot preparations in the United States) are particularly likely offenders because of their tendency to build up to extremely high levels if given too frequently or at too high a dose for a particular patient. It may take weeks at a lower dose of the depot compound for the patient to improve.

   c. **All extrapyramidal** symptoms may be uncomfortable and may contribute to deterioration both directly and often indirectly by decreasing patient acceptance of antipsychotic drugs. Patients should be examined carefully for extrapyramidal signs, such as cogwheeling, rigidity, masklike facies, and choreoathetotic movements.

   d. **Anticholinergic syndromes.** Apparent psychotic relapses may also be due to anticholinergic delirium. Older patients are at particular risk, but high doses of anticholinergic drugs, or polypharmacy with anticholinergic compounds, may produce delirium in any patient. Of the antipsychotics, thioridazine is the most anticholinergic. All of the commonly used antiparkinsonian agents used in psychiatry except amantadine (Symmetrel) are anticholinergic as are all cyclic antidepressants and antihistamines. Patients with anticholinergic delirium will usually, but not always, have some peripheral anticholinergic signs, such as tachycardia; mydriasis; warm, dry skin; dry mucous membranes; ileus; and urinary retention. Confusion, agitation, and inattention are usually prominent; often memory disturbance and visual hallucinations also occur (see Chap. 24).

3. **Drug abuse** commonly complicates the course of schizophrenia.

   a. **Evaluation.** Drug abuse should be suspected when the patient's symptoms take on a new pattern or become relatively treatment-resistant, or whenever a florid psychosis occurs. It is often helpful to get a history from family or other individuals in the patient's environment. If drug abuse is suspected, a drug screen should be obtained at the time of presentation.

   b. Management may be difficult; although it is helpful to explain to the patient that drug abuse may make it impossible to treat his or her symptoms successfully, the patient may be quite resistant to following the physician's advice. It may be necessary to attempt to place the patient in a more structured environment, such as a day program or halfway house in order to diminish opportunities for drug abuse. Follow-up may require repeated drug screens.

4. **Depression and suicidality**

   a. **Evaluation**

      (1) When examining the patient, it is important to ask about symptoms of **depression.** The development of a secondary depression may complicate the course of as many as 25% of schizophrenic patients (Siris, et al., 1987), and depressive episodes are likely to be even more common among chronic schizoaffective patients. Patients may have worsening withdrawal or apathy, lack of energy, worsening self-esteem, decreasing ability to function in major roles, or suicidality.

      (2) Even if not apparently depressed, psychotic patients should be asked about **suicide.** Because schizophrenic patients may not be willing to discuss suicidality in a straightforward manner and because they may act on suicidal ideas that are delusional and unrelated to normal motivations for suicide, the examiner must pay particular care to this part of the interview.

   b. **Management**

      (1) Emergence of depressive symptoms requires that the physician rule out organic causes including drug toxicity, especially subtle antipsychotic drug side effects that may mimic depression. In the absence of an organic cause, depressive symptoms in stable patients may respond to antidepressant therapy, although antidepressants may slow resolution of psychotic symptoms in acutely decompensated patients. One well-controlled study (Siris, et al., 1987) demonstrated significant benefit when full therapeutic doses of imipramine (up to 200 mg/day) were added to the antipsychotic (fluphenazine) in a group of depressed schizophrenic and schizoaffective patients. Significant depression in a chronically psychotic patient is often best treated in a hospital where antidepressant drugs can be begun safely. If the apparent depression is due to demoralization, psychosocial interventions are the best treatment and hospitalization may be counterproductive.

      (2) Serious suicidality on the basis of depression or delusional thinking requires hospitalization because psychotic patients cannot be assumed to have meaningful internal controls protecting them against suicide.

5. **A superimposed medical illness.** Especially if homeless, impoverished, or malnourished, chronically psychotic patients are at high risk for serious complications of medical illness. They frequently do not seek medical help in timely fashion. Thus any chronically psychotic patient presenting with an apparent decompensation must be fully examined for a medical illness

that could be responsible, as well as any coexisting medical illness that could be affecting the patient's overall level of health.

6. Some patients **relapse despite adequate medication** and in the absence of an intercurrent illness or drug abuse.

   a. **Evaluation.** These patients may have more severe illness, may have illness that is medication-resistant, or may have been misdiagnosed. It is important to consider the following possibilities.:

      (1) The patient may not actually be compliant.

      (2) The patient is taking another drug (e.g., an anticonvulsant such as carbamazepine) that alters the metabolism of the prescribed antipsychotic drug.

      (3) The patient has some organic cause of psychosis that has not been discovered—for example, a toxic-metabolic disorder or a neurologic disorder, such as Huntington's or Wilson's disease, or partial complex epilepsy.

      (4) The patient is doing poorly because he or she is overmedicated with resulting akathisia or catatonic-like symptoms.

      (5) The patient is undermedicated and an increase in his or her antipsychotic drug dosage would decrease the number and severity of relapses.

   b. **Management.** If the evaluation suggests that the patient is correctly diagnosed, is being medicated rationally, but has had emergence of psychotic symptoms:

      (1) A careful increase in antipsychotic drug dosage is worthwhile. This should be considered a therapeutic trial, not a life sentence. For patients on depot fluphenazine (Prolixin) or haloperidol (Haldol), temporary oral supplementation (e.g., adding 5 mg/day PO), rather than increasing the dose of the depot preparation, may be the best course unless the pattern of relapses suggests that a permanent dosage increase is warranted. If the relapse was a rare event, the dosage can be decreased again after the patient has returned to baseline and has been stable for several months. If the relapse was severe or relapses have been frequent, a long-term increase in maintenance dosage should be considered (see sec. **IV.A.2**). If a higher dose does not produce improvement in a month, the trial should be reevaluated, with either an even higher dose tried, or with return to a lower dose if side effects were severe despite lack of a therapeutic effect. All too often, treatment-resistant patients are left on heroic doses of antipsychotics with marginal or no benefit; such doses are generally more reflective of physician frustration than good practice. Despite occasional anecdotal reports, it is distinctly uncommon for patients to gain additional benefit from doses greater than haloperidol 20 mg/day or the equivalent and the vast majority of patients need far less.

      (2) Some treatment-resistant patients may be rapidly metabolizing their medication. Unfortunately, the measurement of antipsychotic drug blood levels by various techniques has not been shown to correlate well with therapeutic response, making it difficult to recommend use of blood levels even in treatment-resistant patients. For many drugs the interpretation of levels is rendered impossible by the huge number of possibly active metabolites that are not routinely measured. Some studies suggest that haloperidol levels of 8–10 ng/ml may correspond with a clinical antipsychotic effect, but this is by no means certain. Haloperidol has only one metabolite that may be active, hydroxyhaloperidol.

(3) Truly treatment-resistant patients deserve a thorough diagnostic reevaluation, including a neurologic evaluation, and in many cases an orderly trial of adjunctive medications in addition to antipsychotics. Especially if the patient may be schizoaffective, these may include lithium and carbamazepine. If the patient is agitated a benzodiazepine might be considered. Patients who remain severely impaired after at least two adequate trials of conventional antipsychotic agents and patients who cannot tolerate conventional agents may benefit from a trial of the atypical agent clozapine.

7. **A psychosocial crisis** such as threatened or actual loss of a caregiver or living situation may precipitate an emergency department visit.

   a. **Evaluation.** Chronically psychotic patients are at high risk for social difficulties because they often act with poor judgment, manage their funds poorly, and exhaust their families and other psychosocial supports. Sheltered housing, work programs, and day hospitals are understaffed or unavailable in many areas. The patients may present agitated, confused, or demoralized with no place to go and no resources. In treating such crises the physician will find it helpful to contact family members and personnel of any agencies with which the patient has dealt.

   b. **Management.** Often specialized social service personnel are better able to help with such problems than physicians. Awareness of appropriate local mental health programs, day hospitals, and halfway houses is critical in making a disposition. It is optimal to help the patient establish a long-term relationship with a single clinician. When made from the emergency department, such referrals often fail, however, unless the referring physician follows up to make sure that the patient has kept his or her initial appointment. If possible the patient should be given a written appointment card with all relevant information. While it is not possible to work social miracles in the emergency department, it may be a setting from which helpful referrals and interventions can be made.

8. Lack of a peaceful and accepting **family environment** may contribute to relapse despite the use of medication.

   a. **Evaluation.** When patients have a higher than expected number of relapses despite medication, it is worth looking into the possibility that the family is extremely negative and critical about the patient's psychotic symptoms or lack of initiative (so-called high expressed emotion families).

   b. **Management.** Several studies have now suggested that supportive family therapy to decrease "expressed emotion" in the schizophrenic patient's environment may decrease the rate of relapse. If there is evidence that the family environment may be contributing to a patient's doing poorly, a referral for a family evaluation could prove useful.

IV. Long-term treatment issues

A. Antipsychotic drug therapy is of clear benefit to most patients but is not a panacea. Patients can be expected to have residual symptoms and social difficulties. In addition, antipsychotic medication may cause tardive dyskinesia in 20% of patients treated for more than a year (see Chap. 24, sec. **II.F.**). Social skills training, along with appropriate family therapy and education, can decrease relapse rates among schizophrenic patients when combined with pharmacotherapy. Insight-oriented psychotherapy does not appear to decrease relapse rates.

1. **Choice of antipsychotic drug** depends on the profile of side effects that the patient tolerates best. Low-potency drugs are more sedating and anticholinergic and cause more hypotension. The high-potency drugs have a greater tendency to cause extrapyramidal symptoms (see Appendix I). There is no convincing evidence to suggest that one drug is more effective than another for treatment-resistant patients, with the exception of clozapine.

2. **The optimal maintenance dose** of an antipsychotic drug must be determined individually for each patient. While the evidence is clear that maintenance therapy is effective in decreasing the number and severity of relapses, the effectiveness of medication must be balanced by the side effects suffered by the patient and by the risk of tardive dyskinesia. In general it appears that doses equivalent to 8 mg/day of haloperidol (400 mg/day of chlorpromazine) are adequate in most acute situations and that doses as low as 2–4 mg/day of haloperidol (100–200 mg/day of chlorpromazine) may be effective in long-term maintenance. Throughout therapy it is best to always attempt to use the lowest dose consistent with an adequate therapeutic effect for any particular patient.

3. **Depot preparations.** When repeated problems with compliance threatens the well-being of chronically psychotic patients, consideration should be given to use of depot preparations. In the United States the most commonly used depot preparations are fluphenazine decanoate and haloperidol decanoate. Standard dosages are of fluphenazine decanoate 12.5–25 mg IM every 2 weeks or haloperidol decanoate 150 mg IM every 4 weeks. Doses as low as 10 mg of fluphenazine every 2 weeks have been shown to be effective, although with a higher relapse rate after 1 year than with a 25 mg q2wk regimen (Marder, et al., 1987). There is no evidence that chronic dosing with fluphenazine decanoate above 25 mg q2wk has any therapeutic advantage, although patients clearly suffer worse side effects. One reasonable approach to using depot agents is the following:

   a. Try the patient on an oral dose of the compound to be used to be sure there are no unexpected toxic reactions.

   b. Build up over 2 months to a standard dose (i.e., fluphenazine decanoate 25 mg q2wk or haloperidol 150 mg q4wk) using oral supplementation as needed during this period.

   c. After a stabilization period (e.g., 6–12 months), if the patient has done well, slowly decrease the dose as tolerated.

   d. Rare relapses, especially if mild, can be treated with temporary oral supplementation; if relapses become frequent or are severe, return to a higher dose may be needed.

   e. When patients are on long-acting preparations it is important to be particularly vigilant for side effects.

B. For chronically psychotic patients, **a long-term relationship with a physician** is of great importance as it is in any severe chronic disorder. The physician must monitor medications, side effects, and emergent symptoms of tardive dyskinesia; encourage the patient; help with social problems; and teach the patient's family.

Selected Readings

American Psychiatric Association Task Force on DSM-IV. *Diagnostic and Statistical Manual of Mental Disorders, Fourth Edition, Draft Criteria:* 3/1/93.Washington, D.C.: American Psychiatric Association.

Arana, G. W., et al. Efficacy of anticholinergic prophylaxis for neuroleptic-induced acute dystonia. *Am. J. Psychiatry* 145:993, 1988.

Baldessarini, R. J., Cohen, B. M., and Teicher, M. H. Significance of neuroleptic dose and plasma level in the pharmacological treatment of psychoses. *Arch. Gen. Psychiatry* 45:79, 1988.

Baldessarini, R. J., and Frankenburg, R. Clozapine: A novel antipsychotic agent. *N. Engl. J. Med.* 324:746, 1991.

Breier, A., and Astrachan, B. Characterization of schizophrenic patients who commit suicide. *Am. J. Psychiatry* 141:206, 1984.

Breier, A., et al. National Institute of Mental Health Longitudinal Study of Chronic Schizophrenia: Prognosis and predictors of outcome. *Arch. Gen. Psychiatry* 48:239, 1991.

Carone, B., Harrow, M., and Westermeyer, J. Posthospital course and outcome in schizophrenia. *Arch. Gen. Psychiatry* 48:247, 1991.

Christison, G., Kirch, D., and Wyatt, R. When symptoms persist: Choosing among alternative somatic treatments. *Schizophr. Bull.* 17:217, 1991.

Falloon, I. R. H., et al. Family management in the prevention of morbidity of schizophrenia: Clinical outcome of a two year longitudinal study. *Arch. Gen. Psychiatry* 42:887, 1985.

Hogarty, G., et al. Family psychoeducation, social skills training, and maintenance chemotherapy in the aftercare treatment of schizophrenia. *Arch. Gen. Psychiatry* 48:340, 1991.

Kane, J. M. The current status of neuroleptic therapy. *J. Clin. Psychiatry* 50:322, 1989.

Kay, S. R., and Singh, M. M. The positive-negative distinction in drug-free schizophrenic patients: Stability, response to neuroleptics, and prognostic significance. *Arch. Gen. Psychiatry* 46:711, 1989.

Kramer, M., et al. Antidepressants in "depressed" schizophrenic inpatients. *Arch. Gen. Psychiatry* 46:922, 1989.

Marder, S. R., et al. Low and conventional dose maintenance therapy with fluphenazine decanoate: Two year outcome. *Arch. Gen. Psychiatry* 44:518, 1987.

Shauer, A., et al. Unrecognized cocaine use among schizophrenic patients. *Am. J. Psychiatry* 150:758, 1993.

Siris, S. G., et al. Adjunctive imipramine in the treatment of postpsychotic depression. *Arch. Gen. Psychiatry* 44:533, 1987.

VanPutten, T., and May, P. R. A. "Akinetic depression" in schizophrenia. *Arch. Gen. Psychiatry* 35:1101, 1978.

VanPutten, T., May, P. R. A., and Marder, S. R. Akathisia with haloperidol and thiothixene. *Arch. Gen. Psychiatry* 41:1036, 1984.

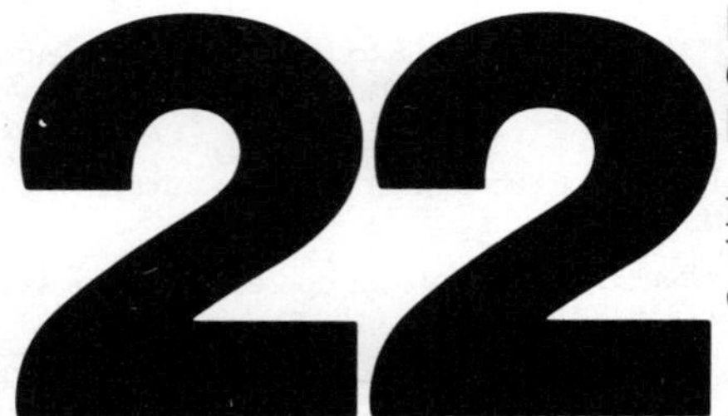

Borderline and Other Personality Disorders

Eugene V. Beresin
William E. Falk
Christopher Gordon

I. Overview of personality disorders

A. Patients with personality disorders are the bane of clinicians who staff psychiatric emergency departments. Not only are they among the most frequent users and abusers of the emergency department, but they present practitioners with perhaps the most complex, confusing, emotionally charged, and time-consuming problems of all psychiatric patients. Only a select group of people with personality disorders arrive at hospital or clinic doorsteps emergently, but those who do tend to lead the most turbulent, chaotic lives, maintain the fewest social supports, teeter on the brink of destroying themselves or others, and as a result, entwine the clinician in evaluations that are often as distressing as they are challenging. It requires critical diagnostic skill in conjunction with careful self-observation to prevent the patient's often disruptive, devaluing or seductive behavior from influencing objective, thoughtful assessment and management.

B. Definition. According to the *Diagnostic and Statistical Manual of Mental Disorders, Fourth Edition, Draft Criteria* (DSM-IV) of the American Psychiatric Association, **personality traits** are enduring patterns of perceiving, thinking about, and relating to oneself and others, exhibited in a wide range of contexts. It is only when a constellation of personality traits are inflexible and maladaptive and produce significant and pervasive distress and impairment that they constitute **personality disorders.** The symptoms of personality disorders are usually first recognized by adolescence and continue throughout most of adult life, though they may diminish by mid-life or old age. Perry and Vaillant (1989) indicate that all personality disorders share the same four characteristics:

1. An inflexible and maladaptive response to stress.
2. A disability in working and loving that is serious and pervasive.
3. Elicitation of problematic responses by interpersonal conflict.
4. A peculiar capacity to "get under the skin" of and distress others.

C. In addition, Perry and Vaillant (1989) observe that the defensive structure of personality disorders tends, in most cases, to cloak anxiety and depression. For people with personality disorders, the interpersonal context is a painful one, in which one both needs but cannot trust or rely on others. A major feature of personality disorders is a **severe lack of empathy,** manifested in part by the patients' inability to see themselves as others see them. As a result, their behavior frequently causes turmoil, since they cannot perceive or take responsibility for the effect they have on others. Of greatest importance to clinicians is to understand that personality structures, even the most disturbing, do not represent voluntary choices. They are not purposely meant to be weapons used against clinicians.

D. Categories of personality disorders. The DSM-IV divides personality disorders into three clusters:

1. **Cluster A** includes patients who appear odd or secretive (paranoid, schizoid, or schizotypal personality disorders).

Table 22-1. DSM-IV draft criteria for borderline personality disorder

A pervasive pattern of instability of interpersonal relationships, self-images, affects, and control over impulses beginning by early adulthood and present in a variety of contexts.

At least five of the following:

1. Frantic efforts to avoid real or imagined abandonment.
2. A pattern of unstable and intense interpersonal relationships, characterized by alternating between extremes of idealization and devaluation.
3. Identity disturbance (i.e., persistent and markedly disturbed, distorted, or unstable self-image or sense of self).
4. Impulsivity in at least two areas that are potentially self-damaging (e.g., spending, sex, substance abuse, reckless driving, binge eating).
5. Recurrent suicidal behavior, gestures, or threats, or self-mutilating behavior.
6. Affective instability due to a marked reactivity of mood (e.g., intense episodic dysphoria, irritability, or anxiety usually lasting a few hours and only rarely more than a few days).
7. Chronic feelings of emptiness.
8. Inappropriate, intense anger or lack of control of anger (e.g., frequent displays of temper, constant anger, recurrent physical fights).
9. Transient, stress-related paranoid ideation or severe dissociative symptoms.

Source: Reprinted with permission from the *Diagnostic and Statistical Manual of Mental Disorders, Fourth Edition, Draft Criteria:* 3/1/93. Copyright 1993 American Psychiatric Association.

2. **Cluster B** includes those who appear dramatic, emotional, or erratic (antisocial, borderline, histrionic, or narcissistic personality disorders). Not surprisingly, Cluster B patients most commonly utilize emergency departments since their lives are most turbulent, erratic, and chaotic. Within this group, **the most common personality disorder seen for emergencies is borderline** (Table 22-1). Tables 22-2, 22-3, and 22-4 delineate the draft DSM-IV criteria for antisocial, histrionic, and narcissistic personality disorders, respectively.

3. **Cluster C** patients are typically anxious or fearful (avoidant, dependent, or obsessive-compulsive personality disorders).

4. There is clearly overlap between the disorders, and patients may meet criteria for more than one personality disorder. Those who do not meet diagnostic criteria for any one specific disorder, but are clearly impaired, are included under the category personality disorder not otherwise specified.

II. Clinical description of borderline personality disorder

A. Etiology. Some understanding of the origins and consequent psychodynamics of the borderline personality is essential for evaluation and treatment. Understanding of etiology is still speculative at this juncture, although increasingly, longitudinal empiric studies are providing a clearer picture. While a wide range of causal variables in biologic, familial, and interpersonal areas may be considered, borderline personality most likely results from complex gene–environment interactions.

1. **Biologic variables.** Temperamental or constitutional factors likely play a role in the vulnerability to borderline personality disorder.

2. **Familial variables.** Epidemiologic studies have demonstrated a cluster of personality disorders in parents of borderline patients, including antisocial, narcissistic, histrionic, and borderline personality disorders. Although such

Table 22-2. DSM-IV draft criteria for antisocial personality disorder

A. Current age at least 18.
B. Evidence of conduct disorder with onset before age 15.
C. A pervasive pattern of disregard for and violation of the rights of others occurring since age 15, as indicated by at least three of the following:
   1. Failure to conform to social norms with respect to lawful behaviors, as indicated by repeatedly performing acts that are grounds for arrest.
   2. Irritability and aggressiveness, as indicated by repeated physical fights or assaults.
   3. Consistent irresponsibility as indicated by repeated failure to sustain consistent work behavior or honor financial obligations.
   4. Impulsivity or failure to plan ahead.
   5. Deceitfulness, as indicated by repeated lying, use of aliases, or conning others for personal profit or pleasure.
   6. Reckless disregard for safety of self or others.
   7. Lack of remorse, as indicated by being indifferent to or rationalizing reasons for having hurt, mistreated, or stolen from another.
D. Occurrence of antisocial behavior is not exclusively during the course of schizophrenia or a manic episode.

Source: Reprinted with permission from the *Diagnostic and Statistical Manual of Mental Disorders, Fourth Edition, Draft Criteria:* 3/1/93.

Table 22-3. DSM-IV draft criteria for histrionic personality disorder

A pervasive pattern of excessive emotionality and attention seeking, beginning by early adulthood and present in a variety of contexts, as indicated by at least five of the following:

1. Is uncomfortable in situations in which he or she is not the center of attention.
2. Interaction with others is often characterized by inappropriate sexually seductive or provocative behavior.
3. Displays rapidly shifting and shallow expression of emotions.
4. Consistently uses physical appearance to draw attention to oneself.
5. Style of speech is excessively impressionistic and lacking in detail.
6. Self-dramatization, theatricality, and exaggerated expression of emotion.
7. Suggestibility, i.e., easily influenced by others or circumstances.
8. Considers relationships to be more intimate than they actually are.

Source: Reprinted with permission from the *Diagnostic and Statistical Manual of Mental Disorders, Fourth Edition, Draft Criteria:* 3/1/93.

Table 22-4. DSM-IV draft criteria for narcissistic personality disorder

A pervasive pattern of grandiosity (in fantasy or behavior), need for admiration, and lack of empathy, beginning by early adulthood and present in a variety of contexts, as indicated by at least five of the following:

1. A grandiose sense of self-importance (e.g., exaggerates achievements and talents, expects to be recognized as superior without commensurate achievements).
2. Preoccupation with fantasies of unlimited success, power, brilliance, beauty, or ideal love.
3. Believes that he or she is "special" and unique and can only be understood by, or should associate with other special or high-status people (or institutions).
4. Requires excessive admiration.
5. A sense of entitlement, i.e., unreasonable expectations of especially favorable treatment or automatic compliance with his or her expectations.
6. Is interpersonally exploitative, i.e., takes advantage of others to achieve his or her own ends.
7. Lack of empathy, i.e., unwilling to recognize or identify with the feelings and needs of others.
8. Is often envious of others or believes that others are envious of him or her.
9. Arrogant, haughty behaviors or attitudes.

Source: Reprinted with permission from the *Diagnostic and Statistical Manual of Mental Disorders, Fourth Edition, Draft Criteria:* 3/1/93. Copyright 1993 American Psychiatric Association.

studies are consistent with a genetic predisposition, there is also increased frequency, compared with control groups, of early parental losses or traumatic separations. Moreover, there is a markedly increased incidence of family violence, alcoholism, physical abuse, neglect, and sexual abuse (see sec. **4**).

3. **Interpersonal/intrapsychic variables.** Most psychoanalytic and developmental theorists have posited deficits in early relationships, resulting in an impaired capacity for self-soothing. Early relationship failures may involve gross assaults on the child, as in sexual or physical trauma, or possibly may stem from more subtle deviations from optimal parenting, such as excessive smothering or enmeshment, often alternating with emotional or actual abandonment. All of this produces in the vulnerable young child and future adult borderline personality, a pervasive sense of emptiness, anxiety, and isolation. The failure to achieve a coherent sense of self provides cold comfort in the face of constant fears of abandonment and aloneness. As these children grow, they strive endlessly to find a person who will satisfy wishes for unconditional nurturing and protection. Since no one can realistically deliver this, interpersonal disappointments easily trigger regression, filled with profound envy, rage, and despair. At these times, the well-recognized defense of **splitting** becomes pronounced as an adaptive measure to preserve the integrity of (and hope for) the loving person always longed for, while differentiating it from the abandoning or smothering person engendering hatred and rage. Other defenses including idealization, devaluation, projection, and denial also come into play. Adult borderline patients maintain these defenses and view the world as a dangerous, hostile place. They feel entitled to the fulfillment of infantile wishes and feel perpetually victimized. Monumental rage emerges, evoking feelings of primitive guilt and worthlessness. Overwhelmed with such emotions, borderline patients often

react impulsively with self-destructive behavior, such as suicide gestures, sexual promiscuity, violent outbursts, or substance abuse. During such regressions there is impaired empathy and an inability to take responsibility for one's feelings or actions.

4. Recent data have underscored the role of **sexual and physical abuse** in the genesis of the borderline syndrome, even when this abuse occurs in developmentally more mature children and adolescents. As many as 70% of borderline patients may have been sexually and physically abused, particularly during latency, with some abuse continuing through adolescence. While these data do not negate the importance of early trauma, they shed new light on the development of the syndrome. Weston et al. (1990) and others view borderline psychopathology as, in part, a consequence of a posttraumatic stress disorder, incorporated into personality structure, even as late as adolescence. According to this thinking, borderline personalities maintain the profile of distrustful, angry victims into adulthood.

B. Clinical presentation

1. **Crisis of aloneness.** Any change in the routine structure of daily life, particularly in relationships, may be sufficient to dislodge a fragile sense of stability and unleash a crisis marked by feelings of terror and frantic attempts to avoid real or perceived abandonment. Virtually all borderline patients present in emergency settings during such a crisis of aloneness. The most common precipitants of this sort include perceived disruptions in therapy, such as a therapist's vacation or change in hours, fees, or location; interpersonal turmoil, such as arguments with a lover, spouse, or friend; major life events, such as unemployment, illness, pregnancy, deaths, or anniversaries of important events; legal problems; or changes in residence.

2. **The great imitator.** When experiencing stress, borderline patients can mimic almost any psychiatric disorder. They may appear agitated, intoxicated, manic, depressed, psychotic, agoraphobic with panic attacks, or delirious. There may be ghastly suicidal gestures, homicidal ideation or intent, or paranoid thinking. They may be angry and assaultive or appear helpless and vulnerable. There may be demands for hospitalization, medications, shelter, or retaliation at uncaring people. Some patients will actively threaten suicide or homicide if their demands are not met. The borderline patient may idealize the hospital staff, expecting unrealistic gratification, which inevitably leads to bitter disappointments and further behavioral deterioration. At the same time, these patients often have a long-standing (often well-founded) pessimism about their chances of being helped. Such conflicting expectations cause them to shift rapidly from primitive idealization to a raging, devaluing, and hateful attitude toward the staff. It is important to note, however, that when not under stress, these patients often exhibit higher-level defenses and strengths, such as intact reality testing, emotional stability, and social adaptability. Such adaptive traits, although not apparent during a regressive episode, may be drawn on during the emergency intervention.

3. **The role of the emergency department service environment.** Borderline patients are highly sensitive to their environment. **The emergency clinician should be acutely aware of the impact of the evaluation setting on the patient.**

   a. Emergency departments in general hospitals are notoriously poor environments for evaluating and treating borderline patients. A setting attuned to promote rapid diagnosis, management of acute medical problems, and triage is not optimal for a calm psychiatric intervention. To the borderline patient, the action-oriented emergency department, with its machinery and white-clad staff, may stimulate the fantasy (and dread) of finally really being taken care of (and possibly engulfed). Often there are long waits and a hostile attitude on the part of medical and nursing staff toward psychiatric patients, both factors underscoring feelings of victimization in the patient. Regression may ensue, compounded by the medical staff's insistence that the psychiatrist "take responsibility" for the patient—a message that may increase regression in "helpless" borderline personality.

b. In other cases, there may be an institutional transference on the part of the borderline patient, who often knows all the secretaries, security guards, and maintenance staff by name. In this situation, the hospital emergency department, despite its medical motif, is a true home, a familiar place of comfort and security. Thus, it is very important for the clinician to understand the **meaning the emergency department environment** plays in the patient's world. This understanding, of course, is easiest for clinicians treating those patients who come frequently to the emergency department. For new patients, on the other hand, it is always wise to consider the effect of the setting on the patient during an assessment and, if possible, make adjustments or even discuss the situation candidly with the patient.

III. Evaluation of the borderline personality disorder

A. Interview technique. Borderline patients and others with poor impulse control require a thorough but **rapid** assessment. Above all, the clinician should conduct the interview in a manner that minimizes decompensation, thwarts regression, and maximizes adaptive defenses and strengths. There are a number of **therapeutic maneuvers** that are important both for psychological stabilization and for obtaining data.

1. **Minimize waiting time.** The longer patients with borderline personality are in the waiting room, the more likely their anger and impulsivity will escalate and interfere with the subsequent interview.

2. Evaluate in a **setting** that is both safe and out of the "limelight."

   a. Both the patient and physician should feel comfortable in the interview room; additional staff should be readily available if necessary.

   b. The patient should not be permitted to disrupt the overall functioning of the emergency department or create public embarrassment for themselves or others.

   c. Friends or family should stay with the patient only if they enhance more adaptive, controlled behavior.

   d. If there is any concern about violence, measures to search and restrain the patient may be necessary (see sec. **IV.C**).

3. **The interviewer's stance.** The first and foremost goal of the interview is to **establish rapport.** This may be challenging. It is important that the clinician act in a concerned, professional manner, despite provocations that induce other feelings.

   a. The best stance is a "down-to-earth" position, in which one assumes an inquisitive role, makes no early assumptions, asks direct questions, and **emphasizes the limitations** of such a brief encounter. This stance paradoxically demonstrates a "powerless" position, almost solicitous in one's sincere effort to gain information, demonstrate concern, but assiduously avoid the "omnipotent doctor" role, which fosters idealized fantasies, greater helplessness, dependency, and regression in the patient.

   b. The interviewer cannot assume any true alliance with a borderline patient. The "emergency alliance" is really placing focus on the current crisis and collecting sufficient data to conduct an appropriate evaluation and intervention.

c. Keep an open mind, in terms of diagnosis, differential diagnosis, an social evaluation. If one prematurely makes the diagnosis of borderlin personality and closes the book on other possibilities, significant medic and psychiatric problems may be neglected. **Keep your index of susp cion for undetected problems high.**

d. Permit the patient to speak first. This may improve the subseque interactions and is preferable to a preemptive reading of the "riot act

e. An offer of food, a cold drink, or an opportunity to make a phone ca can enhance rapport, but the patient should not be allowed to escala requests.

f. The clinician should create an atmosphere of a mature relationship wit the patient, by answering the patient's questions and acknowledgin limitations and difficulties.

g. Always attempt to assess a patient's strengths and not merely psychopa thology. This will be of great benefit in working with the patient o disposition plans.

4. **Determine the patient's overt or covert request** in addition to the chie complaint.

   a. The request will often explain the patient's **reasons for the emergenc** and **facilitate engagement** in the clinical encounter. Ask, "How did yo hope I would help you?" rather than "Why did you come here?"

   b. The request will sometimes reveal wishes or fantasies of diagnostic sig nificance and enhance the clinician's ability to negotiate a treatmen plan and disposition.

5. **Determine the immediate precipitating event.** Many borderline patien decompensate in response to a real or perceived disappointment in an inte personal relationship. Identifying the significant other makes the precip tant clear and opens the door to a productive dialogue, which may be helpfu in determining the treatment plan.

B. History and examination

1. The **medical record and current therapist** are invaluable resources.

   a. They may provide a picture of the patient's long-term functioning, rang of behaviors, and past suicidality.

   b. They may also provide information about previous treatment interven tions and their outcomes.

   c. If the patient is in treatment, it is **critical to contact the therapist fo information** about recent problems in therapy, other stressors, and othe information not in the chart.

2. **Medical history.** If not in the medical record, it is imperative to inquir about previous hospitalizations, use of medications (prescribed and ove the-counter), and **drug and alcohol use** (including detailed informatio about the type of drug/alcohol, quantity, duration, and frequency of use).

3. **Psychiatric history**

   a. A detailed past psychiatric history is essential (see sec. **III.C**). The physi cian must always assess the **degree of suicidality.** It is a common mis conception that personality disordered patients are at low suicide risk One should ask about prior attempts in detail, including intent, means hospitalization, and sequelae (see Chap. 4).

   b. Ask about other forms of impulsive behavior; self-destructive actions homicidal ideation, plans, and attempts; and high-risk behavior—fo example, sexual promiscuity, threatening pregnancy, or transmission of HIV.

c. It is always useful to ask about **previous and current therapy,** particularly the duration, frequency of meetings, focus, goals, use of medications, and attitudes of the patient about the therapist, including what was most and least helpful. Often the answer will clarify the reason for the patient's coming to the emergency department. Moreover, the description of the therapeutic relationship is of great value in making the diagnosis of borderline psychopathology because of the frequent idealization, devaluation, or unrealistic material revealed. Clarification with the current therapist provides the emergency clinician with a degree of reality testing.

4. **Family psychiatric history**

   a. A cursory family psychiatric history may shed light on the risk of comorbid disorders—for example, depression, psychosis, suicide, and alcoholism (see sec. **III.C**).

   b. An often neglected topic, particularly important for but not limited to adolescents, is assessment of **any previous or ongoing physical or sexual abuse.** It is of vital importance, medically, legally, and therapeutically to have an awareness of ongoing trauma and to take appropriate action, if necessary. While one cannot always believe everything said by borderline personality patients in an emergency—some may falsely allege such abuse by family members or lovers—it is crucial to ask about current abuse and seriously consider needs for protection. It is also crucial to consider the fragility of the patient and, in the acute setting, to inquire no farther into past abuse than the patient's level of distress allows.

5. **Social history**

   a. The clinician should evaluate the **social support system.** If someone brought the patient to the emergency department, he or she should be brought into the evaluation. The clinician should inquire about the integrity and role of the family, how effective the social support network has been in the past, and whether members of the system are in crisis now.

   b. **Financial resources** should be assessed.

6. **Mental status examination.** All psychiatric patients seen for emergency evaluation and treatment must have a thorough mental status examination. Since there is no pathognomonic sign or symptom of the borderline personality and the disorder can mimic so many other psychiatric disorders, the diagnosis is partially one of exclusion, and the clinician must rule in or out other major medical or psychiatric conditions. A few important caveats should be kept in mind in making the diagnosis:

   a. **Cognition,** except in cases of intoxication or other organic impairment, is normal in borderline personality disorder. If abnormalities are noted, physical and laboratory evaluation (e.g., toxic screening and other relevant workup) should be initiated.

   b. **Formal thought processes** are generally normal, although some patients may demonstrate transient psychotic thinking. As opposed to schizophrenic patients or others with chronic psychosis, the psychotic-like symptoms of borderline patients are fleeting and highly related to the environment and personal interaction. The patient tends to move in and out of psychotic-like states and lacks a fixed, systematic delusional system. A similar picture, however, may be seen in a delirious or intoxicated patient. Appropriate measures should be taken to rule out these conditions.

c. **Thought content** typical of borderline patients frequently reveals themes of abandonment, aloneness, victimization, anger, and worthlessness, expressed with high drama.

7. **Countertransference responses.** A very useful diagnostic clue available to clinicians is their own emotional reaction to the patient. Affective responses evoked by the patient may reveal his or her defensive structure.

   a. Feelings of rage, aversion, malice, repugnancy, or helplessness may result from a patient's projection, projective identification, or devaluation.

   b. Feelings of being special to the patient and impulses to rescue may arise from idealization.

C. **Differential diagnosis.** A number of other diagnoses may mimic borderline personality disorder or may coexist with it. Consequently, it is important to perform a complete assessment, particularly when deciding to use medication or make recommendations for outpatient pharmacotherapy. The following are the most important disorders in the differential diagnosis:

1. **Mood disorders.** Both depression and mania can present with irritability, hostility, anxiety, negativism, and self-destructive behavior. As many as 20% of patients with borderline personality disorder meet criteria for comorbid major depression.

   a. In general, a history of periods of normal functioning between episodes of illness will differentiate a primary mood disorder from borderline personality disorder.

   b. Hysteroid dysphoria, a subtype of atypical depression, while not an accepted DSM-IV category, is a clinically useful description. It has a number of symptoms that overlap with borderline personality disorder: The patients are predominantly female and are exquisitely sensitive to rejection, which may lead to depressed mood, anergia, anxiety, and neurovegetative symptoms opposite to the usual endogenous pattern (i.e., hyperphagia, hypersomnia). (There is evidence that this subgroup of patients responds preferentially to monoamine oxidase inhibitors and perhaps fluoxetine).

2. **Panic disorder** with agoraphobia, may present with symptoms that mimic borderline personality disorder.

   a. Such patients are often terrified of being alone and, as a result, may become angry, manipulative, depressed, and suicidal to avoid feeling isolated.

   b. Eliciting a history of recurrent panic attacks will help make the diagnosis and point toward specific treatment (see Chap. 18).

3. **Attention deficit hyperactivity disorder (ADHD), residual type**

   a. For patients with a lifelong history of inattention and impulsivity, ADHD should be considered. Obtaining psychological testing performed during school years, if available, may be very useful.

   b. Although ADHD may be the primary problem, secondary borderline or antisocial personality traits may be present due to the impact of ADHD on personality development.

4. **Episodic behavioral dyscontrol** symptoms may result from brain injury or infection and may also occur as the interictal manifestation of complex partial epilepsy.

5. **Alcohol or drug abuse** may result in a history of chronic affective liability, impulsivity, and poor interpersonal relationships. It is critical to obtain history concerning alcohol and drug use.

6. **Posttraumatic stress disorder (PTSD).** A number of borderline patients have comorbid PTSD. Clinical features in common with borderline personality may include irritability or outbursts of anger, poor concentration, hypervigilance, and feelings of estrangement or detachment from others. The diagnosis can be made independently from borderline personality disorder if DSM-IV criteria are met.

IV. Management of the borderline personality disorder

A. Psychotherapeutic interventions

1. It must be realized that **emergency psychotherapeutics** are vastly different from ongoing outpatient psychotherapy in the following ways:

   a. In the emergency setting there is an **absence of a working alliance.** Without the collaboration and trust implicit in such an alliance, it is an error to use the uncovering, interpretive techniques of conventional psychodynamic psychotherapy.

   b. Instead of interpreting defenses or attempting to restructure them, the clinician should **support the most adaptive defenses.**

   c. Provide some semblance of a safe "**holding environment,**" in which the clinician acts as an ancillary ego to foster collaboration aimed at solving the current problem.

2. **Empathic reassurance.** To the distraught borderline patient in crisis there is some comfort knowing the clinician appreciates his or her plight. Repeated empathic comments using psychodynamic themes and beginning early in the interview, such as "It must be terrible to feel so alone" or "I can imagine your pain at feeling so abandoned," may help the patient to feel understood.

   a. The clinician must be aware that such an approach, though intended to reassure the patient that someone understands, may run the risk of engendering omnipotent and omniscient parental fantasies about the clinician, leading to yet another disappointment.

   b. To counter these fantasies, the clinician should be sure the patient appreciates **the reality of the situation, the clinician's limitations,** and the **patient's responsibility in collaborating** to help solve the crisis. Statements such as the following are quite helpful: "Although I've just met you and really know very little about you, I can try to help you work things out in a limited way during this crisis."

3. **Borderline crisis intervention.** The primary goal of crisis intervention with borderline patients is to **thwart regression and ally with the most adaptive ego functions.** Some valuable techniques to achieve this include

   a. **Firm limits.** Borderline patients are prone to confuse feelings with action and behave impulsively in ambiguous situations. The clinician should clearly define the goals and objectives of their encounter and make clear **proscriptions against assaultive or self-destructive behavior** and **the prescription that understanding the situation requires words.** Moreover, it should be stated that while the patient deserves immediate care, the patient's situation is lifelong and **no cures can be expected in the emergency department.**

   b. **No interpretations or tampering with defenses.** The clinician should enhance observing ego capacities by discussing the reality of the crisis situation and limitations of immediate resources in a structured, commonsense dialogue.

c. **Elicit collaboration.** Once the patient can take some responsibility for the origin of the crisis or for its resolution, there is less chance of further regression and maintaining infantile wishes that the clinician will take over.

d. **Use transitional objects.** Many borderline patients need something tangible to demonstrate they received care. These symbolic objects may take the form of written contracts, idea lists generated by the collaboration of clinician and patient, appointment slips, presciptions, or, if indicated, medications judiciously handed out.

4. **Education.** Educating the borderline patient about psychiatric treatment contrasts the function of the emergency department with ongoing outpatient therapy.

   a. **For the patient in psychotherapy,** an emergency department visit usually indicates a crisis or impasse in therapy. The clinician should acknowledge how arduous and at times disappointing psychotherapy is for most patients. This often strikes a clear note of concordance. Once the clinician and patient are allied in this context, the difficulties in current psychotherapy can be explored in a safe and neutral environment. It is always wise to serve as an impartial consultant, but, in most cases, support the current therapy.

   b. **For patients who are not in ongoing psychotherapy,** it is often useful to briefly discuss the process, risks, and potential benefits of psychotherapy, the patient's goals, and where psychotherapy may be obtained. Even at this early juncture, it is wise to explain that psychotherapy is slow, painstaking, and difficult, but the patient deserves the sense of wholeness that may result from the investment.

   c. Stressing the value of ongoing outpatient treatment has another motive: **to thwart unnecessary emergency department abuse.** Many borderline patients become pathologically attached to certain emergency departments, causing undue stress and hardship for the staff. It should be stated that while assistance is always available in a true emergency, the best treatment occurs in regular outpatient visits with a therapist.

   d. A recent dilemma facing many borderline patients is the impact of managed care on long-term outpatient psychotherapy. Numerous insurance companies have placed strict limits on the number of sessions allowed per calendar year. In this new era of health care provision, extended outpatient and day treatment programs are diminishing, resulting in potentially more frequent emergency department visits. The clinician must above all be candid about the limited resources and the resultant deprivation experienced by borderline patients. Highly individualized, creative planning involving not only professional health care centers but also self-help networks (e.g., Alcoholics Anonymous, Alanon), is becoming necessary for each emergency department repeater.

B. Pharmacotherapy

1. The use of medication in patients with borderline personality has only recently been studied in a careful manner. Unfortunately, clear guidelines have not emerged to aid clinicians in the emergency department setting.

2. Dealing with psychological issues may obviate the need for pharmacologic intervention.

3. When talk alone is ineffective, medication is necessary.

   a. Once made, the decision to use medication should be discussed with the patient as fully as circumstances permit.

   b. It must be clear to the clinician that medications are not being administered as part of a negative countertransference reaction, to get the patient out as quickly as possible. It also should be realized that medications may have special, magical meaning to some patients—for example, as a cure for all ills or as an alternative to the painful process of psychotherapy. Such fantasies should be dispelled by a clear explanation of the use and limitations of medications.

   c. The least invasive route of administration is generally preferable; consider oral administration before parenteral routes are used. Although oral preparations have a longer lag before onset of action, they permit patients some degree of control of their situation, provide the message that they are participating in treatment, and promote more mature functioning.

4. **Major psychiatric disorders**

   a. If a patient has symptoms of a superimposed major psychiatric disorder, such as depression or an anxiety disorder, the indicated medical treatment for that disorder can be considered, giving careful consideration to the possibility of concurrent substance abuse.

   b. **If there is no clear emergency, definitive treatment should not be initiated in the emergency department with this type of patient.** Given the impulsivity and instability of these patients, medications that require close monitoring or that can be lethal in overdose (e.g., lithium, tricyclic antidepressants, or monoamine oxidase inhibitors) should only be prescribed in the context of an ongoing treatment relationship.

5. **Symptomatic treatments.** Selection of the class of medication to use acutely remains empiric.

   a. Borderline patients who are **acutely agitated** require sedation. Lorazepam, a benzodiazepine that is available in oral and parenteral forms, is the current treatment of choice.

      (1) Administer 1–2 mg of lorazepam PO or IM initially, then 1 mg every 30–60 minutes until sedation is achieved. Rarely is more than 5 mg required.

      (2) Certain other benzodiazepines, particularly alprazolam (Xanax), may be more likely to cause paradoxical excitement or disinhibition and should be avoided.

      (3) In the unlikely event that disinhibition occurs after administration of a benzodiazepine, haloperidol (Haldol) 2–5 mg IM should prove calming. The dosage can be repeated every 20–30 minutes if needed.

   b. For patients with a history of **episodic dyscontrol** who present with impending loss of control, the oral administration of a rapidly absorbed benzodiazepine, such as diazepam, clorazepate, or lorazepam, can be useful in aborting the full appearance of symptoms.

      (1) If by history the prodrome is brief or if violence seems near, IM or IV lorazepam is a better choice. If there is a history of central nervous system depressant abuse or of benzodiazepine-induced disinhibition, haloperdol 5 mg IM could be used as an alternative.

      (2) Although recent literature suggests that lithium, carbamazepine, serotonergic antidepressants (e.g., fluoxetine), and beta-adrenergic

blockers (e.g., propranolol) may be effective in the long-term treatment of violent behaviors, they are not effective in acute situations.

c. For patients with **affective lability, anger, or psychotic symptoms without marked agitation,** an antipsychotic drug is generally preferable, particularly if there is a history of drug or alcohol abuse.

(1) Low doses of high-potency agents such as haloperidol 2–5 mg PO or IM given every hour as needed for up to three doses have been shown to be of benefit for short-term management of such symptoms. Other high-potency drugs such as thiothixene are probably equally effective, and selection should be based on the physician's familiarity with particular drugs.

(2) At times low-potency agents like chlorpromazine or thioridazine may be preferable because of the lower risk of acute extrapyramidal reactions and the added sedation they provide. A dosage of 25–50 mg of chlorpromazine administered hourly as needed for up to 3 hours is usually effective. Postural hypotension is a potential hazard with low-potency antipsychotics.

(3) If the patient agrees to oral treatment, liquid preparations, when available, are preferable because they are more rapidly absorbed than pills and also diminish the likelihood that the patient will "cheek" the medication.

d. For patients demonstrating **severely disruptive behavior**—that is, those who appear both **agitated and psychotic**—combination treatment with parenteral administration of both a benzodiazepine and an antipsychotic can be useful.

(1) Haloperidol 5 mg with lorazepam 1 mg every hour as needed is quite effective.

(2) Such combination regimens are best avoided if the patient is intoxicated with alcohol or a sedative-hypnotic. In such instances, an antipsychotic alone should be sufficient.

6. Clinical judgment determines the duration of emergency department pharmacotherapy. If the patient is persistently violent, suicidal, or demonstrating severely impaired judgment despite several hours of drug treatment, transfer to an inpatient unit is necessary. Fortunately, many of these patients improve as a new day begins and their feelings of loneliness subside. If acute symptoms have abated, the patient can be discharged after appropriate follow-up has been arranged (see sec. **D**). To guide on-call physicians for the nearly inevitable return visit, it is important to **document drug treatment and the patient's response clearly.**

7. In general, borderline patients should be given very little or no medication on **discharge** from the emergency department. Benzodiazepines can be abused, and antipsychotics can cause neurologic symptoms such as dystonia and long-term side effects such as tardive dyskinesia. In addition, given the impulsivity and instability of these patients, any long-term pharmacotherapy should be carried out only in the context of an ongoing treatment relationship.

C. **Physical restraint** should be avoided unless it is necessary to protect the patient and staff from bodily harm. When needed, the following guidelines should be kept in mind:

1. If the evaluating clinician decides restraints are required, **the decision should be unequivocal.** They should be applied swiftly, without negotiation, taking care not to hurt the patient, but with overwhelming force. Hesitant decisions or half-hearted attempts with a meager staff only increase the likelihood of someone getting hurt.

2. Patients should be told that the restraints were necessary because of their dangerous behavior, and a time limit should be specified when the need for restraints will be reassessed (usually every 15 minutes).
3. Patients should be allowed to vent their rage at the perceived insult.
4. Removal of restraints should proceed in stages—one arm, one leg, the other arm, followed by the last leg. Each stage should be executed at 15-minute intervals.
5. Some borderline patients will provoke a confrontation, necessitating restraints. This may be an attempt to demonstrate how "cruel" the staff are or to reinforce the sense of the patient's own unworthiness or victimization. The clinician, noting escalating behavior, may fend off the need for restraints by indicating clearly that the clinician realizes how desperate the patient feels, but that violent behavior will only result in whatever means are necessary to keep everyone safe, including use of restraints. It is vital to reiterate the prescription that it is far preferable to use words to convey feelings rather than action.

D. Disposition. Arranging a disposition is one of the most difficult tasks for the clinician in the emergency department. This is due to the power struggles that often ensue with a borderline patient who does not want to separate from the emergency department and because of the limited resources available. Disposition should be considered from the beginning of the evaluation of a borderline patient, with attention to both immediate and long-term resources. The assessment of social supports, such as friends, family, or neighbors, can prove invaluable in the short run. Referring a patient for **outpatient treatment** or encouraging the patient in treatment to continue is almost always advisable. Other aspects of disposition include the following:

1. **Hospitalization.** At times acute hospitalization is lifesaving; however, the clinician must recognize that hospitalization may be toxic, promoting serious regression in the borderline patient. Criteria for hospitalization include:
   a. Severe ego disorganization and suicidal ideation resulting from a recent loss.
   b. Inability to contract to continue seeing one's outpatient therapist despite suicidal intent.
   c. Serious suicidal intent with a history of life-threatening suicide attempts.
   d. Homicidal ideation or intent with poor impulse control.
   e. Marked agitation or psychosis, unremitting after an adequate trial of pharmacotherapy.
   f. A diagnostic uncertainty (e.g., a potentially serious comorbid disorder) best evaluated in the hospital.
2. It should be noted that preventing regression in the hospital ideally begins in the emergency department. If the clinician knows or can find out about the ward before transfer, a candid discussion of the rules and structure of the unit should be conducted. It should be emphasized that patients are responsible for their behavior on the ward. Consequences of unacceptable behavior should be explained. Finally, limited goals of the hospitalization should be reviewed prior to admission. This dialogue will vastly improve the quality of hospitalization.
3. **The clinical note.** Management of the borderline patient in the emergency department does not end when the patient leaves. Since the patient is bound to return, **it is critical to write a clear note in the chart** documenting the origins of the crisis, the patient's medical and psychiatric history, and

successful therapeutic interventions. Such a note will clearly help the next clinician manage the patient effectively and consistently.

4. **Educating staff.** Equally important as writing a good note is educating allied health professionals who have had little experience with or understanding of borderline psychopathology. Even in the middle of the night, taking a few minutes to process what happened in the clinical encounter will go a long way in thwarting unnecessary negative or countertherapeutic interventions with borderline patients in the future. An emergency department staff, well educated about the psychopathology and management of the borderline patient, not only will improve the quality of patient care, but also will save the psychiatric clinician time needed to quell the fallout from uneducated staff–patient interactions.

5. **The gold standard of success.** Successful outcome of managing the borderline patient in the emergency department should not be measured by patient satisfaction or total symptom alleviation, although they are always a pleasant gift. Rather, success derives from achieving **psychologic stabilization and getting the patient out of the emergency department safe and sound.**

V. Other personality disorders

A. Many, if not all of the techniques described in this chapter may be used successfully with antisocial, histrionic, or narcissistic personality disorders.

B. **Antisocial personality disorder** (see Table 12-2). Patients with this disorder are notoriously difficult to evaluate and treat because they often lie about their symptoms or come to the emergency ward to avoid incarceration or retaliation from other people they have hurt or offended. A few caveats should be noted regarding their care:

1. Always call referring parties, relatives, court officials, or any identifiable person in the patient's life who can clarify the problem and provide pertinent historical data.

2. Complaints of pain, anxiety, depression, or suicide may conceal attempts to procure drugs. It is not uncommon, after a lengthy history and examination, that the patient becomes furious or threatening when desired medications are not provided. Referral to outpatient self-help groups or an inpatient detoxification program is advisable, though infrequently utilized voluntarily.

3. The clinician should be sure to see the patient in a safe setting if antisocial personality disorder is suspected. Calling for security guards is always in order if one feels threatened.

4. Promises to protect the patient from consequences of antisocial behavior, such as hospitalization, should be avoided. The clinician must remain in control and keep the intervention purely medical in nature.

Selected Readings

American Psychiatric Association Task Force on DSM-IV. *Diagnostic and Statistical Manual of Mental Disorders, Fourth Edition, Draft Criteria:* 3/1/93. Washington, D.C.: American Psychiatric Association.

Bassuk, E., and Gerson, S. Chronic crisis patients: A discrete clinical group. *Am. J. Psychiatry* 137:1513, 1980.

Beresin, E., and Gordon, C. Emergency ward management of the borderline patient. *Gen. Hosp. Psychiatry* 3:23, 1981.

Bick, P. A., and Hannah, A. L. Intramuscular lorazepam to restrain violent patients (letter). *Lancet* 1:206, 1986.

Briere, I., and Zaidi, L. Y. Sexual abuse histories and sequelae in female psychiatric emergency room patients. *Am. J. Psychiatry* 146:1602, 1989.

Brinkley, J. R., Beitman, B. D., and Friedel, R. D. Low-dose neuroleptic regimens in the treatment of borderline patients. *Arch. Gen. Psychiatry* 36:319, 1979.

Cowdry, R. W., and Gardner, D. L. Pharmacotherapy of borderline personality disorder: Alprazolam, carbamazepine, trifluoperazine and tranylcypromine. *Arch. Gen. Psychiatry* 45:111, 1989.

Ellison, J. M., and Adler, D. A. A strategy for the pharmacotherapy of personality disorders. *New Dir. Ment. Health Serv.* 47:43, 1990.

Ellison, J. M., Blum, N. R., and Barsky, A. J. Frequent repeaters in a psychiatric emergency service. *Hosp. Community Psychiatry* 40:958, 1989.

Gerson, S., and Bassuk, E. Psychiatric emergencies: An overview. *Am. J. Psychiatry* 137:1, 1980.

Griffith, J. L. Treatment of episodic behavior disorders with rapidly absorbed benzodiazepines. *J. Nerv. Ment. Dis.* 173:312, 1985.

Gunderson, J. G. Pharmacotherapy for patients with borderline personality disorder. *Arch. Gen. Psychiatry* 43:698, 1985.

Gunderson, J. G. Borderline Personality Disorder. In H. I. Kaplan and B. J. Saddock (eds.), *Comprehensive Textbook of Psychiatry V*. Baltimore: Williams & Wilkins, 1989.

Maltsberger, J. T., and Buie, D. H. Countertransference hate in the treatment of suicidal patients. *Arch. Gen. Psychiatry* 30:625, 1974.

Markovitz, P. J., et al. Fluoxetine in the treatment of borderline and schizotypal personality disorders. *Am. J. Psychiatry* 148:1064, 1991.

Pearlmutter, R. A. The borderline patient in the emergency department: An approach to evaluation and management. *Psychiatr. Q.* 54:190, 1982.

Perry, J. C., and Valliant, G. E. Personality Disorders. In H. I. Kaplan and B. J. Saddock (eds.), *Comprehensive Textbook of Psychiatry V*. Baltimore: Williams & Wilkins, 1989.

Peteet, J. R., and Gutheil, T. G. The hospital and the borderline patient: Management guidelines for the community mental health center. *Psychiatr. Q.* 51:106, 1979.

Salzman, C., et al. Benzodiazepines combined with neuroleptics for management of severe disruptive behavior. *Psychosomatics* 27(Suppl.):17, 1986.

Weston, D., et al. Physical and sexual abuse in adolescent girls with borderline personality disorder. *Am. J. Orthopsychiatry* 60:55, 1990.

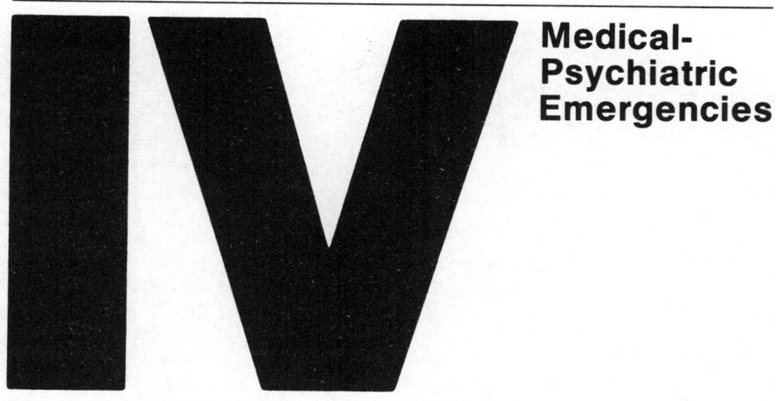

IV Medical-Psychiatric Emergencies

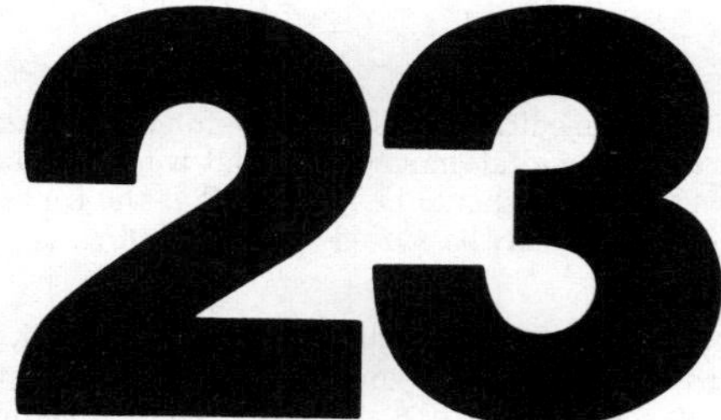

Agitation and Delirium

Steven E. Hyman
George E. Tesar

I. **Agitation** with or without a confusional state is a frequent occurrence among patients seen in the emergency department or on a medical or surgical service. Sequelae of medical illness (e.g., hypoxia), fear, side effects of drugs (e.g., theophylline), major psychiatric disorders, or delirium commonly cause an agitated state in which individuals demonstrate motor hyperactivity, often accompanied by sympathetic activation, anxiety, and disruptive behaviors. **Anxiety and agitation** may be so severe as to impair rationality, causing patients to refuse to comply with treatment or even to try to flee. This can be particularly dangerous if the patient tries to pull out critically important lines and tubes. Even milder anxiety can be threatening to patients with unstable coronary artery disease.

A. **Approach to the patient.** Agitated patients may appear angry, fearful, or confused. Frequently they will have been arguing with members of the staff. Thus it is important to approach the patient politely and in a calm, nonjudgmental way. Physicians should make it clear that they want to hear from the patient what is wrong and that they intend to help. On the other hand, if limits have to be set rapidly because of a medically dangerous situation or risk of violence, they should be set clearly and firmly by the physician; the reasons for such limits (including restraints) should be explained briefly to the patient in a nonpunitive manner.

B. **Evaluation.** Because the agitated state may be the presenting symptom of a wide range of disorders, including some that are life-threatening, a careful evaluation is necessary.

1. Ascertain the patient's **vital signs** before beginning the interview; abnormalities will focus the examination on potential organic causes of the behavioral problems. It is important to decide rapidly whether the problem is a medical emergency.

2. **The safety of the patient and staff** must be the first priority. If there is likelihood of the patient's doing self-harm or harming others, physical restraint will be needed (see Table 5-1).

3. Perform an adequate **mental status examination** to evaluate the possibility of delirium (see sec. **II**), psychosis, or other mental disorder.

   a. It is particularly important to determine whether the patient is paranoid, potentially violent, or suicidal.

   b. If the patient appears to have a personality disorder and has had an outburst because of feeling infantilized and out of control, do not perform a detailed cognitive examination; the patient may experience it as a further insult.

4. If delirium or another acute medical disorder, a major psychiatric disorder, or an intoxication or withdrawal state is ruled out, it is important to find out from these patients what is bothering them and what their wishes are and to develop an idea of the coping mechanisms that they are using.

C. Differential diagnosis

1. **Acute fear or anxiety** about medical illness, loss of function, or loss of control may be enough to cause agitation so severe that it mimics a major psychiatric disorder or delirium. It should be recalled that the converse is also true: Anxiety-like symptoms may be caused by medical illness or drugs (see Table 18-3).

2. In medical patients it is particularly important to consider hypoxia, hypoglycemia, acidosis, arrhythmias, hyperthyroidism, drug withdrawal, or drug administration (e.g., bronchodilators and other sympathomimetics, digitalis, anticholinergics, and antipsychotics and antiemetics [which may produce akathisia]) as possible causes of anxiety or agitation. Even if a treatable medical cause is found, emergency symptomatic treatment may still be needed.

3. A frequently overlooked cause of irritability and irrational behaviors during the first 1–7 days of a hospital admission is **withdrawal from alcohol, benzodiazepines or other sedative-hypnotics, or narcotics.**

4. Acute psychotic disorders, depression, mania, anxiety disorders, posttraumatic stress disorder, and personality disorders may all be associated with severe agitation. Similarly, drugs used to treat these disorders may produce agitation, most commonly akathisia or akathisia-like symptoms caused by antipsychotic drugs or fluoxetine, but also deliria caused by anticholinergic drugs, antidepressants, or lithium.

D. Symptomatic treatment of agitation. Even when a specific cause of agitation is found, symptomatic treatment may be needed to provide comfort and safety. Agitation occurring in the context of acute psychosis should be treated as described in Chap. 19.

1. **Short-acting benzodiazepines** are generally safe and reliable. Lorazepam (Ativan) may be given PO, IV, or IM (of all of the benzodiazepines it has the advantage of being the best absorbed IM). Lorazepam and oxazepam (Serax) are benzodiazepines with no active metabolites, making them relatively safe in the elderly. Oxazepam has the disadvantage of very slow onset after oral administration. Lorazepam may be administered sublingually; however, onset of effect is no more rapid after sublingual administration than after oral administration.

   a. Lorazepam 1–2 mg PO tid–qid or oxazepam 15–30 mg tid–qid is usually effective for mild or moderate anxiety. In extreme panic reactions, lorazepam 1–2 mg can be given **slowly** IV. Slow administration is required because of the risk of respiratory arrest.

   b. In medical patients with questionable respiratory drive or cardiac status, many clinicians prefer to use high-potency neuroleptics in the treatment of extreme agitation or panic. In such situations, haloperidol (Haldol) can be administered either IM or IV (although the latter route is not approved by the Food and Drug Administration). Initial effective doses of haloperidol usually range from 5–20 mg. An initial dose of 5 mg can be given and repeated every 20 minutes until the patient is calm. Once the patient is sedated, haloperidol 5 mg IM or IV can be given as needed. Generally patients require about half of the initially effective dose as maintenance during the next 12-hour period. The dose should be tapered as the patient's symptoms allow. Elderly patients will require lower doses of haloperidol (e.g., 0.5–1.0 mg PO bid) after acute agitation is brought under control. Occasionally a paradoxical response occurs, which is likely to represent akathisia (see Chap. 19). Akathisia often responds to administration of lorazepam 1–2 mg PO tid. Very high doses of haloperidol have been reported to cause torsades de pointes ventricular tachycardia in rare cases.

c. Many patients respond well to combinations of haloperidol and lorazepam with fewer side effects than high doses of either (e.g., haloperidol 2–5 mg PO bid plus lorazepam 1–2 mg PO or IM q4h as needed for anxiety or agitation.

2. **Psychological management.** The availability of effective sedatives should not cause the physician to lose sight of the importance of explanation and reassurance.

   a. With anxious medical patients, it is important to find out what they are afraid of, their conception of their illness, and whether they have ever known anyone else with symptoms like theirs. It is often possible to uncover misplaced fears and misconceptions, which can be corrected.

   b. The physician should emphasize positive aspects of the treatment plan, especially in areas that deal directly with the patient's fears (e.g., that adequate pain medication will be provided). False reassurance should not be given because the physician will lose credibility with the patient.

II. **Delirium, acute confusional states, and toxic/metabolic encephalopathy** are among the many terms that have been used to describe a clinical syndrome consisting of acute global derangement of cerebral function accompanied by abnormalities in arousal.

A. Although some texts make a distinction between acute confusional states and delirium, requiring agitation and hyperactivity for the latter diagnosis, the *Diagnostic and Statistical Manual of Mental Disorders, Fourth Edition, Draft Criteria* (DSM-IV) delirium criteria (Table 23-1) have a more inclusive approach to the diagnosis and includes states in which patients are either hyperactive or hypoactive. This inclusive approach may be justified on the grounds that both types of delirium represent similar pathophysiologic processes differing only by degree.

B. Using the DSM-IV definition, **delirium is among the most common mental syndromes found in a general hospital.** However, its presence is frequently missed both in the emergency department and on the wards.

1. Because it can result from serious medical illness, delirium can be associated with significant morbidity and mortality.

Table 23-1. DSM-IV draft criteria for delirium

A. Disturbance of consciousness (i.e., reduced clarity of awareness of the environment), with reduced ability to focus, sustain, or shift attention.
B. Change in cognition (e.g., memory deficit, disorientation, language disturbance, perceptual disturbance) that is not better accounted for by a preexisting, established, or evolving dementia.
C. The disturbance develops over a short period of time (usually hours to days) and tends to fluctuate during the course of the day.
D. There is evidence from the history, physical examination, or laboratory findings of
   1. A general medical condition, *or*
   2. Substance intoxication or withdrawal, *or*
   3. More than one etiology

   judged to be etiologically related to the disturbance.*

*This criterion permits assignment of the etiology of the delirium to a general medical condition, substance-induced delirium, or to multiple etiologies.
Source: Adapted from the *Diagnostic and Statistical Manual of Mental Disorders, Fourth Edition, Draft Criteria:* 3/1/93. Copyright 1993 American Psychiatric Association.

2. In the elderly, delirium may be the presenting feature of almost any systemic illness, including infections and myocardial infarction, making its recognition particularly important.

3. In younger patients as well as the elderly, delirium often results from prescribed, over-the-counter, or illicit drugs, ingestion or inhalation of toxins, withdrawal states, metabolic derangements, or head injury.

C. Clinical features

1. When mild, delirium may present with impairment only of attention and of higher intellectual functions such as construction and abstraction. As the underlying condition progresses, there may be more dramatic changes in cognitive function, with derangements of speech and praxis along with serious abnormalities in information processing and arousal.

2. By itself, delirium does not produce focal neurologic signs; if present, they require separate investigation and may give clues to the underlying cause of the mental status changes.

3. **Onset** is acute, generally over hours to days.

   a. Acute onset distinguishes delirium from dementia, although the two frequently coexist because dementia is a risk factor for delirium.

   b. In clinical practice, the occurrence of delirium frequently calls attention to a previously undiagnosed dementia.

4. **Mental status examination**

   a. **Attention and concentration** are invariably abnormal.

      (1) Patients are distractible, unable to direct their attention selectively or maintain their focus.

      (2) Tests such as digit span (see Chap. 1) can be used to evaluate attention formally.

   b. Depending on the severity, all other aspects of cognitive function may also be deranged.

      (1) **Abnormalities of memory** may be both anterograde and retrograde, with the result that patients are usually disoriented. Disorientation is not pathognomonic for delirium, however; it may also occur in some acute psychoses, especially acute mania.

      (2) **Thinking and speech** are generally disorganized; speech may be completely incoherent.

      (3) **Constructions** (e.g., the ability to draw a clock) and **praxis** (e.g., the ability to carry out purposeful movements on verbal command) may also be abnormal.

      (4) **Perceptual illusions** or **hallucinations** may occur in any sensory modality, but are most often visual. They may be quite vivid.

      (5) A large percentage of delirious patients have **delusions,** which are usually unsystematized; rarely delusions may be more systematized and stable or recurrent over several days. Persecutory delusions and suspicion are common but are quite different from schizophrenic delusions: persecutory delusions are vague, transient, easily forgotten, inconsistently reported, and highly influenced by the environment.

      (6) Delirious patients may also display **affective lability,** often including rage and fear, which may be a result of their confusion, hallucinations, and delusions.

c. In addition, delirium may cause **abnormalities of arousal,** including derangement of the sleep-wake cycle, motor activity, and autonomic function. In elderly patients, it is very common to have exacerbations of symptoms at night, with prominent agitation and hallucinations.

d. **Hyperactive patients** are primarily agitated and restless with marked sympathetic arousal; this is the typical presentation of withdrawal from ethanol or sedative-hypnotics.

e. **Hypoactive patients** appear sleepy and lethargic, do not initiate conversation, and may need a great deal of stimulation before answering a question. This sort of presentation might occur early in Wernicke's encephalopathy. Many patients fluctuate between hyperactivity and lethargy.

D. **Common causes** of delirium are listed in Table 23-2. **Factors that increase the risk** of delirium include the following:

1. The elderly have decreased rates of metabolism and excretion of many drugs and toxins and may have diminished function in a number of neurotransmitter systems, including cholinergic systems, which increase their risk of delirium.

2. Young children are at increased risk.

3. Risk is elevated in burn patients, cardiac surgery patients, craniotomy patients, and drug abusers.

4. Risk is increased by polypharmacy with anticholinergic drugs, which include atropine, almost all over-the-counter sleeping pills, antihistamines, agents used for bowel spasms and diarrhea, agents used for dizziness and vertigo, preanesthetic agents, all of the cyclic antidepressants, the anticholinergic antiparkinsonian agents, and many neuroleptics (especially thioridazine). In the elderly, polypharmacy with anticholinergic compounds is particularly common and is a frequent contributor to cognitive impairment and frank delirium.

E. **Differential diagnosis**

1. The history is most useful in distinguishing delirium from *dementia*. The onset of delirium is rapid, while in dementia it is slower. Evidence of a new physical illness or drug toxicity should raise the possibility of delirium as a diagnosis.

2. The differentiation of delirium from *depression* may also be difficult because many depressed patients, especially the elderly, may be agitated, may complain of cognitive abnormalities, and may be inattentive on examination. The presence of neurovegetative symptoms (e.g., early morning awakening and anorexia) and the presence of affective symptoms (e.g., feelings of hopelessness, helplessness, or worthlessness) or guilt favor the diagnosis of depression.

3. The distinction of delirium from agitated *psychoses* can be aided by obtaining a history of past psychiatric disorder. Except for formal thought disorder, cognitive deficits in primary psychiatric disorders tend to be inconsistent and often reflect the inability of the patient to pay attention.

F. **Treatment**

1. The cornerstone of treatment for delirium is **good supportive care** while specific therapy for the underlying disorder is given.

2. Because delirious patients are unpredictable and may either harm themselves by falling or by pulling out needed lines and tubes or harm others by striking out, **mechanical restraints** are indicated.

Table 23-2. Common causes of delirium

Medications	Anticholinergic drugs (e.g., atropine, cyclic anti-depressants, many antipsychotics, antihistamines, over-the-counter hypnotics, antivertigo medications, and antispasmodics); sedative-hypnotics (especially those with long half-lives, e.g., flurazepam); decongestants, antiasthmatics, and other sympathomimetics; cimetidine; digitalis; L-dopa; meperidine; methyldopa; gluco-corticoids
Drug abuse	Amphetamines and cocaine; phencyclidine (PCP); hallucinogens; inhaled drugs (glue, nitrous oxide)
Withdrawal syndromes	Alcohol, benzodiazepines (especially alprazolam), barbiturates, and other sedative-hypnotics
Metabolic	Hepatic encephalopathy; uremia; hypoglycemia; hypoxia; hyponatremia; hypo- and hypercalcemia; hypo- and hypermagnesemia; acidosis; hyperosmolar states; porphyria
Vitamin deficiencies	Thiamine (Wernicke-Korsakoff syndrome); vitamin B_{12}; nicotinic acid (pellagra)
Endocrinopathies	Hypo- and hyperthyroidism; hypo- and hyperparathyroidism; Cushing's syndrome and Addison's disease; hypopituitarism
Infections	Any systemic infection in the elderly (especially with a coexisting dementing process); meningitis, encephalitis, and brain abscess; neurosyphilis; AIDS encephalopathy
Neurologic causes	Head injury (post-concussive syndromes, bleeds); stroke; hypertensive encephalopathy; intracranial neoplasms (especially frontal and temporal); complex partial status epilepticus; postictal states
Toxins and industrial exposures	Carbon monoxide; carbon disulfide; organic solvents; heavy metals
Others	Systemic lupus erythematosus (lupus cerebritis); cerebral vasculitis (temporal arteritis, periarteritis nodosa); paraneoplastic syndromes (limbic encephalitis); hyperviscosity syndromes

3. While awaiting the effects of specific therapy for an underlying disorder, while waiting for an offending drug to be metabolized and excreted, or in the case of idiopathic or "nonspecific" delirium, symptomatic use of a **sedating agent** may be necessary. Use of sedatives should be minimized, however, especially in patients in whom the diagnosis is unclear.

4. **Delirium due to ethanol or sedative-hypnotic withdrawal must be treated with a cross-reactive agent.** Alcohol withdrawal is best managed with a benzodiazepine (see Chap. 31). Sedative-hypnotic withdrawal is best managed with phenobarbital, the dose of which is determined with a pentobarbital tolerance test (see Chap. 30).

5. In other patients, especially the elderly, the high-potency neuroleptic **haloperidol** is often used because it has little effect on cardiorespiratory status

and is not very anticholinergic. In older patients, doses as low as 0.5 mg bid may be effective. In younger patients, much higher doses may be required at least initially. Doses of 2–5 mg may be given parenterally every 30–60 minutes as needed. The major liability of neuroleptics, especially in the elderly, is the emergence of parkinsonian symptoms. When elderly patients are given neuroleptics, they should be monitored frequently for cogwheel rigidity, changes in gait, and the development of masked facies. Late re-emergence of agitation while a patient is on haloperidol should raise the suspicion of akathisia. Akathisia can be treated with a benzodiazepine, a beta blocker, or by reduced neuroleptic dosage.

6. **Benzodiazepines** can be a useful alternative to neuroleptics. Lorazepam and oxazepam are two benzodiazepines with short half-lives, no active metabolites, and a route of elimination (glucuronidation) that is relatively preserved in old age and in patients with liver disease. Lorazepam may be more useful than oxazepam in the treatment of agitation because it can be given parenterally and when given orally is absorbed more rapidly than oxazepam. Unlike other benzodiazepines, lorazepam can be given intramuscularly with reliable absorption (best from the deltoid muscle); it can also be given intravenously. Depending on the patient's age and degree of agitation, lorazepam 0.5–2.0 mg can be given **slowly** intravenously. Slow administration avoids the production of high peak levels that could cause respiratory arrest. Nonetheless, especially with medically unstable patients, intravenous benzodiazepines should be given only if personnel trained in cardiopulmonary resuscitation are present. The dose of lorazepam can be repeated every 15–20 minutes until the patient is sedated. Repeat dosing thereafter should be on an as-needed basis, q2h. Combinations of haloperidol and lorazepam may be quite useful in patients with marked hallucinations and delusions who remain hyperactive after large doses of haloperidol or who develop extrapyramidal side effects on higher doses of the drug. In these patients, it is best to give a fixed dose of haloperidol daily and to use the benzodiazepine to titrate the level of sedation. Benzodiazepines will sometimes make the elderly delirious patient more agitated, and a neuroleptic will often be required, at least for a short period of time. Neuroleptics can often be discontinued soon after agitation, delusions, or hallucinations resolve.

7. In addition to pharmacologic interventions, it is helpful to ensure that the patient is getting adequate sleep. An attempt should be made to reassure patients insofar as possible; explanations to the patient should be simple and consistent. It is often helpful to have a consistent physician and primary nurse with whom the patient can identify. Unfamiliar visitors should be limited to avoid overstimulation; however, sometimes the presence of family members can calm a delirious patient. Since delirious patients often confess to imagined crimes or accuse spouses and other family members of transgressions, it is important to warn family members in advance that delirious accusations, threats, and confessions are not related to reality.

Selected Readings

Jenike, M. A. Delirium in Elderly Patients. In *Geriatric Psychiatry and Psychopharmacology: A Clinical Approach.* Chicago: Year Book, 1989.

Lipowski, Z. J. Delirium in the elderly patient. *N. Engl. J. Med.* 320:578, 1989.

Liptzin, B., et al. An empirical study of diagnostic criteria for delirium. *Am. J. Psychiatry* 148:454, 1991.

Smith, L. W., and Dimsdale, J. E. Postcardiotomy delirium: Conclusions after 25 years? *Am. J. Psychiatry* 146:452, 1989.

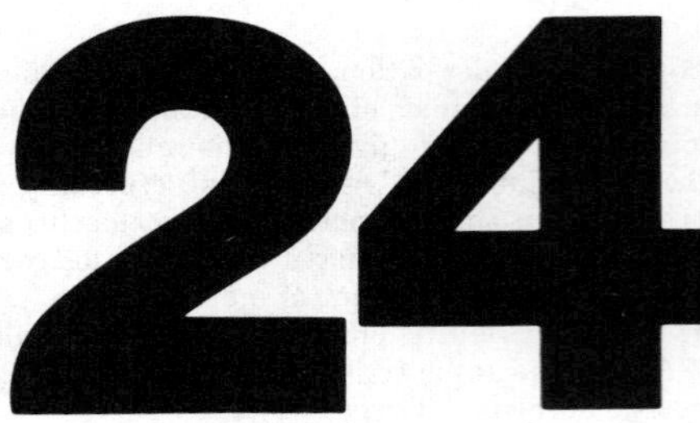

Toxic Side Effects of Psychotropic Medications and Their Management

Steven E. Hyman

I. The major classes of drugs used in the chemotherapy of psychiatric disorders (the neuroleptics, cyclic and atypical antidepressants, monoamine oxidase inhibitors, lithium, and benzodiazepines) can all produce side effects or drug interactions that may cause patients to come for emergency treatment. The side effects of psychotropic drugs are also major contributors to noncompliance with prescribed regimens or reluctance of patients to take adequate therapeutic doses.

II. The **antipsychotic or neuroleptic drugs** are the cornerstone of treatment of psychoses. They are safe, in the sense that it is difficult for patients to kill themselves with these drugs, but they produce a wide variety of toxic effects that may result in discomfort, drug refusal by patients, disfiguring involuntary movements, serious catatonic symptoms, or symptoms that may mimic an exacerbation of the underlying psychiatric disorder. In addition, they can cause the rare but potentially lethal neuroleptic malignant syndrome. A useful generalization about neuroleptic side effects is that those with low potency—for example, chlorpromazine (Thorazine) or thioridazine (Mellaril)—tend to be more sedating and more anticholinergic and tend to cause more postural hypotension than the high-potency agents such as haloperidol (Haldol). The high-potency drugs have a greater tendency to cause extrapyramidal side effects (EPS) (see Appendix I).

A. Mild dose-related side effects of antipsychotics are common including weakness, sluggishness, and apparent apathy. Especially if combined with even mild parkinsonian effects, such as masked facies, these effects may be confused with depression or with the withdrawal and apathy of schizophrenia. Patients who require neuroleptic-antidepressant combinations because of delusional depression may be difficult to evaluate because these neuroleptic effects can mimic the symptoms of depression. (These side effects are one of many reasons that neuroleptics are not indicated in depressions without psychotic features and that fixed antidepressant-neuroleptic combination drugs should not be prescribed.) **Treatment** consists of decreasing the neuroleptic dose to the lowest dose consistent with effectiveness.

B. Anticholinergic side effects such as dry mouth, blurred near vision, and constipation occur with thioridazine and chlorpromazine, and to a lesser extent with other lower-potency neuroleptics. Very high-potency agents (e.g., haloperidol) have only weak anticholinergic properties. It is rare for neuroleptics other than thioridazine to cause severe anticholinergic syndromes by themselves (Table 24-1), except in elderly patients. Such syndromes occur more frequently in the context of polypharmacy with additional anticholinergic agents, such as antiparkinsonian agents, cyclic antidepressants, antihistamines, or over-the-counter sleeping pills. To minimize the risk of an anticholinergic syndrome, high-potency neuroleptics such as haloperidol should be prescribed if concomitant use of an antidepressant is contemplated. When neuroleptics are prescribed together with cyclic antidepressants, additional antiparkinsonian therapy is generally not indicated. **Treatment** is discussed in sec. **III.B.**

C. Cardiovascular effects

1. **Postural hypotension** occurs with low-potency neuroleptics, especially chlorpromazine and thioridazine, and may be severe.

Table 24-1. The anticholinergic syndrome

Systemic manifestations
Tachycardia
Dilated, sluggishly reactive pupils
Blurred vision
Warm dry skin
Dry mucous membranes
Fever
Reduced or absent bowel sounds
Urinary retention
Neuropsychiatric manifestations
Agitation
Motor restlessness
Confusion
Disturbance of recent memory
Dysarthria
Myoclonus
Hallucinations (including visual)
Delirium
Seizures

a. **Prevention** can be accomplished by using high-potency agents, especially in the elderly and patients with cardiovascular disease. If low-potency agents are to be used, they should be started at a low dose and slowly increased. Patients should be warned to get up slowly from recumbency.

b. **Treatment** of acute postural hypotension usually consists of no more than assuming a supine posture; rarely IV fluid resuscitation is needed.

2. **Arrhythmias.** Although cardiac arrhythmias have been reported with very high doses of these drugs, including haloperidol, most of the neuroleptics are extremely safe, even in overdose.

a. The major exceptions to this rule are thioridazine and pimozide (Orap). Like class I antiarrhythmics and cyclic antidepressants, these drugs may **prolong the QT interval** with the rare consequence of producing **torsades de pointes** ventricular tachycardia, an electrocardiographically disorganized-appearing rhythm in which the axis of the QRS complex twists about the isoelectric point.

b. **Treatment** differs from that of typical ventricular tachycardia. It is best treated by overdrive pacing or isoproterenol, which decreases the QT interval and interrupts the reentrant tachyarrhythmia. Agents such as lidocaine, which do not delay repolarization, may also be helpful.

c. Thioridazine and pimozide should not be prescribed to patients with conduction system abnormalities and probably should not be prescribed if there is a history of overdosing and another antipsychotic drug will suffice.

D. Extrapyramidal side effects

1. **Acute dystonias** are tonic contractions that may affect the neck, mouth, tongue, axial musculature, or extremities. Oculogyric crises and opisthotonos may also occur. Dystonias can be frightening and painful and may result in an emergency visit. Laryngeal dystonias rarely occur but may be life-threatening.

a. **Onset** is usually during the first few days of treatment. There is a higher incidence in young males and a higher incidence with high-potency neuroleptics.

b. **Treatment.** Diphenhydramine (Benadryl) 50 mg IM or IV or benztropine (Cogentin) 2 mg IM or IV usually brings rapid relief. The dystonia is likely to recur unless a standing dose of an antiparkinsonian drug is prescribed for at least several days, even if the neuroleptic is discontinued. Benztropine 2 mg PO bid for 7 days should be adequate if the neuroleptic is stopped; if not, the antiparkinsonian agent should be continued with it for several months.

c. **Treatment of laryngeal dystonias** is a medical emergency. Benztropine 2 mg should be given rapidly IV. If there is no response in 5–10 minutes another 2 mg should be given. If that fails, lorazepam (Ativan) 1–2 mg should be given slowly IV. Rarely, endotracheal intubation will be needed.

2. **Drug-induced parkinsonism** may result in bradykinesia, rigidity, cogwheeling, mask-like facies, pill-rolling tremor, stooped posture, festinating gait, and drooling. These symptoms may occur singly or in any combination and differ little from idiopathic parkinsonism. At their most extreme neuroleptic-induced parkinsonian effects may be indistinguishable from **catatonia** (see Chap. 19 for a full discussion). The critical clinical point is that catatonia should never be assumed to be due to a primary psychiatric disorder until a neuroleptic-induced (or other organically based) catatonic syndrome has been ruled out.

   a. **Onset** of parkinsonian effects is more common after several days to weeks of treatment but may occur rapidly if high doses of neuroleptics have been given. The side effects are dose-related and more common with high-potency neuroleptics. The elderly are particularly susceptible to parkinsonian side effects, commonly developing them even on low doses of neuroleptic drugs.

   b. **Treatment.** The neuroleptic should be **decreased to the lowest dose that is therapeutic for the patient.** In addition, a fixed dose of an antiparkinsonian drug should be prescribed—for example, benztropine 2 mg PO bid (see Appendix VI). Some patients will do better on a low-potency neuroleptic, such as thioridazine.

3. **Akathisia** is one of the most troublesome side effects of neuroleptic drugs. It is an intensely unpleasant subjective feeling of needing to move, often accompanied by motor restlessness, pacing, fidgeting, and worsening anxiety or dysphoria. Sleep may be disturbed by an inability to lie down quietly. Mild cases are often misdiagnosed as anxiety. Severe cases may be mistaken for agitation due to the psychosis with the result that the offending neuroleptic is increased rather than decreased in dose. There are reports of suicide associated with akathisia.

   a. **Onset** is variable but is usually several days to weeks after beginning neuroleptic treatment. These are varying estimates of incidence from 20–45% of patients on neuroleptic drugs. Akathisia commonly coexists with other extrapyramidal side effects.

   b. **Treatment.** The key to an appropriate therapeutic response is making the diagnosis: One of the most common errors made in psychopharmacology is to mistake akathisia for a symptom of the underlying disease being treated, with the unfortunate result that more, instead of less, of the offending agent is given. Antipsychotics should be decreased to the minimum effective dose. Several drugs are successful in treating akathisia in particular patients. None of these drugs is clearly superior in all patients; thus an empirical approach is necessary. For patients with other extrapyramidal symptoms not already receiving an anticholinergic drug, an anticholinergic—for example, benztropine 2 mg bid—would be the first choice. For other patients, the choice would be one of the following:

(1) A beta-adrenergic blocker—for example, propranolol 10–30 mg tid (this may be the most widely effective treatment).

(2) An anticholinergic—for example, benztropine 2 mg bid.

(3) A benzodiazepine—for example, lorazepam 1 mg tid or clonazepam 0.5 mg bid.

E. The neuroleptic malignant syndrome (NMS) is an uncommon, but life-threatening reaction to neuroleptic drugs.

1. **Clinical manifestations.** The major symptoms are **delirium, rigidity, fever, and autonomic abnormalities.** Symptoms usually develop over 24–72 hours, with confusion and rigidity commonly developing prior to the fever and autonomic symptoms. The fever may be high, with temperatures greater than 41°C being common. If extrapyramidal symptoms, such as tremor, were previously present, they typically worsen. Course tremor, dystonias, posturing, and rigidity are typical. Rigidity may be severe enough to cause myonecrosis, with myoglobinuria and renal failure. Patients are often stuporous or have a fluctuating level of consciousness; retrospective patient reports suggest that severe anxiety and psychotic symptomatology are common. Patients are often mute; dysphagia and drooling also may occur. Autonomic abnormalities include tachycardia, diaphoresis, and hypertension, hypotension, or wide swings in blood pressure.

2. **Incidence and mortality.** NMS is a clinical diagnosis with a relatively wide continuum of severity. Since there are no clear criteria for making a diagnosis, it is difficult to state an incidence. Estimates have ranged from 0.02–1.9% of patients receiving neuroleptics (the upper end of this range is clearly too high). Although mortality was originally estimated to be as high as 20% (resulting from cardiovascular collapse, renal failure, pulmonary emboli, aspiration pneumonia, or respiratory failure), among patients who receive adequate medical care early in the course, mortality rates are much lower.

3. **Risk factors.** Although NMS may occur with all antipsychotic drugs, even at stable low doses, there is some evidence that the risk is increased with higher total doses or after recent initiation of therapy or dosage increases (Rosebush and Stewart, 1989). Combined therapy with lithium may also increase the risk; most reported cases of NMS with the atypical antipsychotic drug clozapine have occurred with combined therapy with lithium. Although difficult to evaluate because NMS itself causes dehydration, **the major identifiable independent risk factor for NMS appears to be dehydration.**

4. **Laboratory tests.** There are no pathognomonic laboratory findings; however, creatine kinase (CK) is nearly always elevated and may be markedly elevated. Isoenzyme determinations reveal that it is the muscle form of the enzyme (MM) that is affected. Elevated white blood cell counts often occur, but the highest values are generally seen when the patient is also on lithium.

5. **Differential diagnosis**

   a. **Catatonia** may be caused by primary psychiatric disorders or by antipsychotic drugs (see Chap. 19). Rigidity, muteness, and stupor may occur, but the temperature should be elevated by no more than 0.5–1.0°C, and marked autonomic abnormalities are not observed.

b. **Neuroleptic-induced parkinsonism with intercurrent infection.** Except in the case of CNS infection, confusion will not be observed, nor will there be significant worsening of preexisting rigidity and tremor. If there is any reason to suspect meningitis or encephalitis—for example, an onset in which fever is more prominent than extrapyramidal symptoms—a lumbar puncture should be performed. Some clinicians recommend a lumbar puncture in all suspected cases of NMS.

c. **Anticholinergic delirium or coma** must be considered especially because many patients receive both neuroleptics and anticholinergic drugs in combination. The diagnostic picture can be complicated by coexistence of side effects of both neuroleptics and anticholinergics at the same time. In anticholinergic deliria, signs of muscarinic receptor blockade will be prominent (see Table 24-1). Potentially useful differential diagnostic points are that patients with anticholinergic syndromes will have dry skin, whereas patients with NMS are typically diaphoretic. Anticholinergic syndromes are more likely to be associated with hypotension than hypertension or blood pressure fluctuations, which are more likely in NMS. Tachycardia is common in both conditions. An elevated CK favors the diagnosis of NMS.

6. **Treatment** of NMS must commence promptly.

a. Obviously, **neuroleptics must be discontinued.** The effects of neuroleptics last for days to weeks; patients who have received depot preparations of fluphenazine or haloperidol will have drug effect for a minimum of several weeks. Even if the patient is severely psychotic, neuroleptics should not be resumed for at least 2 weeks after resolution of NMS and preferably longer. During the interim, benzodiazepines can be used for sedation.

b. **Meticulous supportive measures** are the key to effective therapy. Cardiac monitoring, adequate hydration, and monitoring of urine output and renal function are critical. High fever should be treated with antipyretics, sponge baths, or hypothermia blankets depending on the severity. Arrhythmias should be treated if they occur; hypotension will require volume expansion and occasionally pressors. The patient should be positioned to avoid nerve compression injuries, aspiration, or decubitus ulcers.

c. **Pharmacologic measures** are difficult to evaluate in a systemic fashion because of the rarity and seriousness of NMS.

(1) **Benzodiazepines**—for example, lorazepam 1 mg IM tid–qid—may be useful in counteracting the hyperadrenergic state and may decrease the severity of the patient's psychological symptoms.

(2) The peripherally acting muscle relaxant **dantrolene sodium** has been used in doses of 0.8–1.0 mg/kg IV q6h. Unfortunately there are no good controls to determine whether it has an overall beneficial effect on the severity or duration of illness. If administered, the duration of therapy is not established. Many clinicians have continued treatment for 2 weeks or longer if a depot neuroleptic was the offending drug. Dantrolene can be given together with bromocriptine.

(3) The centrally acting dopamine agonist **bromocriptine** has been reported to provide relief of rigidity and other symptoms of dopamine blockade in several cases. As with dantrolene, proper controls are lacking. This drug can be started at a dose of 2.5 mg bid and increased to 5 mg tid gradually. Early side effects, such as nausea, usually pass with continued treatment. This drug can be given alone or with dantrolene. The duration of therapy is not established, but 2 weeks or more is common.

F. Withdrawal dyskinesias and tardive dyskinesia are clinically indistinguishable except that the former appear with decrease in neuroleptic dose. The symptoms of tardive dyskinesia are either long-lasting or permanent; withdrawal dyskinesias that persist for more than a few months should be rediagnosed as tardive dyskinesia. Tardive dyskinesia is commonly characterized by oral-buccal-lingual dyskinesias (including masticatory movements, sinuous tongue movements, and tongue protrusion), choreoathetotic movements of fingers, toes, limbs, and trunk, and neck movements including retrocollis. These movements increase with anxiety and stop during sleep. They can be both disfiguring and disabling.

1. **Onset** is typically late in the course of neuroleptic treatment, often after months or years. Abnormal movements often appear after a reduction in neuroleptic dose or discontinuation of the drug. Such movements may be seen, however, even on a constant neuroleptic dose (although they typically worsen transiently if the neuroleptic is then stopped). The movements can be masked by increasing the neuroleptic, but they may reemerge at the higher dose. There is evidence to suggest that higher-potency neuroleptics and long-term adjunctive use of anticholinergic antiparkinsonian drugs put patients at higher risk for developing tardive dyskinesia. It is estimated that 20% of patients on neuroleptics long-term will develop tardive dyskinesia. Additional risk factors are female sex, age greater than 50, and possibly affective disorder. The biologic mechanisms, risk factors, and natural history of this iatrogenic disorder remain poorly understood.

2. Despite occasional optimistic reports, **treatment** is generally not effective. Over time dyskinesias may improve. Generally, further neuroleptic treatment should be avoided in patients with tardive dyskinesia, but in cases where psychotic symptoms are severe and there is no effective alternative, neuroleptic therapy may be necessary.

3. **Prevention**

   a. Neuroleptics should only be used where there are good indications (i.e., psychotic disorders).

   b. The lowest effective dose should be used for the shortest possible time. (Thus in mania, for example, neuroleptics should be used only during acute episodes or if other alternatives fail.)

   c. In chronic psychoses, the need for continued use should be reconsidered every 6 months.

   d. Long-term use of adjunctive anticholinergic agents should be minimized if possible.

G. Other toxic effects

1. Low-potency neuroleptics are **photosensitizers.** Patients on such drugs should use sunscreens.

2. **Agranulocytosis** is a rare, idiosyncratic reaction associated with aliphatic and piperidine phenothiazines; when it occurs, it is usually during the first 6–8 weeks of therapy. During that period the physician should obtain a complete blood count (CBC) if the patient develops any symptoms of infection, such as fever or sore throat, even if the symptoms appear innocuous. There is a substantial incidence of agranulocytosis with **clozapine,** necessitating weekly blood counts.

3. Neuroleptics, especially chlorpromazine, have been associated with **cholestatic hepatitis.** This hypersensitivity reaction usually occurs during the first 2 months of treatment and should prompt discontinuation of the particular drug. If further antipsychotic therapy is necessary, a drug from a different chemical class should be chosen.

III. Cyclic antidepressants commonly produce side effects, even at subtherapeutic doses. The side effects include orthostatic hypotension, anticholinergic (antimuscarinic) effects, and quinidine-like cardiac effects. All of these side effects are dose-related, with lower doses producing toxicity in elderly patients. The incidence and severity of side effects are increased by concomitant administration of neuroleptic drugs.

A. Orthostatic hypotension is probably the most common serious side effect of cyclic antidepressants and of the atypical agent, trazodone (Desyrel). Elderly patients are more prone to this side effect, which may be severe enough to interrupt treatment. Patients should be advised to get up slowly from sitting and lying. Nortriptyline (Pamelor) is the tricyclic least likely to cause hypotension. The hypotensive effects of trazodone can be minimized if it is taken with a small meal. **Treatment** of symptomatic hypotension usually consists of supine posture and adequate hydration.

B. Anticholinergic effects

1. Mild anticholinergic effects are common with therapeutic dosages of these drugs. These effects include dry mouth, blurred near vision, constipation, and urinary hesitancy. There is also a risk of precipitating an attack of narrow-angle glaucoma. More severe anticholinergic effects may occur in older patients even at therapeutic dosages. These include agitation, delirium, tachycardia, ileus, and urinary retention. The most common reason for the appearance of the full anticholinergic syndrome (see Table 24-1) is the concomitant use of more than one anticholinergic drug. Most commonly implicated along with cyclic antidepressants are low-potency neuroleptics, especially thioridazine, antiparkinsonian drugs, antihistamines, antispasmodics, drugs for dizziness, and over-the-counter sleep medication.

2. **Treatment**

   a. If mild to moderate anticholinergic symptoms interfere with treatment, bethanechol (Urecholine), a cholinergic agent that does not cross the blood-brain barrier, may be prescribed. Effective doses range from 10–30 mg PO tid. If long-term treatment is contemplated, corrective glasses may be useful for patients with impairment of near vision.

   b. For **acute urinary retention,** bethanechol 2.5–5.0 mg may be given SQ. Occasionally a urinary catheter will be required temporarily.

   c. If an **anticholinergic delirium or severe anticholinergic syndrome** is suspected, physostigmine salicylate, an acetylcholinesterase inhibitor that crosses the blood-brain barrier, can be diagnostically useful. The therapeutic usefulness of this agent is limited by its toxicity (Table 24-2) and short duration of action. Its only therapeutic use is in otherwise uncontrollable anticholinergic deliria producing life-threatening behaviors. For either diagnostic or therapeutic purposes, it is given IV in doses of 1–2 mg over 2–3 minutes. If there is no response, the dose can be repeated in 20–30 minutes. If a good response occurs, the lowest effective dose can be repeated as the last wears off (approximately 30 minutes). Should a toxic response to physostigmine occur it can be reversed by atropine sulfate 0.5 mg IV for every milligram of physostigmine that was given.

C. The **cardiac toxicity** of the tricyclic and newer tetracyclic antidepressants is due to their quinidine-like effects on conduction and to a much lesser extent to their anticholinergic effects. Patients at highest risk of serious cardiac toxicity are older patients and patients with underlying conduction system disease. Patients with bifascicular block, left bundle branch block, or a prolonged QT interval should generally not receive these drugs. In addition, there would be additive toxicity with class I antiarrhythmics, such as procainamide (Procan) and disopyramide (Norpace). The cardiac toxicities (Table 24-3) occur with all cyclic

Table 24-2. The physostigmine-induced syndrome of cholinergic crisis

Systemic manifestations
- Bradycardia
- Miosis
- Diaphoresis
- Excessive salivation
- Lacrimation
- Copious bronchial secretions
- Dyspnea
- Vomiting
- Biliary colic
- Diarrhea
- Urinary frequency

Neuropsychiatric manifestations
- Confusion (often after initial clearing of anticholinergic delirium)
- Hallucinations
- Myoclonus
- Seizures

Table 24-3. Cardiac toxicity of tricyclic antidepressants

- Sinus tachycardia
- Supraventricular tachyarrhythmias
- Ventricular tachycardia and fibrillation
- Prolongation of PR, QRS, and QT intervals
- Bundle branch block
- First-, second-, and third-degree heart block
- ST- and T-wave changes

antidepressants. Earlier claims that doxepin (Sinequan, Adapin) or maprotiline (Ludiomil) had less cardiac toxicity than the other cyclic agents have not been substantiated. The atypical antidepressants fluoxetine and bupropion appear to be relatively free of adverse effects on cardiac conduction. **Treatment of cardiac emergencies due to cyclic antidepressants** is discussed in Chap. 32, sec. **VI.D.2.**

IV. Atypical antidepressants

A. Fluoxetine is a selective serotonin reuptake inhibitor in wide clinical use because of its efficacy, its lack of anticholinergic or cardiac side effects and its relative safety if taken in overdose.

1. The most problematic side effects of fluoxetine include agitation, neuromuscular restlessness (which may approximate neuroleptic-induced akathisia), and insomnia. These may respond to a dosage reduction or to temporary administration of a benzodiazepine—for example, clonazepam 0.25–0.5 mg bid for akathisia-like symptoms or a benzodiazepine or trazodone 50 mg at bedtime for insomnia. (Some patients receiving both fluoxetine and trazodone complain of cognitive difficulties.)
2. A minority of patients may feel sedated by fluoxetine.
3. Fluoxetine may cause delayed ejaculation in males or anorgasmia in males and females.
4. Other side effects include nausea, headache, and diarrhea.

5. Fluoxetine is a potent **metabolic inhibitor,** raising the blood levels of many drugs including cyclic antidepressants.

6. Fluoxetine should not be used with monoamine oxidase inhibitors (MAOIs); because of its long half-life it should be discontinued 4–5 weeks before starting an MAOI.

B. **Sertraline** is a new selective serotonin reuptake inhibitor. Like fluoxetine, it has little anticholinergic potency. There is little experience with the drug yet, but it also appears to be relatively free of cardiovascular side effects and to be less dangerous than cyclic antidepressants or MAOIs in overdose. The major side effects are nausea, diarrhea, agitation, and sexual dysfunction (delayed ejaculation in males or anorgasmia in males and females). Sertraline should not be used with MAOIs. The recommended washout period before starting an MAOI is 14 days.

C. **Paroxetine** is the most recently approved selective serotonin reuptake inhibitor, which, like other members of its class, is free of anticholinergic effects and appears to be free of significant cardiovascular effects. It is a metabolic inhibitor, inhibiting P-450 enzymes. Its effect on the metabolism of other drugs appears to be less than the effects of fluoxetine, but more than that of sertraline. Major reported toxicities include nausea, drowsiness or insomnia, tremor, sweating, ejaculatory disturbances, and hyponatremia. Paroxetine should not be used with MAOIs.

D. **Bupropion** is also free of anticholinergic effects and does not cause postural hypotension or alter cardiac conduction in a clinically significant manner. Major toxicities reported with bupropion are seizures, ataxia, myoclonus, and dystonias. There are reports of bupropion causing psychotic symptoms, but the incidence appears to be low. Bupropion should not be used with MAOIs.

E. **Trazodone** is also free of anticholinergic effects; it lacks the quinidine-like properties of the cyclic antidepressants and does not appear to have major effects on cardiac conduction. However, trazodone can cause severe postural hypotension. This side effect, as well as nausea, can be minimized if the drug is taken with meals to slow absorption. **Priapism** may occur with trazodone, most commonly early in therapy. Males given trazodone should be instructed to report abnormally prolonged erections to their physician or go to an emergency department for evaluation. Should priapism occur, trazodone should be permanently discontinued.

V. **Monoamine oxidase inhibitors** are an effective class of antidepressant drugs that have significant potential toxicity. The most dangerous side effects are due to interactions with some other drugs and foodstuffs. Side effects are as follows:

A. **Postural hypotension** is dose-related and may limit therapy. For patients with no underlying cardiovascular disease, salt tablets (600–1800 mg bid) or, if those fail, the mineralocorticoid fludrocortisone (Florinef) 0.025–0.05 mg PO qd or bid may alleviate the problem. The physician should be alert for fluid retention, hypertension, edema, or electrolyte abnormalities.

B. **Central side effects** can be troublesome, especially sedation with phenelzine and insomnia with tranylcypromine. Dosing early in the day may improve sleep problems. Occasionally addition of a benzodiazepine will be necessary.

C. **Hyperadrenergic crises** due to ingestion of sympathomimetic substances in drugs or foods are among the most serious toxic effects of MAOIs. A number of amines in foods may induce these sympathomimetic crises, especially tyramine, but also phenylethylamine and others. The inhibition of monoamine oxidase in the gastrointestinal tract, liver, and blood vessels allows these vasoactive amines access, unmetabolized, to sympathetic nerve terminals. All sympathomimetic drugs can lead to crises as can levodopa and tricyclic antidepressants.

1. **Clinical manifestations** include a severe headache, diaphoresis, mydriasis, neuromuscular irritability, hypertension (which may be extreme), and occasionally cardiac arrhythmias.
2. **Treatment** consists of blockade of alpha-adrenergic receptors. The most effective treatment is phentolamine (Regitine) 5 mg IV, repeated as necessary. In milder cases of hypertensive crisis, chlorpromazine 50–100 mg IM can be used. Beta blockers must not be used as initial therapy, because, as in the treatment of pheochromocytoma, their predominant clinical effect may be to intensify vasoconstriction and thus worsen hypertension.
3. **Prevention.** MAOIs are useful drugs but should only be administered to patients who are responsible enough to follow the prescribed tyramine-free diet and to avoid medications with sympathomimetic properties. While cheating on the diet is widely practiced, it should be discouraged because the tyramine content of any given sample of a proscribed food may vary (e.g., it increases as fruits become overripe), and therefore safe consumption on one occasion does not guarantee safety on another. A set of instructions for patients taking MAOIs is given in Table 24-4, which lists foods and medications to avoid.

Table 24-4. Instructions for patients taking monoamine oxidase inhibitors (MAOIs)

1. Take your dose exactly as prescribed.
2. If you visit other physicians or dentists, inform them that you are taking an MAOI. This precaution is especially important if other medications are to be prescribed or if you are to have dental work or surgery where local anesthetics might be used. Physicians may be unaware that the painkiller meperidine (Demerol) interacts dangerously with MAOIs.
3. Take no medications without a doctor's approval, including all over-the-counter medications except plain aspirin or acetaminophen (Tylenol). You must avoid all medications for colds, allergies, and hay fever; all nasal decongestants; cough suppressants; inhalers; and diet pills.
4. Some foods may produce serious reactions. These are all best avoided:
   Aged, ripened, or strong cheeses, such as cheddar, Swiss, Camembert, blue cheeses, Parmesan, and mozzarella (fresh cottage cheese and cream cheese are allowed).
   Sour cream, yogurt.
   Pickles, sauerkraut, and other pickled foods.
   Pickled herrings, anchovies, smoked fish, caviar.
   Liver.
   Fava beans and other broad beans.
   Yeast extracts (Marmite, Bovril).
   All fermented sausages.
   Overripe bananas, canned figs, avocados, raisins (in general, it is best to avoid overripe fruit).
   Chianti and sherry. Some patients will not tolerate beer or any other alcoholic beverages.
   Caffeine-containing beverages—such as coffee, tea, and cola drinks—should be used in moderation.
   Chocolate should be used in moderation. Some patients will not tolerate it.
5. Report promptly any severe headache, nausea, vomiting, chest pain, or other unusual symptoms.

D. Other interactions

1. **Oral hypoglycemics.** MAOIs potentiate hypoglycemia.

2. **Meperidine (Demerol) and dextromethorphan.** MAOIs can interact to produce a syndrome of hypotension, hypertension, central nervous system excitation, neuromuscular irritability, and hyperpyrexia. Interactions with cyclic antidepressants or psychostimulants may occasionally produce a similar syndrome. Treatment is similar to that for MAOI overdoses described in Chap. 32, sec. **VII.**

3. **Interactions with serotonergic drugs** (e.g., clomipramine, L-tryptophan, fluoxetine, and presumably paroxetine and sertraline) may produce a "serotonin syndrome" characterized by delirium, restlessness, tremor, hyperreflexia, myoclonus, fever, diaphoresis, and shivering (Sternbach, 1991). The incidence is not known. The offending agents should be discontinued and supportive measures instituted. Patients should be observed in an intensive care setting. It is important to rule out the possibility of MAOI overdose, which may have many similar features (see Chap. 32).

E. Other side effects

1. **Paresthesias** often respond to pyridoxine 50–150 mg qd.

2. **Edema** may respond to a thiazide diuretic, such as hydrochlorthiazide 25–50 mg bid.

3. Sexual dysfunction may be difficult to manage. Anorgasmia may resolve over time.

VI. Lithium has important dose-related toxicities. Many of its toxic effects may appear during the initiation of therapy because of a rapid rate of rise in blood levels, even if the absolute level is still low. Mild toxicity may occur even at stable therapeutic doses, and severe toxicity may occur with doses not much higher than those that result in safe serum levels. The therapeutic range for lithium therapy is 0.6–1.2 mEq/liter. Patients have widely varying susceptibility to toxic effects, with the elderly being more susceptible to central nervous system toxicity, but in general mild toxicity is to be expected at levels above 1.5 mEq/liter. Severe toxicity may be manifest at levels as low as 2.0 and is almost always evident at levels above 3.0 mEq/liter.

A. Causes of toxicity. Lithium excretion is almost entirely renal and is profoundly affected by sodium balance and dehydration. Any drug or condition that produces a negative sodium balance or dehydration will cause the kidney to reabsorb lithium more avidly and will raise lithium levels. Thus in addition to overdose, the most important causes of lithium intoxication are impaired renal function, dehydration (especially if electrolytes are depleted, such as during prolonged vomiting), sodium restriction, diuretic therapy, childbirth, and nonsteroidal antiinflammatory agents (which alter renal blood flow).

B. Clinical manifestations of toxicity

1. **Neurologic symptoms**

a. **Common at the start of therapy and usually transient, or at mildly toxic levels.** Lethargy, fatigue, muscle weakness, and action tremor.

(1) **Tremor** may be a problem for many patients.

(2) **Treatment.** If still a problem at the lowest effective lithium dose tremor may improve if the patient decreases or eliminates caffeine intake. If not, propranolol (10–80 mg bid) or another beta-adrenergic blocker may help.

b. **With moderate toxicity.** Neuromuscular irritability, including twitching and fasciculations, extrapyramidal symptoms, ataxia, coarsening of tremor, dysarthria, incoordination, difficulty concentrating, confusion, visual disturbance, and altered levels of consciousness.

c. **With severe toxicity** (this is a medical emergency; see Chap. 32, sec. **VIII**). Symptoms include marked neuromuscular irritability or flaccidity, seizures, hallucinations, ataxia, delirium, coma, and death. These symptoms may emerge at levels of 3–4 mEq/liter, although some patients may initially have deceptively mild symptoms at these levels. Without rapid treatment, permanent cerebellar ataxia or memory disturbance may result.

2. **Gastrointestinal symptoms** are common at the start of treatment and are usually transient; they may be minimized by temporarily decreasing the dose or administering lithium citrate (a well-absorbed liquid preparation) instead of lithium carbonate. Patients troubled by nausea even on a stable dose may do better on a sustained release preparation, although these preparations have a greater propensity for causing diarrhea. Gastrointestinal symptoms such as anorexia, nausea, vomiting, diarrhea, and abdominal pain may also emerge later in therapy if toxic levels occur.

3. **Renal toxicity**

a. The most common renal toxicity is **polyuria.** This often emerges after weeks to months of therapy and appears to improve when lithium is stopped (although some patients develop a permanent defect in their urine-concentrating ability). If frequency and nocturia become a problem, despite using the lowest effective lithium dose, the addition of a thiazide diuretic, such as hydrochlorthiazide 50 mg qd may help decrease urine volumes. If this drug is added, lithium levels will rise, so when adding hydrochlorthiazide, the oral dose of lithium should be halved, and the optimal dose reestablished using serum lithium levels. As with all patients on diuretics, potassium levels must also be monitored. The potassium-sparing diuretic amiloride has recently been reported to be effective in treating lithium-induced polyuria with little effect on lithium levels (Battle, et al., 1985). Amiloride is used in doses of 5–10 mg bid.

b. Lithium may rarely cause **interstitial nephritis;** a creatinine clearance should be performed on any patient whose creatinine rises or whose lithium levels rise on a stable oral dose in the absence of dehydration or sodium restriction.

4. **Dermatologic symptoms** include acne and psoriasis. Acne may markedly affect the willingness of adolescents to take lithium unless vigorously treated.

5. **Thyroid toxicity.** The most common symptom is goiter; more rarely hypothyroidism develops with or without goiter. Thyroid stimulating hormone (TSH) should be checked prior to starting lithium therapy and every 6 months thereafter. A goiter may be suppressed with thyroid replacement should it develop; hypothyroidism should be treated in consultation with an internist.

6. **Other toxicities**

a. Clinically significant arrhythmias are rare, except in patients with preexisting SA node dysfunction. Asymptomatic electrocardiographic changes (ST-T wave changes) are common. A baseline electrocardiogram is recommended in patients over 40 years old.

b. Peripheral edema rarely occurs and can be treated with spironolactone.

C. **Treatment of lithium toxicity due to elevated serum levels** is discussed in Chap. 32, sec. **VIII.**

VII. **Benzodiazepines** are relatively safe drugs. Their main problems have to do with abuse, dependency, and withdrawal, rather than side effects. The most important side effect is dose-related oversedation.

A. **Drowsiness, mild impairment of cognitive function, impairment of motor coordination, and memory disturbance** may occur. These effects usually diminish over time with continued use. The development of sedation depends on the sensitivity of the individual, his or her metabolic status, and the presence of other central nervous system depressant drugs. In addition, the degree of central nervous system depression also varies with the intensity of environmental stimuli. Serious **anterograde amnesia** may occur with higher doses of high-potency benzodiazepines, especially triazolam.

B. **Abuse** in the context of prescribed therapy is defined as accelerating daily dosage without indication. Abuse is far rarer than originally reported among patients with proper initial indications (e.g., severe anxiety, temporary treatment of insomnia). Individuals at highest risk for abuse include patients with a history of alcoholism, sedative abuse, or polysubstance abuse and patients with borderline personality disorder.

C. **Withdrawal** symptoms may occur after regular use and are most prominent with high-potency, short-acting agents, such as alprazolam (Xanax). Although withdrawal symptoms are usually mild and self-limited when they occur, more severe symptoms may emerge including irritability, insomnia, rebound anxiety, tachycardia, hypertension, and even psychotic-like symptoms, delirium, and seizures. Withdrawal symptoms from long-acting benzodiazepines may emerge relatively late, as long as 7–10 days after discontinuation. Symptoms from short-acting agents occur earlier and are generally more severe. Symptoms of withdrawal from alprazolam may begin within 24 hours and in the case of psychologic symptoms may respond rapidly only to readministration of alprazolam (rather than other benzodiazepines). Although psychologic dependence can be induced by any benzodiazepine, this problem seems to be most severe in the case of alprazolam. At times a switch to equipotent doses of a longer-acting benzodiazepine may be the only way to withdraw the patient. In the case of alprazolam, replacement with clonazepam (Klonopin) 0.5 mg for every milligram of alprazolam followed by a slow taper has proved successful (Herman et al., 1987).

Selected Readings

ANTIPSYCHOTIC DRUGS

Arana, G. W., et al. The effect of anticholinergic prophylaxis on neuroleptic-induced dystonia. *Am. J. Psychiatry* 145:993, 1988.

Fleischhacker, W. W., Roth, S. D., and Kane, J. M. The pharmacologic treatment of neuroleptic-induced akathisias. *J. Clin. Psychopharmacol.* 10:12, 1990.

Rosebush, P., and Stewart, T. A prospective analysis of 24 episodes of neuroleptic malignant syndrome. *Am. J. Psychiatry* 146:717, 1989.

Sewell, D. D., and Jeste, D. V. Distinguishing neuroleptic malignant syndrome (NMS) from NMS-like acute medical illnesses: A study of 34 cases. *J. Neuropsychiatry Clin. Neurosci.* 4:265, 1992.

Shear, K. M., Frances, A., and Weiden, P. Suicide associated with akathisia and depot fluphenazine treatment. *J. Clin. Psychopharmacol.* 3:235, 1983.

Van Putten, T. The many faces of akathisia. *Compr. Psychiatry* 16:43, 1975.

CYCLIC ANTIDEPRESSANTS

Glassman, A. H., and Bigger, J. T. Cardiovascular effects of therapeutic doses of tricyclic antidepressants. *Arch. Gen. Psychiatry* 38:815, 1981.

Nelson, J. C., et al. Major adverse reactions during desipramine treatment. *Arch. Gen. Psychiatry* 39:1055, 1982.

Pollack, M. H., and Rosenbaum, J. F. Management of antidepressant-induced side effects: A practical guide for the clinician. *J. Clin. Psychiatry* 48:3, 1987.

MONOAMINE OXIDASE INHIBITORS

Rabkin, J., et al. Adverse reactions to monoamine oxidase inhibitors: Part I. A comparative study. *J. Clin. Psychopharmacol.* 4:270, 1984.

Rabkin, J., et al. Adverse reactions to monoamine oxidase inhibitor: Part II. Treatment correlates and clinical management. *J. Clin. Psychopharmacol.* 5:2, 1985.

Sternbach, H. The serotonin syndrome. *Am. J. Psychiatry* 148:705, 1991.

LITHIUM

Apte, N., and Langston, J. W. Permanent neurological deficits due to lithium toxicity. *Ann. Neurol.* 13:453, 1983.

Battle, D. C., et al. Amelioration of polyuria by amiloride in patients receiving long-term lithium therapy. *N. Engl. J. Med.* 312:408, 1985.

BENZODIAZEPINES

Herman, J. B., Rosenbaum, J. F., and Brotman, A. W. The alprazolam to clonazepam switch for the treatment of panic disorder. *J. Clin. Psychopharmacol.* 7:175, 1987.

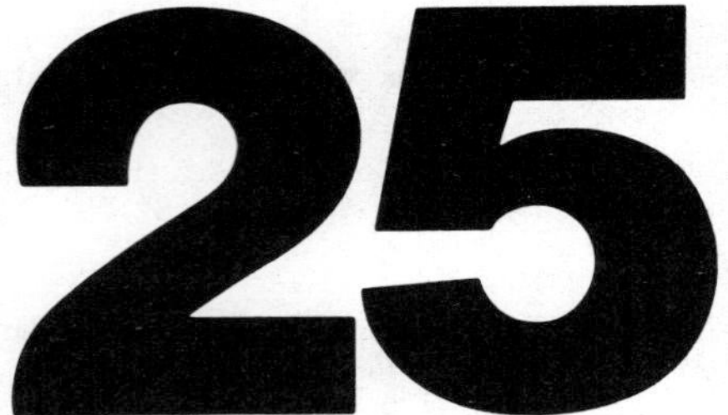

Psychiatric Symptoms of Medical Illness and Drug Toxicity

Michael F. Bierer
Barbara E. Bierer

I. When a patient comes to an emergency department with abnormalities of thought, mood, or behavior, it is incumbent on the evaluating physician to rule out medical etiologies. **Any psychiatric symptom** may be caused or exacerbated by a medical disorder. Thus failure to perform an appropriate medical evaluation, even in cases where the patient already carries a psychiatric diagnosis, may lead to catastrophic results, with unnecessary morbidity, inappropriate dispositions, and, rarely, even death. This chapter presents a general approach to the medical workup, including basic emergency therapy, followed by a more inclusive and detailed discussion of medical conditions that can exacerbate or mimic psychiatric symptoms.

II. **Medical evaluation and basic emergency therapy**

A. The initial **medical evaluation** of psychiatric patients depends on the clinical condition and should be directed toward establishing that the patient is medically stable. Abnormal vital signs or physical findings will focus the examination. If the patient is hemodynamically stable, attention can be turned to those problems that, if neglected, may lead to further deterioration, irreversible deficits, or death. As noted in Chap. 1, all patients with acute psychiatric complaints deserve a full medical as well as psychiatric history, including attention to drug use (prescribed and otherwise). A physical examination including a neurologic examination and detailed mental status examination should be performed. In addition, certain basic laboratory tests should be obtained (Table 25-1). If the patient is being evaluated for the first time, a more complete battery of blood tests will be sent than if the patient has a known history. Certain tests will be obtained only if warranted by the clinical findings (see Table 25-1).

B. **Basic emergency therapy** will depend on the patient's overall medical stability and clinical presentation. If the patient is hemodynamically unstable, delirious, or comatose, certain basic procedures should be followed and emergency medical consultation obtained.

1. Blood tests should be drawn (see Table 25-1) prior to giving the patient any therapy. It is wise to draw two or three extra "red top tubes" at this time.
2. IV access should be established. If the patient is profoundly hypotensive, intravascular volume should be expanded with IV saline.
3. Thiamine 100 mg IV should be given, even in the absence of suspected alcohol use.
4. Fifty milliliters of 50% dextrose should be given IV (see sec. **III.A**). This can be repeated in several minutes if there is no response. The prompt treatment of hypoglycemia may prevent progression to irreversible brain damage. Acute administration of dextrose will not worsen the clinical course of diabetes and therefore should not be withheld while awaiting blood tests.
5. Naloxone (Narcan) 0.4–2.0 mg IV is then administered to reverse possible opioid overdose.
6. Further therapy will depend on the clinical presentation and the underlying cause and should be performed in consultation with specialists.

Table 25-1. Laboratory tests in ambulatory psychiatric patients

Tests to be obtained in all patients with altered mental status:
- Electrolytes, glucose
- Blood urea nitrogen (BUN), creatinine
- Aspartate aminotransferase (AST) or SGOT
- Complete blood count (CBC) with differential
- Urinalysis
- Drug levels; ethanol level; toxic screen

Tests to be sent if clinically indicated:
- Free thyroxine (T_4) triiodothyronine resin uptake (T_3RU), thyroid-stimulating hormone (TSH)
- Liver function tests, including lactate dehydrogenase (LDH), bilirubin, alkaline phosphatase, albumin, amylase
- Prothrombin time, partial thromboplastin time
- Calcium, magnesium
- Arterial blood gases (PO_2, PCO_2, pH)
- Electrocardiogram
- Chest x ray
- Lumbar puncture
- Computed tomographic (CT) scan of the head
- Electroencephalogram (EEG)
- Serum test for syphilis
- Anti-human immunodeficiency virus antibody
- Serum osmolality
- Ammonia level
- Erythrocyte sedimentation rate, and if indicated, antinuclear antibody, rheumatoid factor, lupus band test
- Cortisol level
- Vitamin B_{12} level
- Heavy metal screen
- Urine prophobilinogen and delta-aminolevulinic acid
- Ceruloplasmin, urinary copper, slit-lamp examination
- Urinary vanillymandelic acid (VMA)
- Urinary 5-hydroxyindoleacetic acid (5-HIAA)

III. Toxic and metabolic causes of psychiatric symptoms

A. Hypoglycemia can cause a broad range of symptoms due to sympathetic hyperactivity (e.g., anxiety, sweating, tachycardia, tremor, and restlessness) and neuroglycopenia (e.g., confusion, drowsiness, stupor, coma, and seizures). The manifestations are more severe if the glucose has fallen rapidly or if the low level has persisted for a long time. Irreversible brain damage or death may result. Patients taking beta blockers may lack symptoms or signs of sympathetic hyperactivity.

1. **Etiology** is usually excess insulin. Although there are rare insulin-secreting tumors (insulinomas), almost all clinically significant hypoglycemia occurs in diabetics due to exogenous insulin administration or oral hypoglycemic agents plus a precipitant (such as decreased food intake, exercise, or alcohol abuse). Pentamidine, a drug used for treatment of pneumocystis pneumonia, may cause prolonged hypoglycemia. So-called reactive hypoglycemia rarely if ever causes significant psychiatric symptoms. A small number of individuals, often employed in medically related fields, produce hypoglycemia by surreptitious use of insulin or oral agents.

2. **Diagnosis** is made by the finding of a low blood sugar in the presence of symptoms.

3. **Treatment** should proceed as outlined in sec. **II.B**: IV access is established, blood is drawn, and thiamine and dextrose are administered. Further treatment will require consultation. Hypoglycemia due to excess exogenous insulin can be treated in the emergency department, and the patient can be discharged if alert and able to eat. Hypoglycemia due to most oral agents requires inpatient admission and observation for at least 36 hours because of their long duration of action. Because alcohol ingestion and poor nutrition can cause hypoglycemia and ketoacidosis, chronic inebriates should receive an infusion of glucose while under observation.

B. **Hyperglycemia** produces psychiatric symptoms by two mechanisms, diabetic ketoacidosis and hyperosmolar coma. The former is more likely in insulin-dependent diabetics and the latter in non-insulin-dependent diabetics.

1. **Diabetic ketoacidosis** may or may not result in psychiatric abnormalities. The psychiatric manifestations are due to hypovolemia (on the basis of anorexia and osmotic diuresis), hyperosmolarity, and acidosis. The most common mental symptoms are anxiety and agitation, although delirium may occur. Catatonic-like stupor has rarely been reported.

   a. **Etiology** is insufficient insulin to suppress ketone production by the liver. Usually this results from an intercurrent illness in an insulin-dependent diabetic.

   b. **Diagnosis** is made from the history and the presence of other symptoms such as polyuria, nausea, vomiting, and abdominal pain. Patients may show signs of dehydration and Kussmaul's respirations and have the fruity smell of acetone on their breath. Laboratory tests show an anion gap acidosis, ketones in urine and serum, and usually hyperglycemia.

   c. **Emergency treatment** requires fluid resuscitation, insulin, and intensive medical monitoring. Medical consultation is required.

2. **Hyperosmolar nonketotic coma** occurs typically in older patients, often with mild non-insulin-dependent diabetes. The major central nervous system manifestations are stupor or coma. Focal neurologic deficits and seizures are also reported.

   a. **Etiology** is a relative lack of insulin with enough insulin to suppress ketogenesis but not enough to maintain normal levels of glucose. Glycosuria leads to dehydration and rising osmolality, but often there are contributing factors such as thiazide diuretics, corticosteroids, phenytoin, immobility, or intercurrent illness.

   b. **Diagnosis** is made on the basis of depressed mental status in the presence of a blood sugar > 600 mg/dl and a serum osmolality > 350 mEq/liter in the absence of significant ketonemia or acidosis. Other symptoms and signs include anorexia, nausea, vomiting, and dehydration.

   c. **Emergency** treatment is based on careful volume repletion and insulin. Medical consultation will be needed.

C. **Disturbances of electrolytes, calcium, and magnesium**

1. **Hyponatremia** can produce significant neuropsychiatric symptomatology, depending on the severity of the abnormality, the rate of fall of the serum sodium, and the age of the patient. Acute hyponatremia can produce confusion, lethargy, stupor, coma, and seizures. Focal neurologic deficits can occur. Chronic hyponatremia may produce mild confusion, personality changes, speech abnormalities, and finally also stupor and coma.

   a. **Etiology.** Hyponatremia is due to excess free water for the level of total body sodium. It is difficult to produce hyponatremia on the basis of sodium depletion except at extremes of volume depletion. Usually the problem lies in an inability to excrete a free water load, as occurs in the syndrome of inappropriate antidiuretic hormone secretion (SIADH) and in hypocortisolism, or because of diminished effective plasma volume, as occurs in nephrotic syndrome, liver failure, and congestive heart failure. Hyponatremia on the basis of psychogenic polydipsia occurs only if there is a concomitant stimulus to antidiuretic hormone secretion (usually from a drug) or if the ability of the kidney to excrete free water is exceeded (which, in normal individuals, might require drinking more than 20 liters of free water) (Table 25-2).

b. **Diagnosis** is made on the basis of a low serum sodium. Other diagnostic tests will be necessary to determine the specific cause. It is helpful to obtain simultaneous urine and serum sodium and osmolalities in order to document SIADH.

c. **Treatment** depends on the underlying cause. If dilutional, treatment consists of water restriction. However, emergency treatment will be needed for patients who are in coma or seizing. A diuresis should be initiated with an infusion of furosemide 10–20 mg IV and normal saline (with added potassium). Rarely, hypertonic saline (3%) may be needed, but there is a risk of congestive heart failure; thus hypertonic solutions should be used cautiously (at a rate not exceeding 75 ml/hour), if at all. Frequent monitoring of electrolytes is mandatory. If the cause is hypovolemia, treatment consists of IV saline administration.

2. **Hypernatremia** reflects a deficit of total body water. Its neuropsychiatric manifestations reflect both the severity and rate of onset. The symptoms of all hyperosmolar states are similar (see sec. **III.B.2**) and include lethargy, stupor, coma, and occasionally seizures.

   a. **Etiology** is volume depletion due to diuretic use, vomiting, diarrhea, fever, osmotic diuresis, or an inability to drink water (as may occur in debilitated or delirious patients) (Table 25-3).

   b. **Diagnosis** is based on an elevated serum sodium. Other symptoms and signs typically include postural hypotension, tachycardia, and poor skin turgor.

   c. **Emergency treatment.** If the patient is hypotensive, volume is first expanded with normal saline followed by fluid replacement with hypotonic saline.

3. **Hypokalemia** represents total body depletion of potassium or abnormal intracellular compartmentalization—for example, due to alkalosis. Psychiatric symptoms include apathy, weakness, and confusion.

   a. **Etiology** is due to an imbalance of potassium losses and intake, most commonly due to diuretic therapy (Table 25-4).

   b. **Diagnosis** is made by measurement of the serum potassium. Other cardinal manifestations include muscular weakness, cramping, or tetany. Paresthesias are common. Cardiac arrhythmias are the most serious sequelae, especially for patients on digitalis. Additional laboratory tests should include the other electrolytes, blood urea nitrogen (BUN), creatinine, and if indicated, arterial blood gases.

   c. **Emergency treatment** requires close monitoring and repletion of potassium. If the patient is symptomatic with cardiac arrhythmias, potassium chloride can be given IV no more rapidly than 10–20 mEq/hour with frequent monitoring of levels and electrocardiogram (ECG). Otherwise potassium chloride can be given orally in doses up to 40 mEq tid as needed. Gastrointestinal intolerance is common. If the patient is acidotic, potassium should be given as the bicarbonate or citrate salt. Any abnormalities of pH should also be corrected.

Table 25-2. Causes of hyponatremia

- Extracellular fluid volume excess (mild, no edema)
  - Glucocorticoid deficiency
  - Hypothyroidism
  - Water intoxication
    - Iatrogenic (e.g., IV therapy after surgery)
    - Psychogenic polydipsia
  - Syndrome of inappropriate antidiuretic hormone
    - Malignant neoplasms
    - Pulmonary disease
    - Central nervous system pathology
    - Drugs
      - Amitriptyline
      - Fluphenazine
      - Thiothixene
      - Carbamazepine
      - Barbiturates
      - Nicotine
      - Clofibrate
      - Isoproterenol
      - Acetaminophen
      - Many diuretic agents
      - Chlorpropamide
      - Morphine
    - Stress, pain
    - Idiopathic
- Extracellular fluid volume excess (severe, with edema)
  - Chronic renal failure
  - Nephrotic syndrome
  - Hepatic cirrhosis
  - Congestive heart failure
- Extracellular fluid volume depletion (hypovolemia)
  - Renal losses
    - Diuretic therapy
    - Adrenal insufficiency
    - Mineralocorticoid deficiency
    - Salt-losing nephritis
    - Osmotic diuresis (glucose, mannitol)
  - Extrarenal losses
    - Vomiting
    - Diarrhea
    - Burns
    - Pancreatitis
- Pseudohyponatremia (euvolemic)
  - Hyperglycemia
  - Hyperlipidemia
  - Hyperproteinemia

Table 25-3. Causes of hypernatremia

- Free water deficit, normal total body sodium (Rx: water replacement)
  - Renal losses
    - Nephrogenic diabetes insipidus
      - Congenital
      - Drug-induced: lithium, demeclocycline, propoxyphene
    - Central diabetes insipidus
      - Central nervous system lesions (tumor, infection, neurosurgery)
      - Drug-induced: alcohol, phenytoin
      - Trauma
      - Idiopathic
  - Extrarenal losses (skin, respiratory losses)
- Free water deficit, low total body sodium (Rx: hypotonic saline)
  - Osmotic diuresis (glucose, mannitol)
  - Children and elderly with unreplaced losses from gastrointestinal and respiratory tracts
- Excess total body sodium (Rx: water replacement; diuretics, if needed)
  - Cushing's syndrome
  - Primary hyperaldosteronism
  - Hypertonic saline infusion

Table 25-4. Causes of hypokalemia

- Increased potassium losses
  - Renal
    - Diuretic therapy
    - Excessive glucocorticoids
    - Excessive mineralocorticoids
    - Osmotic diuresis (glucose, mannitol)
    - Renal tubular acidosis
    - Metabolic alkalosis
    - Magnesium deficiency
    - Drugs: penicillin, carbenicillin
  - Extrarenal losses
    - Vomiting
    - Diarrhea
    - Laxative abuse
    - Bowel and biliary fistula
    - Ureterosigmoidostomy
- Decreased potassium intake
- Redistribution
  - Alkalosis, metabolic and respiratory
  - Administration of glucose and insulin
  - Hypokalemic periodic paralysis

4. **Hyperkalemia** is due to impaired renal excretion or shift of potassium out of the intracellular compartment by acidosis. It has few psychiatric manifestations, but weakness and paresthesias may occur.

5. **Hypocalcemia** may result from hypoparathyroidism, lack of vitamin D, or malabsorption. The **etiologies** are presented in Table 25-5. Psychiatric symptoms depend on the susceptibility of the individual, the severity of the disorder, and the rate of fall in serum Ca^{2+}. Patients may have anxiety, agitation, depression, confusion, weakness, and memory disturbances. If mild, these symptoms may be confused with a primary affective or anxiety disorder (Table 25-6).

   a. **Diagnosis** is based on a low serum calcium in the presence of a normal albumin (which binds calcium in the blood). For each 1 gm/dl that the albumin is low, the serum calcium will be decreased by 0.8 mg/dl. Thus, if the measured Ca^{2+} is 6.2 but the albumin is only 2.0 (normal 4.0), the corrected serum calcium is 7.8. Measurement of ionized calcium is unaffected by serum proteins. Cardinal symptoms and signs include paresthesias, muscle cramping, and tetany (including carpopedal spasm and laryngospasm). Chvostek's and Trousseau's signs may be present. Other electrolytes and serum Mg^{2+} should also be measured, and if

Table 25-5. Causes of hypocalcemia

Cause	PTH	25-OHD_3
Hypoparathyroidism	Low	Normal
Postsurgical		
Infiltrative		
Familial		
Idiopathic		
Pseudohypoparathyroidism	High	Normal
Hypomagnesemia	Variable	Variable
Malabsorption	High	Low
Vitamin D deficiency	High	Low
Liver disease		
Drug-induced		
Phenobarbital		
Phenytoin		
Alcohol		
Glutethemide		
Renal disease		
Hereditary		
Acute hyperphosphatemia	Variable	Variable
Acute pancreatitis	High	Variable
Rhabdomyolysis	High	Variable
Drug-induced	Low	Variable
Mithramycin		
Calcitonin		
Diuretic agents		
EDTA		
Factitious	Normal	Normal
Hypoalbuminemia		
Alkalosis		

EDTA = ethylenediaminetetraacetic acid; 25-OHD_3 = 25-hydroxyvitamin D; PTH = parathyroid hormone.

Table 25-6. Symptoms and signs of hypocalcemia

Psychiatric	Nervousness, agitation, weakness, confusion, depression, memory loss
Neurologic	Headache, paresthesias (circumoral and acral), muscle stiffness and cramps, tetany, carpopedal spasm and laryngeal spasm
	Chvostek's sign: elicitation of facial twitch by tapping over facial nerve
	Trousseau's sign: elicitation of carpal spasm by inflation of blood pressure cuff above systolic blood pressure for 3 min
Gastrointestinal	Abdominal pain
Cardiovascular	Hypotension, decreased myocardial contractility, QT prolongation on electrocardiogram, ventricular arrhythmias

indicated, vitamin D and parathyroid hormone (PTH) levels should be checked.

b. **Treatment.** Acute hypocalcemic symptoms, such as laryngospasm, should be treated with IV calcium gluconate in consultation with a specialist. For patients with carpopedal spasm who are hyperventilating, rebreathing into a paper bag should be instituted to stop respiratory alkalosis (since alkalosis will further decrease the ionized calcium).

6. **Hypercalcemia** commonly produces neuropsychiatric symptoms. If the onset of hypercalcemia is gradual, these may be the only symptoms, commonly mimicking those of functional major depression. Delirium with paranoid ideation and other psychotic symptoms have been reported. With worsening hypercalcemia, confusion, stupor, coma, and death may ensue.

   a. **Etiologies** are presented in Table 25-7.

Table 25-7. Causes of hypercalcemia

Cause	PTH
Hyperparathyroidism	High
Hyperplasia	
Adenoma or adenocarcinoma	
Malignancy	Normal or low
Skeletal metastases	
Hematologic malignancies	
Humoral factors	
Granulomatous diseases, especially sarcoid	Low
Thyrotoxicosis	Normal or low
Adrenal insufficiency	Normal or low
Drug-induced	Normal or low
Lithium	
Thiazide diuretics	
Hypervitaminosis A or D	
Immobilization (with Paget's disease, fractures)	Low
Milk-alkali syndrome	Low
Familial hypocalciuric hypercalcemia	Normal

PTH = parathyroid hormone.

b. **Diagnosis** depends on elevation of the serum calcium that is not due to hyperalbuminemia (see sec. **5.a** above for correction factor). The symptoms and signs include mental status abnormalities, constipation, polyuria, polydipsia, renal concentrating abnormalities, nausea, and vomiting. The ECG reveals a shortened QT interval in many cases.

c. **Treatment** is a medical emergency when severe symptoms are present. Brisk infusion of normal saline should be begun, as the patient's status allows. Furosemide may be given to prevent fluid overload. Consultation with an internist or emergency physician should be obtained.

7. **Hypomagnesemia.** Magnesium levels are regulated by gastrointestinal absorption and renal excretion. Hypomagnesemia may lead to irritability, depression, apathy, and personality changes. In addition, hypomagnesemia predisposes to seizures, especially during alcohol withdrawal.

   a. **Etiology.** Hypomagnesemia results from poor nutritional status (e.g., in alcoholism or malabsorption). It may also occur because of renal wasting or prolonged diarrhea.

   b. **Diagnosis** is by low serum level. There is often concurrent hypocalcemia (Mg^{2+} is necessary for PTH release). Systemic symptoms are similar to those of hypocalcemia, and the two syndromes may be clinically indistinguishable. Symptoms include muscle weakness, muscle spasm (including carpopedal spasm), paresthesias, and seizures. Chvostek's sign may be present. Other laboratory values to check are calcium, albumin, phosphate, and electrolytes.

   c. **Treatment** is magnesium replacement. For seizures or tetany, magnesium should be repleted IV. Magnesium sulfate 2 gm can be given IV rapidly over 2 minutes in an emergency, no faster than 150 mg/minute. Further therapy will depend on blood levels of magnesium. Chronic replacement, if necessary, will depend on the underlying cause.

8. **Hypermagnesemia** occurs in the setting of renal failure. The neuropsychiatric symptoms include drowsiness, lethargy, and eventually coma and respiratory depression.

   a. **Diagnosis** is confirmed by a high serum magnesium level. Renal function should be evaluated. Systemic manifestations include muscular weakness; deep tendon reflexes are diminished or absent. Cardiac findings include bradycardia and heart block. Asystole may occur.

   b. **Emergency treatment.** Acute cardiac disturbances may require calcium gluconate. Therapy for renal failure, including emergency dialysis, should be undertaken if necessary.

D. Disturbances in acid-base balance

1. **Metabolic acidosis** is frequently encountered in the emergency room and may produce a wide variety of psychiatric manifestations. Metabolic acidoses may present with an anion gap that is either elevated (> 12) or normal (Tables 25-8 and 25-9). The symptoms will partly reflect the underlying disorder. Psychiatric symptoms include irritability and restlessness. As acidosis becomes more severe, cognitive impairment occurs, and acute confusional states and delirium may develop. Finally, seizures and coma may result.

   a. **Diagnosis** is made from the laboratory values of the electrolytes, arterial blood gases, osmolality, BUN, blood glucose, and serum ketones. The anion gap is equal to $Na - (Cl + HCO_3)$ and should equal 12 or less. Systemic symptoms will reflect the underlying illness.

   b. **Therapy** is directed at the underlying condition. Agitation and restlessness should not be treated with a sedative-hypnotic drug, which could

Table 25-8. Metabolic acidosis with an increased anion gap

- Ketoacidosis (AG> 25)[a]
  - Diabetic ketoacidosis
    - Symptoms: altered mental status, agitation, stupor
    - Findings: hyperglycemia, positive nitroprusside test
  - Alcoholic ketoacidosis
    - Symptoms: nausea, vomiting, withdrawal symptoms
    - Findings: hyperosmolar, blood sugar normal or slightly elevated
  - Starvation
    - Symptoms: altered mental status
- Hyperosmolar hyperglycemic nonketotic coma
  - Symptoms: change in mental status, coma
  - Findings: serum osmolality > 350, blood sugar > 650 mg, ketones negative
- Ingestions (AG> 25)
  - Paraldehyde
    - Symptoms: nausea, vomiting, paraldehyde odor, intoxication, stupor
  - Methanol
    - Symptoms: nausea, vomiting, mental status changes, seizures, coma
    - Findings: ocular changes, unexplained measured osmolality greater than the calculated osmolality[b]
  - Ethylene glycol
    - Symptoms: nausea, vomiting, mental status changes, seizures, coma
    - Findings: unexplained measured osmolality, urine positive for oxolate/hippurate crystals
  - Salicylates
    - Symptoms: nausea, vomiting, altered mental status, tinnitus, mania, confusion, lethargy, seizures, coma
    - Findings: high salicylate level, respiratory alkalosis, urine ferric chloride test positive
- Uremia (AG 15–20)
  - Symptoms: lethargy, depression, confusion, memory loss, delirium
  - Findings: BUN> 40; serum creatinine> 4; GFR< 20 ml/minute
- Lactic acidosis (AG> 25) (congestive heart failure, hypotension, shock, sepsis, hypoxia, hemorrhage)

AG = anion gap; BUN = blood urea nitrogen; GFR = glomerular filtration rate.

[a] $AG = Na^+ - (Cl^- + HCO_3^-)$; normal = ≤ 12.

[b] The measured osmolality should equal the calculated osmolality:

$$\text{Osmolality} = 2(Na^+ + K^+) + \frac{BUN}{2.8} + \frac{\text{glucose}}{18}.$$

Table 25-9. Metabolic acidosis with a normal anion gap

- Compensation for respiratory alkalosis
- Renal tubular acidosis
- Interstitial nephritis
- Diarrhea
- Ureterosigmoidostomy or obstructed ileal loop
- Drug-induced
  - Acetazolamide
  - Acidifying salts
  - Cholestyramine

decrease respiratory drive. Low doses of haloperidol are safe. Because the symptoms cannot be distinguished from hypoglycemia, as the initial response in the emergency setting blood samples should be drawn, followed by IV fluid replacement, thiamine 100 mg IV, and 50 ml of a 50% glucose solution. If the $pH < 7.0$, $NaHCO_3$, one or more ampules, should be given IV, pending transfer to an acute care facility.

2. **Respiratory acidosis,** or hypercapnia, results from alveolar hypoventilation. Psychiatric symptoms may herald a life-threatening decompensation. The earliest psychiatric symptoms are memory disturbance and impaired cognitive skills. With chronic hypercapnia, lethargy and somnolence are common. Eventually confusion, agitation, and delirium may occur. Hallucinosis may be part of the delirium. Ultimately, respiratory failure leads to seizures, coma, and death.

   a. **Etiologies** include overdoses with central nervous system depressant drugs, primary pulmonary disease, and central nervous system lesions.

   b. **Diagnosis.** Respiratory acidosis is suggested by the finding of a high PCO_2. Compensatory metabolic alkalosis may cause an elevation of the serum bicarbonate and normalize the pH. A chest x-ray, drug screen, and other workup are indicated.

   c. **Treatment** is directed at the underlying cause. Oxygen or administration of bicarbonate may result in a further decompensation by depressing central respiratory drive and therefore is contraindicated. The patient must be attended during transfer (if necessary) to an acute care hospital because intubation and assisted ventilation may prove necessary.

E. **Hypoxia,** or decreased oxygen content of the blood, results in decreased tissue oxygenation. Regardless of the etiology, it may lead to profound neuropsychiatric symptoms. These include fluctuating sensorium, agitation, confusion, delirium, seizures, and death. Chronic hypoxia may produce irritability, cognitive impairment, and personality changes. The sequelae of a hypoxic or anoxic episode (postanoxic encephalopathy) may clear slowly or may be permanent. Severe hypoxia of even a few minutes duration may result in defects in memory and cognition and personality changes. Anoxia or severe hypoxia lasting more than 3 minutes may result in global dementia, prolonged or irreversible coma, or death. Neurologic manifestations of postanoxic encephalopathy include tremors and myoclonus. If hypoxia is coupled with hypotension, watershed cerebral infarcts may occur.

1. **Diagnosis.** Hypoxia is diagnosed if the PO_2 is less than 60 mm Hg in arterial blood. The patient may appear cyanotic.

2. **Treatment** requires restoration of adequate oxygenation and then treatment of the underlying disorder. Arterial blood gases must be followed.

F. **Other metabolic disturbances**

1. **Hepatic encephalopathy** is a common feature of both acute and chronic liver insufficiency. A variety of neurologic and psychiatric changes accompany deterioration of liver function, possibly related to circulating toxins or altered cerebral metabolism. Early in the disorder psychiatric manifestations may dominate the clinical picture. Liver failure is often irreversible and carries a grim prognosis.

   a. **Psychiatric manifestations** generally depend on age, the chronicity of the disorder, and to some extent the premorbid personality of the patient.

      (1) **Acute hepatic encephalopathy** may present, especially in younger patients, with agitation, restlessness, euphoria, disinhibited behav-

iors, and psychosis. The patients may have a clinical appearance that is indistinguishable from intoxication or mania. Features of the mental status examination that suggest organicity may be subtle or absent early on.

(2) **Mild chronic encephalopathy** may present with features similar to acute encephalopathy or, alternatively, with a gradual deterioration in concentration, cognitive function, and personal care that can be misdiagnosed as depression or dementia. This presentation is often accompanied by somnolence and reversal of the normal diurnal sleep pattern.

(3) **Severe chronic encephalopathy** produces depressed mental status and dementia. Confusion may be prominent. Without successful treatment patients become progressively stuporous and comatose. It has been estimated that a third of patients with hepatic failure die in coma due to encephalopathy.

b. **Etiologies.** Encephalopathy occurs with progressive liver failure from any cause, but often there is a precipitant for the encephalopathy that is correctable if recognized early. Causes are given in Table 25-10.

c. **Diagnosis** is made on the basis of a history of liver disease and abnormal liver function tests. Often in end-stage cirrhosis the hepatocellular enzymes will be in the normal range, but failing hepatic synthetic function will be reflected by an elevated prothrombin time and a decreased serum albumin. The ammonia level is characteristically elevated when encephalopathy is present. The symptoms and signs of hepatic dysfunction may be subtle but are almost always present by the time encephalopathy occurs.

Table 25-10. Common precipitants of hepatic encephalopathy

Infection

Azotemia
- Dehydration
- Dietary protein load
- Gastrointestinal bleeding
- Transfusion of packed red cells

Constipation

Neurologic disease
- Subdural hematoma
- Wernicke-Korsakoff syndrome

Superimposed metabolic disorder
- Hyponatremia
- Hypoglycemia
- Acidosis
- Hypoxia
- Hypothyroidism

Superimposed surgery

Drug-induced
- Sedative-hypnotics
- Narcotic analgesics
- Tranquilizers
- Diuretic agents
- Anesthetic agents
- Paraldehyde

Progressive hepatocellular disease

(1) **Asterixis,** a transient repetitive loss of tone in voluntary motor movements, is an important but nonspecific sign. It also occurs in uremia, sedative overdose, hypoxia, and hyperviscosity syndromes.

(2) **Other neurologic signs** include ataxia, dysarthria, tremor, spasticity, hyperreflexia, and clonus. Seizures may occur.

(3) **Systemic signs** include spider angiomata, palmar erythema, and ecchymoses. In acute hepatic disease the liver is often enlarged, but in end-stage disease it may be small due to fibrosis and scarring. Signs of portal hypertension, such as splenomegaly or ascites, may be present. Gynecomastia, testicular atrophy, and loss of pubic hair also may occur.

d. **Therapy** for encephalopathy should commence in the emergency department. Thiamine, glucose, lactulose, antacids, and vitamin K should be given as indicated, as well as any specific therapies required by the etiologic disease process. Use of narcotics or sedative-hypnotics is to be avoided. If agitation and delirium are severe, physical restraint will be needed. Short-acting benzodiazepines, such as lorazepam, should be used in low doses if sedation is necessary. Start with lorazepam 1 mg IV for severe agitation. Wait as long as possible before repeating. **With all sedatives there is high risk of precipitating coma.**

2. **Acute pancreatitis** may present with delirium. Exacerbations of recurrent pancreatitis may be accompanied by hallucinations, cognitive impairment, and agitation. The preponderance of these patients use alcohol; thus the syndrome may easily be confused with that of alcohol withdrawal. In such patients, the presence of abdominal pain, steatorrhea, and diabetes suggests chronic or recurrent pancreatitis. The serum amylase is almost always, but not invariably, elevated. Calcification on an abdominal plain film may suggest chronic pancreatitis. The psychiatric symptoms usually resolve over 7–10 days with treatment of the pancreatitis. Haloperidol or lorazepam may be given parenterally to control dangerous behaviors (see Chap. 23, sec. **II.F** for regimens useful in the treatment of delirium).

3. **Uremia.** Renal failure from any cause may produce mental status changes. Clinically these are often indistinguishable from other metabolic encephalopathies. The major psychiatric features are lethargy, apathy, and depression. Abnormalities of concentration and memory may simulate depression or dementia. Acute delirium may occur. Occasionally patients present with irritability, agitation, and restlessness. If renal failure worsens, seizures, stupor, and coma may supervene.

a. **Diagnosis** is based on accompanying clinical findings and typical laboratory data. The BUN and creatinine will be significantly elevated. Neurologic signs may include myoclonus, fasciculations, and asterixis. Peripheral neuropathy and muscle cramps are common. The EEG shows diffuse slowing.

b. **Treatment** of uremia requires correction of metabolic disturbances such as acidosis, hyperkalemia, hyponatremia, and hyperphosphatemia. An acute deterioration of mental status is an indication for dialysis.

4. **Dialysis dementia** or encephalopathy is a potential complication of long-term hemodialysis. The diagnosis is suspected because of the clinical setting. The etiology is unclear, although aluminum toxicity has been implicated. Subtle changes in personality occur and may proceed to more florid symptoms including memory deficits, emotional lability, withdrawal, and irritability. Visual hallucinations may occur. Depression that is unresponsive to pharmacotherapy has been reported. Late in the course, speech disturbances, myoclonus, ataxia, and seizures occur. Treatment has been relatively unsuccessful; renal transplantation and dialysis with deionized water

have been tried. Benzodiazepines at low doses may be of symptomatic benefit for agitation.

G. **Vitamin deficiencies and malnutrition.** Severe malnutrition is associated with psychiatric and neurologic symptoms such as memory disturbance, listlessness, apathy, irritability, personality changes, and psychotic symptoms. Although uncommon in the United States, malnutrition should be suspected in alcohol-dependent individuals, the chronically mentally ill, and the elderly. In addition to the general symptoms of malnutrition, specific psychiatric symptoms may result from vitamin deficiencies. Diagnosis is made by specific blood levels.

1. **Thiamine deficiency** occurs most frequently in alcoholics. In its early stages it may result in malaise and headaches. Later, neuropathy, cardiomyopathy, and the Wernicke-Korsakoff syndrome may result (the Wernicke-Korsakoff syndrome is discussed in Chap. 31, sec. **VII**).

2. **Nicotinamide (niacin) deficiency, or pellagra.** In its early stages, pellagra may present principally with neuropsychiatric manifestations including weakness, irritability, and insomnia. Later symptoms include depression, confusion, memory loss, and psychotic symptoms. In its advanced state, the syndrome is characterized by dementia, diarrhea, and an erythematous dermatitis in a stocking and glove distribution. Rapid improvement should occur with administration of niacin 500 mg PO every day for 10 days followed by 100 mg PO every day.

3. **Pyridoxine (vitamin B_6) deficiency** is commonly iatrogenic, caused by administration of medications that affect metabolism of vitamins. Isoniazid and D-penicillamine are common offenders. Psychiatric symptoms include apathy, weakness, irritability, and mild memory impairment. Seizures may occur. Pyridoxine 50 to 100 mg PO every day should be given when antagonistic drugs are administered.

4. **Vitamin B_{12} deficiency** may be due to pernicious anemia or other causes, such as strict vegetarianism. Usually hematologic and neurologic abnormalities are present by the time psychiatric symptoms occur, but occasionally psychiatric symptoms are the sole manifestation of the vitamin deficiency. Thus, a B_{12} level should be obtained in any unexplained dementia or delirium. Psychiatric symptoms range from mild irritability and inattentiveness to dementia and psychosis. Typically, a megaloblastic anemia is present and is responsible for fatigue, pallor, and dizziness. Neurologic findings include peripheral neuropathy and dorsal column signs. These result in paresthesias, diminished position sense, anesthesia, and ataxia. Workup includes a B_{12} level, and if abnormal, a Schilling test. Therapy usually requires parenteral B_{12} replacement, such as 100 μg IM for 7 days followed by 1000 μg IM monthly. The degree of reversibility is quite variable.

H. **Industrial toxins** are infrequent causes of mental disturbance but have serious sequelae if not properly identified.

1. **Carbon monoxide poisoning** is responsible for many accidental deaths and suicides. It binds hemoglobin with high affinity, forming carboxyhemoglobin, with resulting tissue hypoxia. The earliest symptoms are headache, irritability, and confusion; occasionally nausea, vomiting, and visual symptoms occur. Delirium is reported. Finally central nervous system hypoxia may result in seizures, coma, and death. If the diagnosis is suspected, a carboxyhemoglobin level must be drawn. Arterial blood gases will not reflect the degree of hypoxia. Patients should be treated with 100% oxygen. If respiratory depression or seizures are present, intubation with assisted ventilation is required.

2. **Carbon disulfide** is used as a rubber solvent. Exposure may result in personality changes or an acute psychosis that can resemble mania, although the degree of confusion is usually suggestive of an organic etiology. Emo-

tional lability may occur, characterized by outbursts of anger and irritability, alternating with apathy and profound fatigue. Headache, insomnia, and nightmares are common. Cognitive deficits often occur. Other symptoms include nausea, conjunctivitis, and pulmonary disease. High doses may cause coma, respiratory depression, and death.

I. Heavy metal poisoning. In each of the following, blood tests and urine tests are needed to make the diagnoses.

1. **Lead poisoning** most commonly occurs in children who chew peeling lead paint. It is also an occupational hazard for deleaders and radiator workers. It can produce encephalopathy with lethargy and confusion. Delirium and symptoms resembling mania may occur with more severe poisoning. Eventually seizures and coma occur. Other symptoms include abdominal cramps, peripheral neuritis, ataxia, and mild anemia. Treatment involves limiting exposure and, in severe cases, the administration of chelating agents.

2. **Chronic arsenic poisoning** may present with memory impairment, apathy, fatigue, and mild confusion. Myalgias, paresthesias, dermatitis, and anorexia also occur. The diagnosis is made by analyzing the urine for arsenic. Treatment is with chelating agents.

3. **Mercury poisoning.** Acute intoxication causes severe gastrointestinal symptoms with vomiting and bloody diarrhea. Delayed effects include agitation, tremor, and renal and hepatic injury. Chronic mercury poisoning may present with subtle personality changes. Patients may become withdrawn, easily embarrassed, and timid. (This constellation of symptoms, called erythism, is most vividly depicted by the Mad Hatter in *Alice's Adventures in Wonderland*). Patients may also exhibit emotional lability and, later, fatigue and depression. Other symptoms include gingivitis with loosening of the teeth, peripheral neuritis, tremors, colitis, and renal damage. Treatment involves limiting exposure and use of chelating agents. Symptoms can improve dramatically.

4. **Chronic manganese poisoning** results from inhalation of industrial fumes. Early symptoms include headache, fatigue, lassitude, irritability, and arthralgias. If exposure continues, personality changes become prominent. Emotional lability may occur, with spells of laughter, tearfulness, impulsive behavior, and aggressive outbursts. Insomnia and hallucinosis are usually also present at this stage. Confusion may occur intermittently; acute psychosis may be seen. Prolonged manganese toxicity results in lesions of the basal ganglia, resulting in parkinsonian symptoms. Treatment is limited to termination of exposure. The psychiatric symptoms usually improve, but parkinsonian symptoms, if present, do not.

5. **Thallium poisoning** results from ingestion of thallium-containing pesticides. Initially headache, paresthesias, abdominal pain, vomiting, and diarrhea develop, but these clear after several days. Psychiatric symptoms occur later and include paranoia, delusions, depression, and suicidality. Cranial nerve palsies, choreiform movements, tremor, seizures, and delirium occur with severe poisoning. Alopecia occurs approximately 10 days after the exposure and may be an important clue to the diagnosis.

IV. Endocrinopathies

A. Hypothyroidism may be either primary (due to failure of the thyroid gland) or secondary (due to failure of the pituitary). Women are affected more frequently than men. Psychiatric symptoms commonly occur and may be the presenting symptoms. They include lethargy, difficulty in concentrating, and depressed affect. With severe hypothyroidism (myxedema) there are often personality changes, including a sarcastic "myxedema wit"; rarely, psychosis may occur, with paranoia and hallucinations. The psychosis may be difficult to distinguish from mania.

1. **Etiologies** are listed in Table 25-11.
2. **Diagnosis** is made on the basis of the clinical picture and is confirmed by laboratory tests. Symptoms may include weight gain, cold intolerance, dry skin, and constipation. Muscle weakness and peripheral neuropathy may occur. Examination may reveal a goiter (e.g., if Hashimoto's thyroiditis is present). The relaxation phase of the deep tendon reflexes may be prolonged. Brittle hair and scaling skin may be observed. With more severe disease, peripheral edema and bradycardia may be present. Myxedema coma rarely occurs, but presents with stupor, hypothermia, hypoventilation, hypotension, and hypoadrenalism. Laboratory diagnosis is based on the free thyroxine (T_4) index and thyroid stimulating hormone (TSH). The free T_4 index is calculated by multipling the total T_4 by the tri-iodothyronine resin uptake (T_3RU), which corrects for bound (and therefore inactive) T_4. The T_4 is uninterpretable without the T_3RU. In primary hypothyroidism, the TSH will rise and is the the most sensitive test.
3. **Treatment** requires thyroid hormone replacement. Until treatment is initiated, the clearance of many drugs, including most psychoactive drugs, may be impaired. Thus, smaller doses than usual should be used if psychotropic drugs are needed.

B. **Hyperthyroidism** is almost always primary, due to Graves' disease, hyperfunctioning thyroid nodules, or thyroiditis. Cases of hypersecretion of TSH by pituitary tumors are rare. Psychiatric manifestations may be prominent. The most common are anxiety, emotional lability, and poor concentration. Although some patients become restless, hyperactive, and euphoric, others, especially the elderly, may become withdrawn, depressed, and lethargic (so-called apathetic hyperthyroidism). In elderly patients this may be the only presenting feature. Rarely, delirium or organic psychoses resembling mania may occur.

1. **Etiology.** Symptoms are due to overproduction of T_4 and T_3. Rarely, T_3 toxicosis may occur with normal T_4 levels. The causes are listed in Table 25-12.
2. **Diagnosis.** Typical systemic symptoms include tachycardia, weight loss, heat intolerance, and diarrhea. Fine tremor, sweating, and proximal muscle

Table 25-11. Causes of hypothyroidism

Primary hypothyroidism (TSH high)
Hashimoto's thyroiditis
Subacute thyroiditis
Ablative
Surgery
Irradiation
Iodine 131
Drug-induced
Lithium
Iodides
Thionamides
Amiodarone
Congenital
Iodide deficiency
Biochemical defects (e.g., hypomagnesemia)
Secondary hypothyroidism (TSH low)
Pituitary disease
Hypothalamic disease

TSH = thyroid stimulating hormone.

Table 25-12. Causes of hyperthyroidism

Primary thyroid disease
- Graves' disease
- Subacute thyroiditis
- Toxic nodular adenoma
- Multinodular goiter
- Thyroid carcinoma (rarely)
- Exogenous iodine (jodbasedow)
- Hydatidiform mole
- Ovarian carcinoma (struma ovarii)
- Amiodarone
- Excessive exogenous thyroid replacement
  - Iatrogenic
  - Surreptitious self-administration (factitious hyperthyroidism)

Secondary disease
- Pituitary tumors (extremely rare)

weakness may also be seen. If Graves' disease is reponsible for the thyrotox icosis, ophthalmopathy and pretibial myxedema may also be present. Th thyroid examination may reveal a diffuse goiter, an isolated nodule, or multinodular goiter. Laboratory diagnosis is based on an elevated free T index, which is calculated by multiplying the T_4 and the T_3RU. A total T should also be ordered if the diagnosis is suspected but the T_4 is in th normal range. In questionable cases a thyrotropin-releasing hormone (TRH stimulation test is diagnostic.

3. **Treatment.** Propranolol 10–40 mg PO qid, or another beta blocker in appro priate doses, will help with peripheral symptoms such as tachycardia tremor, and often with anxiety. Anxiety unresponsive to a beta blocke should respond to a benzodiazepine. Definitive therapy aimed at the thyroi depends on the patient's diagnosis, age, and the severity of the illness Thyroid storm is a major medical emergency.

C. **Adrenocortical insufficiency** of any etiology results in symptoms because o cortisol deficiency. Early neuropsychiatric symptoms include lethargy, fatigue and depression. Untreated, delirium, organic psychosis, and finally stupor an coma may occur.

1. **Etiology.** The illness may be either primary (due to adrenal failure) o secondary (due to a lack of adrenocorticotropic hormone [ACTH] from th pituitary). Primary adrenal insufficiency may be due to autoimmune adre nal failure (Addison's disease) or destructive processes such as granuloma tous diseases or infections, especially tuberculosis. Secondary hypoadre nalism is due to pituitary destruction of any cause or, more rarely, t hypothalamic disease. Iatrogenic hypoadrenalism may be caused by with drawal of therapeutic doses of exogenous corticosteroids, which have sup pressed adrenal activity.

2. **Diagnosis** should be suspected if nausea, vomiting, anorexia, and hypoten sion occur that are otherwise unexplained. Primary hypoadrenalism ma also result in hyperpigmentation. Laboratory abnormalities often includ hyponatremia, hyperkalemia, and eosinophilia. A screening test can be per formed by drawing a baseline cortisol and then stimulating with adrenocor ticotropic hormone (Cortrosyn) 0.25 mg IV. A repeat cortisol is drawn hour later. The cortisol should rise by at least 8 μg/dl and have an absolut level of at least 18 μg/dl. If this proves abnormal, a more definitive worku is required.

3. **Treatment** requires steroid replacement. Hypotension may herald an addi

Table 25-13. Causes of Cushing's syndrome

Excess ACTH
Pituitary adenoma (Cushing's disease)
Ectopic ACTH by malignancies
Adrenocortical excess
Adrenal adenoma
Adrenal carcinoma
Exogenous corticosteroids
Factitious
Iatrogenic

ACTH = adrenocorticotropic hormone.

sonian crisis, a medical emergency requiring fluid resuscitation and high doses of parenteral glucocorticoids.

D. **Cushing's syndrome** may be endogenous or caused by administration of high doses of corticosteroids. It has prominent neuropsychiatric symptoms that may differ depending on the cause. In endogenous Cushing's syndrome the most common psychiatric symptoms are depression and insomnia, with sleep disturbance an almost universal feature. Other symptoms include emotional lability, agitation, difficulty in concentrating, and decreased energy. Suicidality is common, and in untreated cases suicide accounts for more than 10% of all mortality. Delirium or psychosis may occur. The psychosis may be symptomatically indistinguishable from functional affective psychoses. Exogenous Cushing's syndrome more commonly results in euphoria, mania, or delirium, although depression may occur.

1. **Etiologies** are listed in Table 25-13.
2. **Diagnosis** may be difficult. Specific systemic features include central obesity (with thin limbs), deep purple striae, proximal muscle weakness, osteoporosis, thin skin, and easy bruising. Hypertension and poor glucose tolerance are common. Hirsutism and plethora reflect an increase in adrenal androgen production. Laboratory diagnosis is often difficult. A screening dexamethasone suppression test may yield false-positive results in depressed or stressed patients.
3. **Treatment** depends on the etiology. Patients should be evaluated for depression and suicidality. Psychosis and delirium may be treated with neuroleptics and sedatives (see Chap. 23). If due to exogenous steroids, the dose should be held or decreased if possible.

E. **Hyperparathyroidism** results in the clinical manifestations of hypercalcemia (see sec. **III.C.6**). **Hypoparathyroidism** produces the syndrome of hypocalcemia (see sec. **III.C.5**).

F. **Hypopituitarism** results in symptoms referable to specific hormone deficiencies, such as hypothyroidism, hypoadrenalism, and hypogonadism.

G. **Pheochromocytoma** is a rare tumor of the adrenal medulla that secretes norepinephrine and epinephrine. Although the symptoms are classically paroxysmal in nature, many patients also have sustained symptoms of catecholamine excess. Psychiatric features are anxiety and apprehension. During a paroxysm there is often a feeling of impending doom that simulates a panic attack. Acute attacks may be precipitated by stress. Panic disorder may be misdiagnosed in these patients.

1. **Diagnosis** is suspected when there are paroxysms of hypertension, tremulousness, diaphoresis, headache, and tachycardia. Half of all patients have

sustained hypertension. Laboratory confirmation requires demonstration of elevated catecholamines or their metabolities in serum or urine. Typically there is elevation of vanillylmandelic acid (VMA) in a 24-hour urine specimen, but repeat testing may be necessary.

2. **Treatment** requires surgical removal of the tumor in a medically prepared patient.

V. Infectious causes of psychiatric symptoms

A. **Meningitis and encephalitis** may present with acute delirium or with more subtle psychiatric symptoms, such as confusion or irritability. The diagnosis is suggested by the presence of fever, leukocytosis, and, in the case of meningitis, signs of meningeal irritation, such as stiff neck. **In immunocompromised patients, any or all of these symptoms may be absent.**

1. **Diagnosis.** It is critical to make a rapid diagnosis of meningitis or treatable encephalitis because the success of therapy usually depends on its rapidity. If there is any sign of a central nervous system infection, a computed tomographic (CT) scan, if available, followed by a lumbar puncture must be performed. **Herpes simplex encephalitis** is the most common sporadically occurring encephalitis. Its presenting manifestations include change in personality or behavior, psychotic-like symptoms including hallucinations, and memory disturbance along with fever and leukocytosis on the blood count. Treated early with antiviral agents, herpes encephalitis may respond; the course is otherwise often devastating. Therefore, if suspected, a CT scan with contrast or a magnetic resonance imaging (MRI) scan should be performed, looking for typical signs of temporal involvement. If there is any question about the diagnosis, some clinicians advocate an emergency brain biopsy.

2. **Treatment** of meningitis or encephalitis depends on the presumed causative agent. Appropriate antibiotics or antiviral agents should be started promptly in the emergency department.

B. **Acquired immunodeficiency syndrome (AIDS).** At least two-thirds of patients with AIDS have neuropsychiatric symptoms. The human immunodeficiency virus (HIV), the causative agent of the disease, infects a population of lymphocytes, which leads to profound immunosuppression and susceptibility to central nervous system (CNS) and systemic infection. Additionally, HIV is neurotropic and produces primary infections of the nervous system.

1. In as many as one-third of AIDS patients, the presenting symptoms are neuropsychiatric and may precede any other signs of the disease. The most common CNS presentations are a subacute encephalitis and progressive dementia. Termed the AIDS dementia complex (ADC), this must be a diagnosis of exclusion because the patient with HIV is susceptible to multiple toxic, metabolic, and infectious processes. ADC is a progressive dementia that usually starts with impaired memory, concentration, or libido, but may progress to frank psychosis and mutism. Neurologic signs are legion; ataxia and incontinence are not uncommon in advanced cases. The degree of encephalopathy does not correlate with any specific neuropathologic finding.

2. In addition to the HIV-specific dementia, many other systemic processes in AIDS may compromise the CNS, the most common being infectious.

   a. A number of protozoan and fungal infections of the CNS, including *Toxoplasma gondii, Cryptococcus neoformans,* atypical mycobacteria, and *Mycobacterium tuberculosis* are more frequently seen in the immunocompromised patient with HIV infection than in any other population. CNS viral infections such as cytomegalovirus, herpes simplex, and herpes zoster may be seen. Papovaviruses may cause progressive multifocal leukoencephalopathy, a rare process that may cause blindesss, ataxia, and dementia. There may be increased incidence of bacterial CNS infection as well.

b. Cryptococcal meningitis is common in patients with AIDS. The majority of patients with cryptococcal meningitis will have fever and headache. Meningismus is rare (less than 20%). Many patients will have no specific symptom or sign of infection other than low-grade fever; the only positive finding might be the presence of cryptococcal antigen in the cerebrospinal fluid (CSF) or a positive CSF culture.

3. Neoplastic processes are common in patients with AIDS. Kaposi's sarcoma may metastasize to the brain. Primary CNS lymphoma and CNS involvement of aggressive systemic lymphoma are more common in patients with AIDS.

4. **Psychiatric morbidity and mortality** are high. People with AIDS carry a higher risk of suicide than matched samples of the general population. The suicide rate may be no higher than that for other chronically ill people such as those on renal dialysis. Depression may mimic the organic psychiatric symptoms caused by AIDS or ADC. There may be a heightened risk for atypical manic episodes. Severe anxiety states are particularly common when patients first learn of infection and later as debility progresses.

5. **Diagnosis**

a. The **diagnosis** should be suspected in anyone with mental symptoms who has a history of behavior that has made infection with HIV possible or who has any of the criteria for the diagnosis of AIDS. Additionally, any young person with a dementing illness should have an appropriate workup. The HIV antibody screen is sensitive and specific. Examination of the CSF is nonspecific but may show a monocytic pleocytosis, elevated protein, normal to low glucose, and oligoclonal IgG bands. HIV may be isolated from CSF. CT scan may show atrophy. Focal or diffusely increased signal by MRI is often evident in subcortical white matter.

b. Patients with **infectious or neoplastic** involvement of the CNS may present with fever, generalized or temporal lobe seizures, and focal findings, suggesting primary CNS pathology. However, patients may also present with subtle findings such as poor concentration, impaired memory, or personality changes. Weight loss and low-grade fever may raise the index of suspicion, and a careful neurologic examination may reveal a focal deficit. If fever is of recent onset, then infection is more likely than ADC to be the cause of psychiatric symptoms. The workup should include appropriate blood work, CT or MRI scan, lumbar puncture, and CSF and blood cultures.

6. **Treatment.** Zidovudine (ZDV), didanosine (DDI), and dideoxycytidine (DDC) are all approved by the Food and Drug Administration for certain patients with HIV infection. They all inhibit retroviral reverse transcriptase and thus replication. These antiretroviral agents are now being used both in combination and serially to combat the emergence of resistance. In some studies, the neurologic deficits in AIDS appear to respond to ZDV. The success of therapy for secondary infections and complications of AIDS will depend on the specific pathology. Prompt diagnosis, however, is critical to the outcome.

7. **Confidentiality.** The clinician is faced with several competing and urgent agendas. Balancing the issues of confidentiality, partner notification, and contact tracing is complicated, and there are no universally accepted guidelines.

a. **Patient confidentiality and the right to privacy** must be protected at the risk of eroding the hard-won trust that physicians and patients expect. Many states confer extraordinarily stringent protection of confidentiality about HIV testing and information. The law and the public perception of the HIV epidemic are evolving quickly on this front, and it is possible that current prohibitions against contact tracing will diminish. (We must remember that at the dawn of the epidemic, in the early 1980s, homosexuality was illegal in 24 states.)

b. The physician has a duty to prevent the spread of disease, and one might consider direct **partner notification** to be an appropriate method. The **"duty to warn"** may counterbalance the patient's right to privacy in the case of a potentially fatal infection. Relying on the patient voluntarily to inform those at risk can be of low efficacy. There is empiric evidence that people infected with HIV often fail to inform their contacts of the risk of infection.

c. To **protect the public health,** still a third approach has historically been adopted for sexually transmitted diseases: voluntary **contact tracing** both ensures confidentiality and permits public health departments to contact individuals at risk. Only about 10% of people who are notified through partner notification programs know that they might have been exposed prior to official notification. This shows that contact tracing actually provides new information for unsuspecting patients. Ethical positions and laws supporting the notion of **permitting the breech of confidentiality but not requiring it,** and of employing public health personnel in the task rather than the physician have been introduced.

d. There is no uniform standard from state to state on the physician's responsibility to inform in cases where sexual or needle-sharing partners of HIV-positive individuals may be ignorant of their risk. Similarly different professional groups have different stances on the duty to warn and on the degree to which a patient's confidentiality need be protected Physicians behave inconsistently. There are data showing that physicians will disclose names of infected patients to health departments at differing rates depending on the patient's sexual preference, gender, and race. Therefore, uniform practices should be encouraged.

e. We recommend urging patients to inform their sexual or needle-sharing partners voluntarily. How far individual physicians are willing to go to transmit that information is a highly variable matter determined by personal preference and local law. Some states have contact-tracing programs in place by which the patient can consent voluntarily to give public health personnel the names of people at risk of having been infected. This approach partly removes the physician from the loop, confers protective information to people at risk, but at the same time maintains a high level of confidentiality. Professional societies have issued guidelines, but these are inconsistent.

C. Lyme disease is an illness transmitted to humans by certain ticks infected with *Borrelia burgdorferi,* a spirochete. It is the most common tick-borne illness in the United States. Although the most common manifestations of the human infection is a rash called erythema chronicum migrans (ECM), untreated Lyme disease may progress to later stages, and neurologic abnormalities are characteristic of stage II Lyme disease. Stage II also includes cardiac conduction abnormalities. Stage III is characterized by chronic arthritis. These stages occur days to months after the rash. Stage II neurologic manifestations (neuroborreliosis) commonly include headache, stiff neck, and photophobia. Lyme encephalitis is characterized by emotional lability, ataxia, depressed mood, and sleep disturbance. Cranial nerve palsies, radiculoneuritis, or transverse myelitis may occur. CSF examination may show a mild lymphocytic pleocytosis with normal glucose and protein, making the syndrome difficult to distinguish from other aseptic meningitides. *B. burgdorferi* is cultured rarely from CSF.

1. **Diagnosis** is facilitated if the patient can give a history of exposure to the tick or of an episode of ECM, or if the patient has been in endemic areas during the likely season (summer to fall on the East Coast and spring to summer in the West). Usually tests of serum antibody will be positive. There will typically be circulating IgG to *B. burgdorferi* by the time neurologic abnormalities develop.

2. **Treatment** of neurologic Lyme disease requires intravenous penicillin or ceftriaxone (or other third-generation cephalosporin) for 10 days.

VI. **Collagen vascular diseases** may produce a wide variety of psychiatric symptoms. Occasionally the psychiatric symptoms precede other manifestations of the illness.

A. **Systemic lupus erythematosus (SLE)** is a multisystem disease of presumed autoimmune etiology. Women are affected more commonly than men. The clinical course is highly variable; neuropsychiatric symptoms occur in about half of patients. The psychiatric symptoms include mood disturbances, especially depression. Delirium or acute psychosis that is not due to steroid therapy may occur. Delusions and hallucinations are common during these episodes. The most common CNS symptoms are seizures.

1. **Diagnosis of SLE** is based on the presence of a variety of symptoms with laboratory confirmation. Symptoms include fever, weakness, photosensitivity, a butterfly rash, alopecia, arthralgias and arthritis, glomerulonephritis, pleural effusions, pleurisy, pericarditis, anemia, seizures, headaches, focal neurologic findings, anemia, thrombocytopenia, and psychiatric disturbances. The antinuclear antibody (ANA) is positive in 90% of patients. The LE test is less sensitive, but more specific. Antibodies to double-stranded DNA are found in 50% of patients. Recently it has been reported that autoantibodies to ribosomal P proteins may be found in a high proportion of patients with lupus psychosis.

2. **Treatment** is largely supportive. Corticosteroids are useful for some indications but their use for CNS disease is controversial. Delirium, pyschosis, and seizures should be treated as outlined elsewhere in the manual.

B. **Mixed connective tissue disease (MCTD)** is a rheumatologic disorder that occurs 80% of the time in females. Neuropsychiatric features are similar to those of SLE. Renal disease is less common. The ANA may be positive, often in a speckled pattern. Antibodies in RNase-sensitive extractable nuclear antigen are positive in 75% of patients. Treatment is supportive. Delirium or psychosis is treated as outlined in Chap. 23.

C. **Vasculitis**

1. **Necrotizing vasculitis** defines a group of inflammatory disorders of blood vessels. One of these, polyarteritis nodosa, affects small and medium-sized vessels of brain, liver, heart, skin, kidneys, and gastrointestinal tract. It is more common in men. Psychiatric symptoms vary greatly from mild cognitive impairment to confusion, hallucinosis, delirium, and coma. Psychiatric symptoms are rare in the absence of other systemic manifestations such as headache, weakness, fever, skin lesions, abdominal complaints, renal disease, pericarditis, and mononeuritis multiplex. The disease is rapidly fatal unless treated. The diagnosis is made by angiography and biopsy of affected vessels. Treatment with corticosteroids and immunosuppressive agents may result in dramatic improvement.

2. **Giant cell (or temporal) arteritis** is an inflammatory disorder of large and medium-sized vessels that occurs in older patients. Clinical symptoms include fever, fatigue, weight loss, and headaches. Listlessness and depression are common and may be the presenting complaints. If untreated, blindness may result within days. If clinically suspected, the diagnosis is supported by an elevated erythrocyte sedimentation rate (ESR). The diagnosis is con-

firmed by the finding of segmental arteritis on biopsy of affected vessels. Dramatic improvement occurs with corticosteroids.

3. **Polymyalgia rheumatica** is related to giant cell arteritis, but the arterial biopsy is negative. In addition to listlessness and depression, patients may complain of proximal muscle weakness. The ESR is elevated, and the disorder responds to low-dose corticosteroids.

VII. **Neoplastic diseases** are the second leading cause of death in the United States. It is estimated that 15–20% of patients with malignancies will have neuropsychiatric symptoms at some time in their course. Reactive depression is the most common of these, but other important syndromes occur. Intracranial neoplasms may cause psychiatric symptoms by local mass effects. Other psychiatric symptoms are produced, however, by remote effects of neoplasms.

A. **Paraneoplastic syndromes** are tumor effects not due to direct invasion or compression of organs by the tumor.

1. **Nonspecific systemic symptoms** are common and include lethargy, anorexia, cachexia, and occasionally fever.

2. **Ectopic hormone production** may result in hypercalcemia, Cushing's syndrome, SIADH, and other syndromes.

3. **Dementia** with memory impairment and confusion may occur rarely with most types of carcinoma. Symptoms are progressive. This paraneoplastic syndrome must be considered a diagnosis of exclusion. A CT scan and lumbar puncture should be performed to exclude cerebral metastases, carcinomatous meningitis, or infection. Possible metabolic causes should also be investigated thoroughly before this diagnosis is made.

4. **Limbic encephalitis** occurs in association with carcinoma, most commonly of the lung. This paraneoplastic syndrome may have an autoimmune component. It is characterized initially by affective symptoms, especially depression and severe anxiety. Hallucinosis and seizures often follow. Cognitive impairment is often prominent. Other possible causes of altered mental status should be investigated. The EEG is often abnormal, especially in the temporal leads. Treatment of the underlying tumor may bring about a remission. Acute psychosis and delirium should be treated as outlined in Chap. 23.

5. **Cancer of the pancreas** may result in depression that often precedes the discovery of the cancer by months. Weight loss and abdominal pain suggest the diagnosis but in the context of depression may be thought to be functional.

B. **Hyperviscosity** results from either plasma protein in high concentration or of large size (macroglobulinemia) or from polycythemia, which is an abnormally high number of circulating red cells. Symptoms that are common to both macroglobulinemia and polycythemia include confusion, fatigue, headache, visual disturbances, and transient focal neurologic findings. In both, coma may occur.

1. Increased serum viscosity is usually the result of **macroglobulinemia** and less commonly of multiple myeloma. A bleeding diathesis, retinopathy, and hypervolemia develop when the viscosity rises above 4. Urgent treatment is plasmapheresis. If this is not available, IV fluid administration may be used as a temporizing measure.

2. **Polycythemia** is an abnormally high red cell mass and number. Secondary polycythemia is marked by an elevated erythropoietin level. This may occur in chronic hypoxia or, rarely, secondary to certain neoplasms thought to secrete an erythropoietin-like factor. Primary polycythemia is marked by a low erythropoietin level and is termed polycythemia vera. This is a chronic, slowly progressive disease marked by increasing red cell mass. In either

case, the hematocrit is usually greater than 50 and thus confers an elevated blood viscosity. This in turn produces decreased cerebral perfusion and can cause thrombotic or hemorrhagic events. Bleeding is common. Symptoms include pruritus, urticaria, and splenomegaly with left upper quadrant pain. Rarely secondary gouty arthritis may occur from the increased turnover of red cells.

a. **Diagnosis.** A common cause of secondary polycythemia is hypoxemia and is easily identified by an arterial blood gas. Dehydration will result in a falsely elevated hematocrit. Diagnosis of polycythemia vera is made by the measurement of a red cell mass using ^{51}Cr-labeled red cells.

b. **Therapy** for polycythemia is directed initially toward reducing the hematocrit to the 40–45% range by serial phlebotomy. Therapy of polycythemia vera may include marrow suppression with chemotherapeutic and other agents.

C. **Carcinoid syndrome** results from the release of bioactive mediators, such as serotonin, histamine, bradykinin, and corticotropin from tumors containing argentaffin cells. The clinical syndrome reflects the mediators released by the particular tumor. Symptoms are often paroxysmal and may be mistaken for panic attacks or somatization. Typically there are vasomotor paroxysms characterized by flushing, tachycardia, watery diarrhea, abdominal cramping, and occasionally hypotension. The diagnosis is confirmed by the finding of elevated 24-hour urinary 5-hydroxyindoleacetic acid (5-HIAA). Therapy is directed at the underlying tumor.

VIII. **Cardiovascular disorders** such as hypotension, arrhythmias, and congestive failure may produce psychiatric symptoms. Arrhythmias can produce anxiety. Hypotension may produce agitation, confusion, seizures, and coma. Congestive failure may result in the psychiatric symptoms of hypoxia. Even angina or myocardial infarction may present with anxiety or, very rarely, delirium. The cardiovascular disorder that most often presents with psychiatric symptoms is hypertensive encephalopathy.

A. **Hypertensive encephalopathy** (usually with a diastolic blood pressure greater than 130 mm Hg) is a medical emergency. The patient may be confused and agitated or acutely delirious. Headaches, nausea, vomiting, seizures, stupor, and coma may all occur. Retinal hemorrhages, exudates, and papilledema are often present. Renal and cardiac symptoms are common. Treatment should take place in an intensive care unit.

B. **Stroke** may produce specific syndromes discussed in Chap. 26. Dominant hemisphere strokes commonly produce tricyclic-responsive depression.

IX. Psychiatric symptoms are commonly the result of **prescribed and over-the-counter medications.** The psychiatric effects of medications are given in Table 25-14 and their effects in causing **sexual dysfunction** are given in Table 25-15.

Table 25-14. Psychiatric symptoms caused by medications

Medication	Symptoms
Analgesics	
Acetaminophen	Delirium (overdose), drowsiness or toxic psychosis (in the elderly)
Pentazocine	Sleep disturbance, hallucinations, depression, paranoia, panic
Propoxyphene	Confusion, auditory hallucinations
Salicylates	Confusion, delirium, hallucinations (overdose), anxiety
Antiasthmatic drugs	
Aminophylline, theophylline	Anxiety, restlessness, insomnia, seizures
Beta-agonists	Anxiety, tremor, insomnia
Anticholinergics	All may produce anxiety, agitation, confusion, and delirium
Atropine	
Belladonna	
Antiparkinsonians	
Scopolamine	
Anticonvulsants	
Carbamazepine	Fatigue, drowsiness, ataxia, confusion
Clonazepam	Depression, confusion, insomnia, psychosis
Ethosuximide	Irritability, insomnia, aggressiveness, depression (may be suicidal), psychosis
Phenobarbital	Irritability, depression, hallucinations, dangerous withdrawal syndrome
Phenytoin	Anxiety, confusion
Primidone	Fatigue, irritability, depression
Valproic acid	Sleepiness, depression, agitation, psychosis
Antihistamines	All may produce drowsiness, restlessness, confusion, or agitation; delirium or psychosis
Anti-infective agents	
Antibiotics	
Aminoglycosides	Lethargy, depression, confusion or delirium (rarely)
Amphotericin	Delirium
Cephalosporins	Confusion, paranoia, hallucinations
Penicillins	Agitation, panic, confusion, hallucinations, myoclonus, seizures
Quinolones	Delirium, depression
Sulfonamides	Anxiety, depression, insomnia, hallucinations
Antimalarials	
Chloroquine	Agitation, nightmares, delirium
Antiparasitic drugs	
Thiabendazol	Hallucinations
Antituberculous drugs	
Cycloserine	Anxiety, depression, confusion, hallucinations, paranoia (mental effects common)
Isoniazid	Depression, agitation, delirium, paranoia, hallucinations
Rifampin	Drowsiness, poor concentration, confusion

Table 25-14 (continued)

Medication	Symptoms
Anti-infective agents (continued)	
Antiviral drugs	
Amantadine	Visual hallucinations, nightmares
Vidarabine	Hallucinations, confusion, psychosis
Acyclovir	Fatigue, insomnia, confusion, hallucinations
Zidovudine (ZDV)	Agitation, restlessness, insomnia
Antineoplastic drugs	
Methotrexate	Irritability, confusion, dementia
Procarbazine	Anxiety, agitation, mania
Vinblastine	Depression
Vincristine	Hallucinations
Cardiovascular drugs	
Antiarrhythmics	
Disopyramide	Panic reactions, depression, hallucinations
Procainamide	Drowsiness, paranoia, psychosis
Quinidine	Apprehension, agitation, confusion, delirium
Lidocaine	Confusion (seizures are common)
Antihypertensives	
Hydralazine	Depression, confusion, psychosis (rare)
Methyldopa	Drowsiness, depression, paranoia, hallucinations
Reserpine	Depression (common)
Others	
Beta blockers	Lassitude, fatigue, depression, confusion, hallucinations, nightmares
Digitalis	Apathy, weakness, hallucinations, paranoia, delirium, psychosis, euphoria
Calcium channel agents	Hallucinations, depression, irritability
Decongestants	
Ephedrine or pseudoephedrine	Agitation, insomnia, anxiety
Histamine H_2 antagonists (e.g., cimetidine)	Confusion, delirium, depression (especially in the elderly)
Nonsteroidal anti-inflammatory drugs	Paranoia, depression, confusion, anxiety
Other drugs	
Levodopa	Confusion, depression, mania, hyperactivity, psychosis
Bromocriptine	Depression, manic symptoms, hallucinations, paranoia, nightmares
Corticosteroids and anabolic steroids	Depression, euphoria, confusion, mania, psychosis
Cyclosporine	Delirium
Interferon alpha	Delirium, anxiety, depression

Table 25-15. Drugs associated with sexual dysfunction

Drug	Impotence	Decreased libido	Decrease in ejaculate	Delayed ejaculation	Decreased orgasm
Psychotropics					
Cyclic antidepressants					
Amitriptyline	x	x	x		
Amoxapine[a]	x	x	x		
Clomipramine	x	x		x	x
Desipramine[b]	x	x			
Doxepin[c]	x	x			
Imipramine	x	x		x	x
Maprotiline	x	x			
Nortriptyline	x	x			
Protriptyline	x	x			
Monoamine oxidase inhibitors					
Isocarboxazid	x			x	x
Pargyline			x		
Phenelzine	x		x	x	x
Tranylcypromine[d]	x				x
Fluoxetine				x	x
Trazodone[e]					
Neuroleptics					
Chlorpromazine[e]	x	x			
Chlorprothixene[e]			x	x	
Clozapine[e]					
Mesoridazine[e]			x		
Molindone[d]				x	
Perphenazine			x		
Piperacetazine			x		
Thioridazine[a,e]			x	x	
Thiothixene[f]					

Lithium	x	x			
Sedative-hypnotics					
Chlordiazepoxide		x			
Diazepam		x		x	
Psychostimulants					
Fenfluramine	x	x			
Drugs of abuse					
Amphetamine	x			x	x
Cocaine		x			x
Ethanol	x				
Heroin	x	x	x	x	x
Marijuana	x	x			
Nitrous oxide	x				
Phencyclidine	x	x	x		
Anticholinergic agents					
Homatropine methylbromide	x				
Meperizolate bromide	x				
Methantheline bromide	x				
Propantheline bromide	x				
Anticonvulsants					
Phenytoin		x			
Primidone		x			
Cardiovascular agents					
Antiarrhythmics					
Disopyramide	x				
Mexiletine	x	x			
Antihypertensives					
Beta-adrenergic blocking agents (propranolol and others)	x	x			
Clonidine	x				
Diuretic agents					
Acetazolamide	x	x			
Chlorthalidone	x	x			

Table 25-15 (continued)

Drug	Impotence	Decreased libido	Decrease in ejaculate	Delayed ejaculation	Decreased orgasm
Cardiovascular agents (continued)					
Diuretic agents					
Spironolactone	x	x			
Thiazide diuretics	x				
Guanethidine[a]	x		x		
Hydralazine	x				
Methyldopa	x	x	x	x	
Phenoxybenzamine			x		
Prazocin	x				
Reserprine	x	x	x		
Histamine H_2 blockers (cimetidine and others)	x	x			
Other medications					
Clofibrate	x	x			
Disulfiram	x				
Hormonal agents					
Estrogens		x			
Methandrostenolone		x			
Norethandrolone	x	x			
Norethindrone	x	x			
Progesterone	x	x			
Levodopa			x		
Muscle relaxants					
Baclofen	x		x		
Omeprazole[g]					

[a]Retrograde ejaculation.
[b]Difficult, painful ejaculation.
[c]Ejaculation dysfunction
[d]Spontaneous erection.
[e]Priapism.
[f]Spontaneous ejaculation.
[g]Painful nocturnal erections.

Selected Readings

Ayers, J. C., Olivero, J. J., and Fromer, J. P. Rapid correction of severe hyponatremia with intravenous hypertonic saline. *Am. J. Med.* 72:43, 1982.

Beck, L. H. (ed.). Body fluid and electrolyte disorders. *Med. Clin. North Am.* 65:251, 1981.

Brennan, T. A. AIDS and the limits of confidentiality. *J. Gen. Intern. Med.* 4:242, 1989.

Drugs that cause psychiatric symptoms. *Med. Lett. Drugs Ther.* 31:113, 1989.

Drugs that cause sexual dysfunction. *Med. Lett. Drugs Ther.* 34:73, 1992.

Hollander, H. Neurologic and psychiatric manifestations of HIV disease. *J. Gen. Intern. Med.* 6:324, 1991.

Hollander, H., and Levy, J. Neurologic abnormalities and recovery of human immunodeficiency virus from cerebrospinal fluid. *Ann. Intern. Med.* 106:692, 1987.

Lishman, W. A. *Organic Psychiatry* (2nd ed.). Oxford: Blackwell, 1986.

Navia, B., et al. The AIDS dementia complex: II. Neuropathology. *Ann. Neurol.* 19:525, 1987.

Navia, B. A., Jordan, B. D., and Price, R. W. The AIDS dementia complex: I. Clinical features. *Ann. Neurol.* 19:517, 1987.

Rubenstein, E., and Federman, D. D. (eds.). *Scientific American Medicine.* New York: Scientific American, 1992.

Schrier, R. W. *Renal and Electrolyte Disorders* (4th ed.) Boston: Little, Brown, 1992.

26 Neurologic Illness Mimicking Psychiatric Disorder

Steven E. Hyman

I. The scientific boundary between disorders traditionally considered neurologic ve sus psychiatric is becoming increasingly unclear. The traditional concept that ne rologic disorders are caused by anatomically based neuropathology, while psychia ric disorders are "functional"—that is, caused by transient chemical abnormaliti or by learning—is clearly inadequate. For example, there is now little doubt th schizophrenia is associated with anatomic abnormalities, at a minimum includin ventricular enlargement. Despite the uncertainty of the boundary and the existen of many disorders treated by both neurologists and psychiatrists (e.g., Alzheimer disease and temperolimbic epilepsy), in practice much of neurology can still b distinguished from psychiatry by neurology's focus on disorders with demonstrab neuropathology. Many disorders traditionally within the purview of neurology pr duce mental symptoms. It is critical to identify neurologic or medical causes psychiatric symptoms because the treatments are likely to differ considerably. is important not to be misled by prior psychiatric diagnoses or psychologic descri tors used by patients, but to evaluate each patient with an open mind.

A. **Evaluation.** To differentiate neurologic and psychiatric disorders it is useful consider certain differential diagnostic points:

1. **In the history,** onset of new mental symptoms late in life or acute ons from an asymptomatic baseline increases the likelihood that the proble is neurologic as do association of the symptoms with fever, headache, dizz ness, ataxia, nausea, vomiting, focal weakness or sensory loss, or reporte loss of consciousness. A prior history of head injuries with loss of consciou ness, seizures, or central nervous system (CNS) infections should also b ascertained.

2. **In the mental status examination** (see Chap. 1) abnormalities in level consciousness, memory, and higher cortical function are particularly like to reflect a medical or neurologic disorder. Although lack of orientation often said to reflect organicity, many patients with acute psychoses, esp cially mania, but also schizophreniform patients and patients with so-calle brief reactive psychosis, may not be oriented to time or place. Indeed, suc patients may appear quite perplexed at the height of their symptoms. Ce tain other findings on the mental status examination may be deceptive first but must be interpreted correctly if the right diagnosis is to be reache

   a. **Lack of normal inflection** during speech may initially suggest depre sion to the examiner but could also result from organic processes inclu ing drug-induced or idiopathic parkinsonism or dysprosody from a foc nondominant hemisphere lesion. It is important to entertain all of thes possibilities and to look for associated findings that may confirm one these diagnoses.

   b. Isolated vascular lesions of **Wernicke's area** may occur, resulting i fluent nonsensical speech laced with neologisms but not accompanied b any other focal neurologic findings. In addition to their aphasia suc patients occasionally appear euphoric or alternatively paranoid an combative. Unless the physician systematically examines languag function, noting lack of comprehension, paraphasic errors (word substitutions), and impaired repetition, the patient might be incorrectly diagnosed as having a psychotic disorder or delirium (see Chap. 1). Potentially disastrous errors of this sort are entirely avoidable with a careful mental status examination.

c. **Apathy** with delayed responses to questions and commands, a paucity of spontaneous speech, and blunted affect are consistent with depression or schizophrenia but also with frontal lobe syndromes, and idiopathic or neuroleptic-induced parkinsonism. It is important to look for features that help differentiate these states—for example, guilt, poor self-esteem, or hopelessness in the case of the depressive; perseveration and other findings (see sec. **II**) in the frontal lobe patient; and masked facies and cogwheel rigidity for drug-induced or idiopathic parkinsonism.

3. **In the physical examination,** abnormalities of vital signs or other physical findings may suggest an organic disorder. Fever should always raise the question of central nervous system infection. Focal neurologic deficits are particularly important, although a normal neurologic examination is still consistent with an organic brain syndrome. The neurologic examination should include cranial nerve, motor, sensory, and cerebellar testing, and testing of reflexes including frontal release signs (such as grasp, snout, and suck). In addition, if the patient apears to have abnormal involuntary movements, the Abnormal Involuntary Movements (AIMS) test (Fig. 26-1) should be performed to document them so that the effects of medication on them can be judged and their progression over time followed. If the patient is too agitated to comply with full neurologic testing, it should be accomplished as soon as the patient's condition permits.

   a. When a left hemisphere lesion is suspected, testing of language should be particularly careful and tests of praxis, left-right discrimination, and finger identification should be included.

   b. When a right hemisphere lesion is suspected, constructional ability and the possibility of hemisensory neglect should be tested carefully.

B. **If a neurologic disorder is suspected,** it is important to focus on aspects of the history that will be informative and will allow the physician to generate diagnostic hypotheses—for example, the nature and acuteness of onset of symptoms (vascular disease often presents with acute onset of the maximal deficit, whereas tumors often progress insidiously, but relentlessly). It is important also to differentiate new deficits from old ones. **In obtaining neurologic consultation** it is best to present specific hypotheses and to discuss with the neurologist which symptoms and other aspects of the case are not typical of a primary psychiatric disorder. This approach is more likely to yield a successful interaction among colleagues than global requests to "rule out organicity."

C. **Diagnostic tests.** As with any patient who has an acute alteration of mental status, certain laboratory tests are necessary (see Chap. 25), including a complete blood count, electrolytes, calcium, glucose, blood urea nitrogen (BUN), creatinine, and, if indicated, a toxic screen. If there are focal findings on the neurologic examination or suggestions of focal lesions on the mental status examination, a computed tomographic (CT) scan is indicated. Most physicians also prefer to obtain a CT scan prior to performing a lumbar puncture unless it would entail undue delay. **A lumbar puncture is indicated if there is any possibility of CNS infection.** Finally, an electroencephalogram (EEG) may be helpful in the diagnosis of epilepsy, although it frequently fails to detect an abnormality in complex partial seizures due to deep limbic foci.

II. **Frontal lobe disorders.** Patients with bilateral frontal lobe disease will often have personality changes without any obvious cognitive, motor, or sensory deficits. Thus the diagnosis may be quite difficult to make.

Either before or after completing the examination procedure, observe the patient unobtrusively at rest, e.g., in the waiting room.

The chair to be used in this examination should be hard and firm without arms.

Ask the patient whether there is anything in his or her mouth, and if there is to remove it.

Ask the patient about the condition of his or her teeth. Ask the patient if he or she wears dentures and to what extent they are currently bothering him or her.

Rate movements on a scale of 0–4: 0 (none), 1 (minimal), 2 (mild), 3 (moderate), and 4 (severe).

( ) Have patient sit in chair with hands on knees, legs slightly apart, and feet flat on floor. Look at entire body for movements while in this position.

( ) Ask patient to sit with hands hanging unsupported—if male, between legs, if female and wearing a dress, hanging over knees. Observe hands and other body areas.

( ) Ask patient to open mouth. Observe tongue at rest within mouth. Do twice.

( ) Ask patient to protrude tongue. Observe abnormalities of tongue movement. Do twice.

( ) Ask the patient to tap thumb, with each finger, as rapidly as possible for 10–15 seconds, separately with right hand, then left. Observe facial and leg movements.

( ) Flex and extend patient's left and right arms, one at a time.

( ) Ask patient to stand up. Observe in profile. Observe all body areas again, including hips.

( ) Ask patient to extend both arms in front with palms down. Observe trunk, legs, and mouth.

( ) Have patient walk a few paces, turn, and walk back to chair. Observe hands and gait. Do twice.

Figure 26-1. Abnormal Involuntary Movements (AIMS) test.

A. Clinical manifestations. The patients often have impairments in complex traits, such as loss of interest in the environment, apathetic blunting of intellect and emotion, and loss of foresight, planning, and social drive. Some patients lose their mental flexibility; they have a tendency to perseveration and to become concrete and stimulus-bound. Others may show loss of normal socialization with resulting disinhibition of emotions and intellect. The generalization is often made that patients with lesions of the basal orbital regions are likely to be euphoric, disinhibited, and jocular (but in a brittle manner that easily deteriorates into irritability), whereas patients with dorsal-lateral lesions are most often apathetic, with deficits of mental flexibility. Clinically, patients are usually more complex than this dichotomy allows, with their actual symptoms depending on the exact size, location, and bilaterality of the lesion.

B. Causes of frontal lobe syndromes are listed in Table 26-1.

C. Examination of patients with frontal damage may reveal deficits in concentration (as tested by digit span), but memory is preserved. Because of their tendency for perseveration (lack of mental flexibility) they may perform poorly on certain tests, such as the visual pattern completion test (Fig. 26-2). Normal individuals should be able to complete this task without difficulty. A similar test, developed by Luria, is the following: The patient is told to hit the top of a table, first with his or her fist, then with the palm open, and then with the side

Table 26.1 Causes of frontal lobe syndromes

Tumors (gliomas, subfrontal meningiomas, pituitary adenomas)
Head injury
Normal pressure hydrocephalus
Stroke
Surgery
Multiple sclerosis
Dementias (Pick's disease; late stages of Alzheimer's disease)

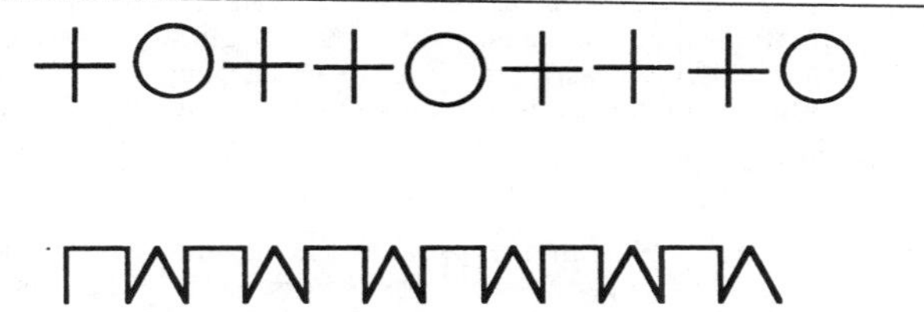

Figure 26-2. Visual pattern completion test. The patient should be asked to reproduce and complete each figure. Loss of sequence or perseveration suggests frontal lobe problems.

of the hand. The physician should demonstrate once. Patients with frontal lobe damage often fail within 10–20 seconds. With extensive lesions frontal release of grasp reflexes, incontinence, akinesia, and mutism may be seen. With the largest lesions, motor deficits may also be in evidence. Given the possible causes, it is obviously important to differentiate frontal lesions from nonorganic disorders.

III. Psychiatric symptoms accompanied by a movement disorder

A. Because of neuroleptic treatment, many psychiatric patients have symptoms of an extrapyramidal movement disorder, either drug-induced parkinsonism or tardive dyskinesia (described in Chap. 24, sec. **II.D.2** and **F**, respectively). Because psychiatrists have become inured to seeing mentally ill patients with abnormal movements, it is common to pay inadequate attention to them. This may result in suboptimal treatment or in missing neurologic disorders altogether. It is critical that any patient with a movement disorder be asked in detail both about the nature, onset, and duration of his or her motor symptoms and about prior neuroleptic usage. If the patient manifests abnormal involuntary movements, as AIMS scale (see Fig. 26-1) should be recorded.

B. Specific disorders

1. **Parkinsonism.** Patients who appear parkinsonian (e.g., with bradykinesia, rigidity, tremor, festinating gait, and masked facies) should be carefully questioned about prior neuroleptic exposure. If it cannot be established that the symptoms were drug-induced, the patient should be observed for at least several days neuroleptic-free. If sedation is needed, a short-acting benzodiazepine can be used.

2. **Huntington's disease** is an autosomal dominant genetic disorder that produces movement disorder, psychiatric symptoms, and dementia. Early in the course psychiatric symptoms may be more prominent than movement disorder and may mimic mania, depression, or schizophrenia. Rigidity (espe-

cially in juvenile cases) or choreoathetoid movements and a positive family history usually make the diagnosis fairly obvious. Treatment of the psychiatric problem is symptomatic, based on the treatment of the most similar psychiatric disorder (e.g., tricyclics for depression). Neuroleptics may suppress some of the abnormal movements.

3. **Wilson's disease** (hepatolenticular degeneration) is a rare autosomal recessive disorder of copper metabolism that results in deposition of copper in liver, brain, cornea, and kidneys. It often presents in adolescence or early adulthood with neuropsychiatric or hepatic symptoms. Despite its rarity, it is discussed here because it is treatable if discovered early.

   a. **The psychiatric symptoms** often mimic schizophrenia or an affective disorder. The hepatic abnormalities may be insidious. Thus the diagnosis is rarely thought of and often missed. The failure to diagnose this treatable illness is catastrophic, but some authorities estimate that more than half of all cases are missed. A broad range of psychiatric symptoms occur, including delusions, hallucinations, and affective abnormalities.

   b. **The diagnosis** may be suspected because of an atypical psychiatric course, or because of the presence of other manifestations of the disease:

      (1) **Kayser-Fleischer rings** are pathognomonic for the disease. They appear as golden brown deposits forming crescents around the cornea. Early in the disease a slit-lamp examination may be required. Kayser-Fleischer rings are almost invariably present by the time neuropsychiatric manifestations occur.

      (2) **Neurologic findings** include resting or intention tremor, dysarthria, choreoathetoid movements, rigidity, clumsiness, and gait disturbance. Unfortunately, these may mimic the extrapyramidal effects of neuroleptic drugs; thus, once neuroleptics are begun Wilson's disease may no longer be suspected. It is therefore imperative that patients with psychosis and any of these neurologic findings have a slit-lamp examination and laboratory tests for Wilson's disease before a psychiatric diagnosis is made and neuroleptic treatment begun.

      (3) **Hepatic involvement** may take several forms. Acute hepatitis, simulating viral hepatitis, may occur and even become fulminant. Alternatively, findings more like that of chronic active hepatitis may be present.

      (4) **Laboratory tests** show a decreased serum ceruloplasmin (less than 20 mg/dl), increased urinary excretion of copper (more than 100 μg/24 hours), and increased copper deposition in the liver on biopsy.

   c. **Therapy** is most likely to be successful if started early. Early treatment of asymptomatic patients may prevent the onset of symptoms. Thus all family members must be screened if a patient is identified. Penicillamine, a copper chelator, is the drug of choice.

IV. **Complex partial epilepsy,** also called temporolimbic epilepsy, may cause acute psychiatric symptoms under a variety of circumstances. Those that could masquerade as symptoms of a primary psychiatric disorder in the emergency department setting include confusion, psychosis, and, rarely, violence. The diagnosis and treatment of complex partial epilepsy are fully discussed in Chap. 27.

A. The **ictus** of a complex partial seizure may present as a dissociative state. If there are associated premonitory hallucinations, sensory distortions, or other aurae, or if there are motor automatisms during the ictus, the diagnosis is usually clear. The diagnosis may be difficult, however, if these are absent. Often the episodic pattern of symptoms is the best clue that they may be due to epilepsy, but partial complex epilepsy should be considered in the differential diagnosis of all dissociative states. Rarely complex partial status epilepticus occurs, in which patients have prolonged dissociative states or unresponsiveness mimicking catatonia. In the **postictal phase** patients may be confused or belligerent or may exhibit bizarre behavior. If the ictus is brief or goes unnoticed, these symptoms may occasionally be the only manifestation of the problem.

B. Psychosis

1. Although this issue is controversial, it appears that brief psychotic episodes can occur in the absence of confusion as a subictal or interictal manifestation of both temporal lobe and generalized epilepsy. The diagnosis should be considered whenever episodic psychotic symptoms occur in a pattern not typical for primary psychiatric disorders. The relationship between the psychotic symptoms and EEG differs from case to case, suggesting a heterogeneous etiology of the psychotic symptoms (Ramani and Gumnit, 1982). If the psychosis occurs as a subictal or ictal symptom, it might respond to an anticonvulsant alone (i.e., without addition of a neuroleptic). In other cases neuroleptics will be necessary. Unfortunately, good treatment studies of such patients are lacking.

2. Many studies have found an increased incidence of chronic psychotic symptoms in patients with partial complex seizures, although these findings have been disputed. Patients with chronic psychotic symptoms in the context of epilepsy typically require neuroleptic treatment in addition to anticonvulsant treatment. Because anticonvulsants, including carbamazepine (Tegretol), may increase the metabolism of antipsychotics, higher than usual doses of the antipsychotic may be needed in some patients.

C. Violence. Violence is uncommon during complex partial seizures, and when it occurs, it is typically poorly directed—that is, patients generally do not carry out apparently planned acts of violence during seizures. When violence does occur in such patients it may be an interictal manifestation associated with the deepening of emotions (Devinsky and Bear, 1984) that may form part of the interictal syndrome. Since it is not usually ictal, violence may not respond, at least in the short term, to anticonvulsants, although a trial of carbamazepine would be worthwhile.

V. Transient global amnesia (TGA) is characterized by abrupt onset of bewilderment with inability to form new memories. TGA lasts for several hours up to two days, with lasting amnesia for the period and occasionally retrograde amnesia. There is no associated loss of consciousness or higher cognitive functions; by definition there are no associated seizures or motor abnormalities. TGA is most common after the age of 50. About a quarter of patients have recurrent episodes but do not appear to be at higher risk for subsequent strokes or dementia than unaffected individuals. There is no treatment necessary. A recent study found that a third of cases followed exertion, intense emotion, or sexual intercourse. Unlike complex partial seizures, there is no disruption of other higher cognitive functions and no abnormality (such as a confusional state) detectable once the attack ends. Unlike dissociative and fugue states, personal identification is always intact in TGA.

VI. Another neurologic disorder that can masquerade as a primary psychiatric disorder is **acute intermittent porphyria (AIP).** This is an inherited (autosomal dominant) disorder of heme biosynthesis characterized by recurrent episodes of neurologic and psychiatric disturbances and abdominal pain. The disease often presents in the second to fourth decades of life and is more common in women. The manifestations can be extremely variable. Acute attacks last from days to weeks and typically begin with abdominal pain. Nausea, vomiting, and constipation may occur. Fever and leukocytosis may also be found; thus the presentation can mimic a surgical abdomen. Psychiatric symptoms occur in the majority of cases. The patients may become acutely depressed or restless and agitated. Visual hallucinations and paranoia may occur. When psychiatric symptoms predominate, an acute functional psychosis may be misdiagnosed.

A. Diagnosis is made on the basis of family history, laboratory tests, and the

Table 26-2. Drug use in acute intermittent porphyria

Known to be safe	Known to be unsafe
Antihistamines	Alcohol
Atropine	Barbiturates
Beta-adrenergic blocking agents	Griseofulvin
Chloral hydrate	Imipramine
Chlorpromazine	Phenytoin
Digoxin	Steroids
Diphenhydramine	Sulfonamides
Ether	Tolbutamide
Nitrofurantoin	
Guanethidine	
Neostigmine	
Nitrous oxide	
Opiates	
Oxazepam	
Penicillins	
Promethazine	
Reserpine	
Salicylates	
Streptomycin	
Succinylcholine	
Tetracyclines	

overall clinical picture. In addition to abdominal symptoms, tachycardia and diaphoresis may occur. Neurologic symptoms include weakness and peripheral neuropathy. Paralysis may occur and may even involve respiratory muscles. Reflexes may be diminished or absent. Rarely, seizures or coma ensue.

B. Laboratory findings confirm the diagnosis. During acute attacks delta-aminolevulinic acid and porphobilinogen are increased in the urine. Certain drugs can provoke an attack and should be avoided (Table 26-2). Fasting, dehydration, stress, and high estrogen levels (as in third trimester pregnancy) may also precipitate attacks.

C. Treatment of acute attacks involves hydration, supportive measures, and a high carbohydrate diet (which suppresses delta-aminolevulinic acid formation in the liver). Pain may be effectively controlled with chlorpromazine 50 mg IM q4h prn. Psychosis may be treated with neuroleptic drugs as needed. Depressed patients must be screened for suicidality. Electroconvulsive therapy (ECT) is probably the best treatment for severe depression because imipramine, and probably other tricyclics, may worsen the underlying disorder. Diazepam should be used for seizures, as phenytoin and barbiturates are contraindicated.

Selected Readings

Delgado-Escueta, A. V., et al. The nature of aggression during epileptic seizures. *N. Engl. J. Med.* 305:711, 1981.

Dening, T. R., and Berrios, G. E. Wilson's disease: Psychiatric symptoms in 195 cases. *Arch. Gen. Psychiatry* 46:1126, 1989.

Devinsky, O., and Bear, D. Varieties of aggressive behavior in temporal lobe epilepsy. *Am. J. Psychiatry* 141:651, 1984.

McKenna, P. J., Kane,. J. M., and Parrish, K. Psychotic syndromes in epilepsy. *Am. J. Psychiatry* 142:895, 1985.

Mesulam, M. M. *Principles of Behavioral Neurology*. Philadelphia: Davis, 1985.

Miller, V., et al. Transient global amnesia: Clinical characteristics and prognosis. *Neurology* 37:733, 1987.

Ramani, V., and Gumnit, R. J. Intensive monitoring of interictal psychosis in epilepsy. *Ann. Neurol.* 11:613, 1982.

Zubenko, G. S. Progression of illness in the differential diagnosis of primary dementia. *Am. J. Psychiatry* 147:435, 1990.

27 Seizures

M. Elizabeth Ross

I. The recognition and management of epilepsy in its many forms are two of the major areas of overlap between neurology and psychiatry. Epilepsy is common, estimated to occur in 6–34 per 1000 people.

A. The psychiatrist can expect to encounter problems in the acute care of patients with seizures in a variety of clinical settings including:

1. Withdrawal from alcohol or other central nervous system (CNS) depressants (including prescribed agents, e.g., short-acting benzodiazepines).

2. Acute abuse of epileptogenic drugs—for example, cocaine.

3. Seizures caused by psychotropic agents that lower the seizure threshold—for example, tricyclic and other cyclic antidepressants, low-potency neuroleptics.

4. Seizures caused by metabolic abnormalities (e.g., hyponatremia in polydipsia, primary or induced hypoglycemia).

5. Psychiatric patients who also have epilepsy.

6. Patients whose psychiatric symptoms could be due to epilepsy (see Chap. 26).

B. This chapter deals primarily with the most pressing clinical problem, the acute management of grand mal seizures and status epilepticus. Also discussed are diagnostic considerations leading to the correct identification and appropriate treatment of epilepsy in the practice of acute care psychiatry. Table 27-1 lists the major categories of seizures, adapted from the Commission on Classification and Terminology of the International League Against Epilepsy.

II. **Generalized seizures.** Seizures in which the electroencephalogram (EEG) is diffusely abnormal, without localization to a specific brain region, are classified as generalized seizures. Clinically, there are no signs or symptoms implicating a specific area of the brain from which the epileptic discharges emanate. Generalized seizures always produce loss or impairment of consciousness.

A. **Tonic-clonic (grand mal) seizures.** Generalized tonic-clonic seizures are the most common form of epilepsy encountered in the emergency department. Although only 10% of epileptic patients have tonic-clonic seizures as their sole manifestation, grand mal episodes occur secondarily in more than half of patients with other forms of seizure.

1. **Clinical features.** Typically, grand mal seizures begin with a **tonic phase** in which the patient stiffens, becomes rigid, and rapidly loses consciousness. There may be arching of the back or opisthotonus with deviation of the eyes upward or to either side followed by head turning in the same direction. In some cases the seizure may begin with a cry due to contraction of thoracoabdominal muscles. The respiratory rate may become irregular and the patient may become cyanotic. Pupils nearly always dilate at the onset of the

Table 27-1. Classification of seizure types

I. Generalized seizures
  A. Tonic-clonic (grand mal) seizures
    1. Primary—idiopathic or familial
    2. Secondary to a definable structural lesion (e.g., tumor, arteriovenous malformation, old infarct)
    3. Secondary to infection (e.g., meningoencephalitis, abscess)
    4. Secondary to drug intoxication (e.g., cocaine)
    5. Secondary to metabolic imbalance (e.g., hypoglycemia, hyponatremia)
    6. Grand mal status epilepticus
  B. Absence seizures
    1. Typical absence—electroencephalogram (EEG) with 3 per second spike and wave, impairment of consciousness only
    2. Complex or variant absence—with one or more additional components of myoclonus, atonic episodes (drop attacks), automatisms, autonomic phenomena (e.g., enuresis), or tonic episodes.
  C. Myoclonic seizures
    1. Infantile spasms (West's disease: myoclonic seizures in children, Lennox-Gastaut), EEG with "hypsarrhythmia"
    2. Adult generalized myoclonic seizures (following cerebral anoxia or familial)
  D. Atonic seizures—isolated or part of an absence seizure
  E. Tonic seizures—uncommon in adults
  F. Clonic seizures—uncommon in adults
II. Partial (focal) seizures
  A. Simple partial seizures—consciousness not impaired
    1. Motor: focal, jacksonian (focal, with a march), versive (usually contraversive), postural, phonatory (with vocalization or speech arrest)
    2. Sensory: somatosensory, visual, auditory, olfactory, gustatory, vertiginous
    3. Autonomic
    4. Psychic (e.g., déjà vu, jamais vu)
  B. Complex partial seizures—consciousness impaired; encompasses temporal lobe or psychomotor seizures
    1. Simple partial onset followed by impairment of consciousness
    2. Impairment of consciousness at onset, with or without automatisms
  C. Partial seizures evolving into secondarily generalized tonic-clonic seizures

tonic phase. In the **clonic phase** the limbs make a rhythmic jerking movement. This usually begins as a small twitch that increases in amplitude and force with time. Often rhythmic eye blinking and jaw movements that may result in tongue biting also occur. Bladder or bowel incontinence commonly occurs during the ictus. The duration of the **postictal phase** is often roughly proportional to the duration of the seizure. In this phase the patient is typically disoriented, confused, and somnolent to some degree. This phase may last from 20 minutes to several hours. After prolonged seizure or status epilepticus, however, the patient may be obtunded, requiring 24–48 hours to become fully alert and oriented. Complaint of headache, fatigue, and muscle soreness is common during the postictal phase. One should consider the possibility of pseudoseizure if the patient recovers from a grand mal episode with no postictal symptoms (see Chap. 28, sec. **IV.C.5**).

2. **Treatment.** The emergency management of a grand mal seizure depends on whether the patient is still actively seizing or has recently seized, but has stopped. If the patient is actively seizing, the objective is to stop the seizure in progress. If the patient has already stopped, the objective is to prevent further seizures. Accomplishment of these objectives requires swift determination of the cause of the ictus. Choice of anticonvulsant therapy is determined by practical concerns of efficacy, time required to achieve therapeutic blood levels, and duration of action. A broader range of anticonvulsants can be considered when circumstances permit a more leisurely attainment of therapeutic levels. In such cases drug choice depends on selection appropriate to seizure type, balanced by consideration of the relative toxicity of available medications (see sec. **IV**).

   a. **Tonic-clonic seizure in progress**

      (1) **Ensure adequate oxygenation.** The patient should be positioned to avoid injury during the ictus. An adequate airway must be maintained. This may be accomplished using a plastic oral airway only if it can be inserted without trauma. The lay practice of inserting a pen or spoon in the mouth can break teeth during masseteric contraction and tooth fragments can be aspirated. Similarly, a wooden tongue depressor may break and splinter. Oxygen should be administered via nasal cannula or face mask. Intubation will not be necessary for most grand mal seizures; however, this option should be exercised if the patient is unconscious and vomiting or if the seizure is refractory to initial therapy. In the latter case, multiple drug therapy will have to be employed, which may cause respiratory depression, necessitating assisted ventilation.

      (2) **Establish venous access and draw initial blood studies.** A large-bore IV catheter should be placed and blood samples collected for electrolytes, blood urea nitrogen (BUN), creatinine, glucose, calcium, magnesium, and liver function tests. A complete blood count (CBC) and erythrocyte sedimentation rate may be helpful in assessing the possibility that an infection or collagen vascular disease precipitated the seizure. A toxic screen should be obtained if there is any reason to suspect alcohol or drug abuse or a drug overdose. The IV fluid administered should be 0.9% saline in anticipation of giving phenytoin (Dilantin), which precipitates in water or 5% dextrose.

      (3) **Drug therapy.** Immediately after drawing the blood tests, 100 mg of thiamine followed by 50 ml of 50% glucose in water should be given IV. If the patient continues to seize during these initial measures, a benzodiazepine, lorazepam (Ativan) 2 mg, or diazepam (Valium) 5–10 mg, should be given slowly IV. These agents can be repeated in 5 minutes if the seizure continues. If the tonic-clonic movements have stopped spontaneously there is no need to give benzodiazepines as their half-life is brief and they will not prevent seizures over the long term. (Lorazepam has a longer duration of action than diazepam because of its smaller volume of distribution.) A first-line anticonvulsant should then be administered, phenytoin is most often used because it can be given IV and therapeutic levels can be achieved within 20 minutes. The loading dose of phenytoin is 1000–1500 mg (15 mg/kg) diluted in 0.9% saline, which should be infused **slowly** with a maximum rate of 50 mg/minute. During infusion of phenytoin the blood pressure should be measured every few minutes and the electrocardiogram (ECG) should be monitored continuously. The

incidence of hypotension and arrhythmia increases with faster rates of infusion. Should hypotension occur, the infusion must be slowed or stopped until blood pressure returns to normal. Following the full loading dose, maintenance phenytoin is started within 18–24 hours, usually 300–400 mg a day given in divided doses. Where compliance is a problem, phenytoin may be given as a single daily dose, but at the risk of developing toxic side effects at peak and breakthrough seizures at trough levels.

(4) Cause of the seizure. Once the seizure is under control it is imperative that the cause be identified and treated. One must consider the following:

(a) Does the patient have a history of seizure disorder?

(b) If so, what anticonvulsants does the patient take? Is the patient compliant with his or her regimen? What are his or her blood levels of anticonvulsant?

(c) Does the patient have a febrile illness that will lower seizure threshold?

(d) If so, what is the cause of the fever? (If not immediately obvious, a lumbar puncture is necessary to evaluate the possibility of meningoencephalitis.)

(e) Is the patient taking any other drugs or alcohol that might interfere with the metabolism of the anticonvulsant or lower his or her seizure threshold? (Table 27-2).

(f) Are there any metabolic abnormalities detected by the patient's blood tests that could have precipitated seizures?

(g) If there is no history of previous seizures or the seizure patient has never been evaluated fully, a computed tomographic (CT) scan of the brain with contrast should be obtained in the emergency department or a magnetic resonance imaging (MRI) scan should be obtained shortly thereafter, to determine whether a tumor or other structural lesion is the cause of seizure. The evaluation of a new-onset seizure should also include an EEG on admission or as an outpatient.

b. Treatment of a tonic-clonic seizure in the postictal phase. If the postictal patient is awake at the time he or she comes to medical attention, one has the option of giving a 15 mg/kg load of phenytoin orally in divided doses of 200–400 mg at 2-hour intervals. Alternatively, another first-line anticonvulsant such as carbamazepine or sodium valproate may be chosen (see sec. **IV**). For rapid oral loading, valproic acid (Depakene) should be administered as it reaches peak plasma levels in 1 to 4

Table 27-2. Effects of psychotropic drugs on seizure threshold*

Psychotropic drugs known to lower the seizure threshold
- Tricyclic and tetracyclic antidepressants (especially maprotiline in doses above 200 mg and clomipramine in doses above 250 mg); bupropion
- Low-potency neuroleptics (especially chlorpromazine)

Drugs known not to affect the seizure threshold
- Monoamine oxidase inhibitors

*Data are incomplete on many psychotropic drugs; data on lithium carbonate are conflicting.

hours. Divalproex sodium (Depakote) requires 3 to 4 hours to reach peak levels. However, if the postictal patient is lethargic and confused when first encountered in the emergency department, it is likely that he or she has had a prolonged seizure; since another convulsion may be imminent, the more rapid IV load of phenytoin is recommended.

c. Treatment of tonic-clonic status epilepticus

(1) Grand mal status epilepticus is defined as continual tonic-clonic seizure activity or recurrent seizures without a conscious interval, lasting for more than 30 minutes. This is truly a medical emergency as the mortality rate from status epilepticus is 6–20% and the risk of permanent brain damage increases with the time required to stop the seizure. The majority of patients with status epilepticus have a preexisting seizure history. Among these, noncompliance with anticonvulsants, alcohol withdrawal, and drug abuse are most often implicated as precipitants. Other causative factors such as metabolic imbalance, CNS infections, mass lesions, and medication overdose must be considered.

(2) It is essential to establish IV access rapidly with a large-bore catheter; if necessary, a central line should be placed. The patient should be intubated to protect the airway. Blood samples should be drawn for electrolytes, glucose, BUN, creatinine, CBC, drug toxicology screen, and anticonvulsant levels. Arterial blood gases should also be obtained. Immediately after drawing venous samples, 100 mg of thiamine and 50 ml of 50% dextrose in water should be administered IV. Lorazepam 2–4 mg or diazepam 10–20 mg should be given IV. The drug should be repeated in 5 minutes if the first dose was ineffective. Although they are short-acting and therefore not definitive treatment for status epilepticus, benzodiazepines reach therapeutic levels in plasma and brain rapidly, halting seizures within 5 minutes in 80% of cases. Immediately after the benzodiazepine is given, infusion of a loading dose of phenytoin, diluted in 0.9% saline, should be started. Therapeutic levels can be attained in as little as 20 minutes, giving 15 mg/kg at a maximum rate of 50 mg/minute. Infusion must be slower if hypotension develops.

(3) Seizures will be refractory to treatment if the patient is acidemic. Thus 1 ampule of $NaHCO_3$ should be given to the patient who has been seizing continuously for longer than 5 minutes. This should be done while awaiting results of the first arterial blood gas, which will dictate further adjustments to correct acid-base balance. Blood gases and pH should be followed periodically as the seizure is being treated.

(4) If seizures persist after phenytoin has been loaded, phenobarbital should be administered (the patient has already been intubated so that respiratory depression from the combined effects of benzodiazepine and barbiturate administration is not an issue). The loading dose of phenobarbital is typically 6–20 mg/kg given IV at a rate not to exceed 60 mg/minute. If all attempts to stop the ictus fail and the patient is seizing after 90 minutes, general anesthesia should be instituted using pentobarbital to produce electrical inactivity of the EEG. This may be done using 3 mg/kg pentobarbital as an IV loading dose followed by 100–200 mg/hour given in IV bolus doses. Transfer of these patients to a suitable acute care facility is mandatory.

B. Absence (petit mal) seizures. Absence seizures are common only in children between the ages of 6 and 16 years. The EEG classically shows a 3/second spike and wave pattern. Attacks usually begin in childhood, decline in late adolescence, and seldom occur after age 30. Thirty-two percent of patients who begin their illness with pure absence later develop tonic-clonic seizures while 14% of absence patients begin their illness with both petit and grand mal seizures.

1. **Clinical features.** Absence seizures begin and end abruptly with the major feature being an alteration in consciousness. There is never an aura or warning. Spells seldom last longer than 20 seconds. A blank stare may be accompanied by automatisms involving lip smacking, eye blinking, or chewing movements. The end of the seizure is abrupt. Occasionally a patient will resume conversation as if uninterrupted. There is no postictal confusion. The EEG in absence seizures often begins with 4–6/second diffuse multispike activity, which may evolve into the classic 3/second spike and wave pattern. Several independent investigators have reported that 79–95% of children with classical absence seizures alone can be cured of attacks when treated early in the course of illness. For those with a mixed absence–tonic-clonic seizure history in childhood, seizures often persist into adulthood and are replaced by grand mal or partial complex seizures. It should be mentioned that complex or variant absence seizures include an abrupt change in level of responsiveness with one or more additional components of myoclonus, atonic episodes (sometimes called "drop attacks"), autonomic phenomena such as enuresis, or tonic episodes.

2. **Treatment.** The treatment of choice for pure absence seizures without history of grand mal or partial complex episodes is ethosuximide (Zarontin). Therapy is usually started with 250–500 mg/day, to be increased over 10–14 days to a dose of 15–40 mg/kg body weight. Therapeutic blood levels range from 40–100 μg/ml. Side effects include gastrointestinal symptoms, drowsiness, lethargy or hyperactivity and irritability. There may be alterations in mood. Toxicity includes blood dyscrasias, urticaria, and rashes. Patients with a mixed disorder of petit and grand mal attacks should be treated with valproic acid (Depakene). The starting dose is 250 mg/day with weekly increments of 5 mg/kg/day to a maintenance dose of 20–30 mg/kg/day. The therapeutic level is 50–120 μg/ml. Common side effects include gastrointestinal disturbance and ataxia. Hepatic complications may occur and have occasionally proved fatal. Therefore liver function tests should be monitored every 2 weeks during the first 6 months and every 2 months thereafter. Hyperammonemia may occur as well, associated with encephalopathy, so that serum ammonia levels should also be followed (see sec. **IV.A.3**).

C. **Myoclonic seizures.** There are numerous seizure disorders in which myoclonic episodes occur, possessing a wide variety of etiologies and prognoses. They do not as a rule fall under the purview of acute care psychiatry and therefore will only be briefly mentioned here. The single common characteristic of these seizures is the series of brief, repetitive, bilaterally synchronous movements of face, arms, and legs. Truncal movements are rare. The treatment for benign forms (e.g., juvenile myoclonus) is valproic acid. Treatment of other forms of myoclonic epilepsy can be difficult and, when suspected, a referral should be made to a neurologist.

III. **Partial (focal) seizures.** Seizures in which clinical and EEG manifestations can be anatomically localized to a specific brain region are termed *partial* or *focal* epilepsies. They comprise the most common forms of seizure disorder; it has been estimated that 67% of adults and 40% of children with epilepsy are afflicted with partial seizures. They usually begin in one focus in a hemisphere and may or may not spread. The EEG may be focally abnormal, or, if the focus is located deep in the hemisphere, the tracing may appear normal. When consciousness is not impaired during the ictus, the seizure is classified as *simple partial* and when consciousness is impaired, it is classified as *complex partial*. Complex partial seizures have also been referred to as *psychomotor epilepsy, temporal lobe seizures,* and *fugues epileptiques.*

A. Simple partial seizures

1. **Clinical features.** Simple partial seizures are epileptic discharges arising from a single focus or functional unit of the brain. The patient remains conscious and aware of his or her surroundings throughout the ictus. The epileptic discharge may involve the motor cortex, resulting in:

   a. Tonic-clonic movement of a single digit or limb.

   b. Jacksonian seizures in which a twitch beginning in the face or distal extremity "marches" along the motor homunculus to involve the entire limb or generalize into a grand mal seizure.

   c. Versive seizures in which the patient turns, usually away from the side of the abnormal electrical discharge.

   d. Phonatory seizures in which the patient may cry out or suffer speech arrest. Sensory seizures may include tactile sensations or visual (formed or unformed), auditory, olfactory, or gustatory hallucinations. Though rare, partial seizures may be comprised of autonomic symptoms such as stomach cramping, tachycardia, diaphoresis, or incontinence. These autonomic symptoms should not be regarded as due to seizure until other more common causes are excluded. Psychic seizures may also occur in which the patient experiences feelings such as déjà vu, jamais vu, unfounded fear, alarm, or fixed intrusive ideas.

2. **Treatment.** The majority of simple partial seizures are caused by focal structural disease. It is therefore particularly important to pursue a careful diagnostic evaluation in such cases. A contrast enhanced brain CT scan will reveal a lesion in up to 50% of cases. In those instances in which the initial CT is negative, MRI should be obtained. Should these studies fail to reveal a lesion, scanning should be repeated at 6-month intervals for at least 1 year. Cerebral angiography should be considered to rule out the possibility of a small arteriovenous malformation causing an irritative focus. **First-line drugs** for the treatment of the partial epilepsies are carbamazepine and phenytoin. Carbamazepine has gained wide acceptance as the drug of choice for this class of seizure disorder. Alternative medications include sodium valproate, phenobarbital, and primidone (see sec. **IV**).

B. Complex partial seizures

1. **Clinical features.** In complex partial seizures, often heralded by an aura, the patient's level of consciousness and responsiveness to stimuli are impaired. The aura consists of symptoms, often those of a simple partial seizure, that precede the impairment of consciousness that occurs as the seizure spreads. If abnormal, the EEG shows a discrete focus of aberrant discharge. The most common interictal pattern is one of epileptiform spikes or sharp waves while the most common ictal pattern is comprised of rhythmic 16–30 per second low-voltage potentials. Complex partial seizures are readily distinguishable from absence seizures. In contradistinction to absences, complex partial seizures usually last longer than 10–20 seconds and typically last 3 (though usually not more than 5) minutes. Forty-five percent of epileptics with complex partial seizures have an aura, whereas no aura occurs in petit mal seizures. There is a period of postictal confusion and lethargy in complex partial seizures, while in absence seizures the return to full alertness is abrupt. Automatisms in complex partial seizures are often more elaborate than in absences. For example, there may be head and eye deviation, clonic facial jerks, sudden walking or running, or perseverative motions of the limbs such as kicking and defensive combativeness. One should be immediately suspicious of patients, ostensibly in the throes of

a complex partial seizure, who perform elaborate and purposeful actions. Occasionally one will hear of a patient with complex partial seizures who, for example, is able to continue driving during an ictus but overshoots his or her exit and subsequently realizes that time has passed for which he or she cannot account. However, deliberate actions that are neither repetitious nor "automatic" cannot be carried out during a complex partial (psychomotor or temporal lobe) seizure. Partial complex seizures may mimic primary psychiatric disorders (see Chap. 26).

2. **Treatment.** As noted in the preceding section, the drug of choice for partial seizures is carbamazepine. Phenytoin is another first-line medication while alternatives include phenobarbital and primidone.

IV. Use of anticonvulsants in the treatment of epilepsy. The choice of anticonvulsants to be used in the treatment of epilepsy is governed by the practical considerations of the speed with which one must attain therapeutic levels and the efficacy of a given medication for a specific seizure type; these must be balanced by consideration of the relative toxicities of these medications. In the setting of acute management of status epilepticus or prolonged grand mal seizures, phenytoin should be the first anticonvulsant used because it can be given rapidly and parenterally, unlike carbamazepine or valproate. If necessary, phenytoin can be followed by an IV load of phenobarbital (see sec. **II.A.2.c.(4)**). When there is not a pressing emergency, the choice of anticonvulsants is not constrained. The goal of therapy is to obtain control of seizures with a single medication, because combined therapies entail greater toxicity for the patient. The chosen antiepileptic should be adjusted until seizures are controlled or a high therapeutic or toxic level is achieved. If seizures continue to occur, a second drug is added. Once a therapeutic level of the second drug is reached, the first medication is discontinued. If seizures still occur with a high therapeutic or toxic level of the second medication, a third is introduced and crossed over, and so on. If control cannot be achieved with a single medication, combination therapy must be employed.

A. **Primary generalized seizures.** Medications of choice for the treatment of generalized tonic-clonic and absence seizures are phenytoin, carbamazepine, and sodium valproate. Because of its abuse potential, possibility of lethality in overdose, and tendency to cause excessive sedation, phenobarbital (and primidone, whose active metabolite is phenobarbital) is generally avoided whenever possible. Increasingly, sodium valproate is being used as the first drug of choice in the treatment of both primary generalized tonic-clonic seizures and associated absence seizures. Primary absence not associated with grand mal seizures may also be treated with ethosuximide.

1. **Phenytoin** is effective, but its use is limited by its many side effects. Side effects include possible cognitive impairments, which may interfere with learning. Nystagmus is common and at higher concentrations, ataxia, drowsiness, and diplopia may occur. Gingival hyperplasia, hirsutism, and coarsening of facial features also may occur. Allergic reactions range from a fairly common morbiliform rash to exfoliative dermatitis and Stevens-Johnson syndrome. Other reported adverse effects include a lupuslike syndrome, hepatic granulomas, hepatitis, lymphadenopathy, pseudolymphoma, megaloblastic anemia, pulmonary infiltrates, peripheral neuropathy, osteomalacia from interference with vitamin D metabolism, and depression of serum folate and vitamin K levels. Congenital abnormalities and retardation have occurred in infants born to mothers taking phenytoin during pregnancy.

2. **Carbamazepine.** This drug has a more favorable side effect profile than phenytoin. Its main disadvantages are the lack of a parenteral form, and rare, but potentially lethal blood dyscrasias. Excessively rapid increases in dose can produce sedation, dizziness, and diplopia; these side effects may also emerge at toxic levels. Such side effects can generally be avoided by

starting at a low dose of 200 mg bid and increasing the dose slowly as needed, using increments of 200 mg/day added at weekly intervals. The usual therapeutic dosage is 600–1200 mg/day in three divided doses. Reversible, mild leukopenia is well documented, but agranulocytosis and aplastic anemia can occur (reported indicence: 1 in 20,000 patients). Also reported are Stevens-Johnson syndrome, cardiac toxicity, hypoosmolality due to inappropriate secretion of antidiuretic hormone, and hepatitis, which is sometimes fatal. Carbamazepine is teratogenic in rats, but this is not established in humans.

3. **Sodium valproate.** Serious adverse effects are uncommon but pancreatitis has occurred as well as fatal hepatic failure, most notably in children under the age of 3 years who were taking more than one anticonvulsant. Chronic liver disease or hyperammonemia without hepatic enzyme abnormalities can occur. Hyperammonemia can be associated with lethargy or obtundation. Other adverse reactions are nausea and vomiting, weight gain, hair loss, rash, tremor, headache, insomnia, leukopenia, red blood cell aplasia, and thrombocytopenia. Neural tube defects have been reported in infants born to women who were taking valproate during pregnancy.

4. **Phenobarbital.** The half-life of this drug is 100 hours, so that steady-state concentrations require weeks to obtain. Sedation and behavioral-cognitive disturbances including hyperactivity, inattention, and depression are the most common side effects. Barbiturate overdose is always a potential risk.

B. **Partial (focal) epilepsies.** Carbamazepine is the drug of choice for the treatment of simple and complex partial seizures as well as partial seizures with secondary generalization. Although clinical trials have failed to show a significant difference in efficacy for carbamazepine over phenytoin or primidone, the relative lack of serious side effects of carbamazepine has led to the recommendation that it be used in the initial management of these seizures. Carbamazepine has essentially no deleterious effects on cognitive function, does not decrease libido or produce impotence, and has no dysmorphic effects. Phenytoin should be used when carbamazepine fails.

Selected Readings

Browne, T. R. Therapy of status epilepticus. *Compr. Ther.* 8:25, 1982.

Browne, T. R., and Feldman, R. G. *Epilepsy: Diagnosis and Management.* Boston, Little Brown, 1983.

Cascino, G. D. Complex partial seizures: Clinical features and differential diagnosis. *Psychiatr. Clin. North Am.* 15(2):373, 1992.

Cascino, G. D. Intractable partial epilepsy: Evaluation and treatment. *Mayo Clin. Proc.* 65:1578, 1990.

Chadwick, D. W. Valproate monotherapy in the management of generalized and partial seizures. *Epilepsia* 28(Suppl. 2):S12, 1987.

Commission on Classification and Terminology of the International League Against Epilepsy: Proposal for the classification of the epilepsies and epileptic syndromes. *Epilepsia* 26:268, 1985.

Delgado-Escueta, A. V. The Epilepsies: New Developments of the 1980's. In S. H. Appel (ed.), *Current Neurology.* Vol. 6, 1986. Pp. 235.

Pippenger, C. E., and Lesser, R. P. An overview of therapeutic drug monitoring principles. *Clev. Clin. Q.* 151:241, 1984.

So, E. L. Update on epilepsy. *Med. Clin. North Am.* 77(1):203, 1993.

Wilder, B. J. Antiepileptic drugs used in the emergency management of seizures and introduction of phenytoin prodrug. *Epilepsia* 30(Suppl. 2):S1, 1989.

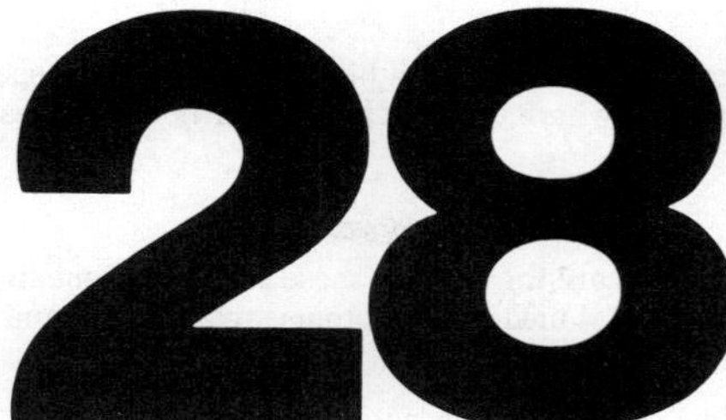

Malingering, Factitious Illness, and Somatization

Theodore A. Stern

I. Most individuals who come to an emergency department do so for the diagnosis and treatment of physical symptoms. Occasionally there are no demonstrable organic findings or known physiologic mechanisms to account for these symptoms. To treat such patients successfully, a broad differential diagnosis must be considered, an appropriate interview must be conducted, and clinically indicated diagnostic tests must be performed. Failure in any of these areas may result in continuation of the individual's symptomatology and in initiation of needless and, often, invasive procedures. The physician should also pay attention to his or her own reactions to the patient, because these may provide clues for the evaluation and if unrecognized may interfere with the diagnostic workup and subsequent treatment.

II. Evaluation of the patient with somatic symptoms of psychiatric origin. A wide spectrum of psychiatric disorders is associated with the manifestation of somatic symptoms. Some symptoms are so profound that the presence of serious or even life-threatening illness must be considered. As a consequence, the search for the correct diagnosis is often made under pressure of time. The situation may be complicated by the presence of concomitant medical illness or by a real organic lesion from the past that has led to some genuine physical signs on which the patient may elaborate a convincing story.

A. General recommendations

1. Symptoms must be investigated initially as though they were caused by a medical disorder, even if the clinician suspects that there is little or no organic basis for the symptoms. This is especially important if the symptoms might herald a serious illness.

2. Physicians tend to believe what they are told by their patients; this trait often helps them establish a therapeutic relationship. However, a healthy skepticism should be maintained, especially when aspects of the clinical presentation are unconvincing or unusual.

3. Be aware of countertransference reactions stimulated by the patient. When the physician is unduly irritated, fascinated, or angry, it may be a warning that he or she is being manipulated or duped.

4. It is helpful to remember that psychiatric disorders causing somatic symptoms fall on a continuum from the totally willful invention of symptomatology to the involuntary production of symptoms.

5. It is important to make the diagnosis of somatization when it is present and to rule it out when it is not. Diagnostic impressions should be recorded in a nonjudgmental fashion in the patient's chart.

6. The physician should not be dismayed when fooled by a patient. These disorders are unique in medicine because they violate the normal relationship between patient and physician. Moreover, the somatoform disorders and malingering are diagnoses of exclusion; it is only when the physician is reasonably certain that an organic illness is not present that these diagnoses are invoked. Both when symptoms are due to unconscious psychologic

conflicts and when the patient has lied outright, proof is difficult, especially in the emergency department where the physician usually feels pressure to work rapidly.

B. Medical history

1. Complicated medical histories are the rule for these patients. Time invested in accruing a complete history of medical symptoms, evaluations, and treatments will be well spent.
2. Medical records should be obtained when possible.
3. Contact with other physicians and hospitals (with the consent of the patient) offers similar benefits. Knowledge of previous presentations and medical evaluations will hasten the assessment and help avoid needless procedures and testing. Suspicion should be raised when a patient prevents the physician from obtaining records or speaking with other physicians about his or her care or when information turns out to be false.

C. Interview

1. After it is clear that no medical crisis is in progress, the physician should proceed with an interview that attempts to be empathic and engenders trust.
2. Patients should be screened for the presence of a major psychiatric disorder (e.g., panic disorder, depression, or a psychosis). Unrealistic beliefs or interpretations of physical symptoms may be due to hypochondriasis or, if delusional, to a psychosis.
3. When psychologic conflicts are suspected, they should not be disregarded; such conflicts may exacerbate the symptoms of a physical condition or may be the cause of somatic complaints in the absence of a physical condition.

D. Examination of the patient. Inconsistencies among the history, the physical examination, and laboratory data should not be passed off to laboratory error or to an inadequate examination. Even small discrepancies are noteworthy and may guide the physician to the proper diagnosis.

III. Psychiatric differential diagnosis of somatization. When a patient complains of a physical symptom, a search must first be made for demonstrable organic findings or a pattern of illness that is suggestive of a physical disorder.

A. Physical conditions. A thorough history and physical examination must be performed. If a specific condition is found, it obviously should be treated.

B. Psychologic factors affecting physical conditions. On occasion, psychologic factors may be uncovered and implicated in the initiation or exacerbation of a physical condition (e.g., tension headache or irritable bowel syndrome).

C. Specific conditions and psychiatric disorders

1. **Malingering and factitious illness.** If there is insufficient evidence to warrant a diagnosis of a physical condition by virtue of a lack of organic findings or an absence of a typical pattern of illness, and if the symptoms are apparently under the individual's control, the diagnosis of malingering or factitious illness should be entertained. Because this is a common problem in the emergency department it is discussed in detail in sec. **IV.**
2. **Somatoform disorders.** These are a group of disorders, which according to the *Diagnostic and Statistical Manual of Mental Disorders, Fourth Edition, Draft Criteria* (DSM-IV), have as their essential features physical symptoms for which there are no demonstrable organic findings or known physiologic mechanisms, and for which there is positive evidence, or a strong presumption, that the symptoms are linked to psychologic factors or conflicts. Unlike

malingering or factitious disorders, the person does not experience the sense of controlling the production of symptoms.

a. **Somatization disorder** is the DSM-IV name for what might have been called hysteria in the past, or Briquet's syndrome by some authors. Individuals with this disorder manifest recurrent and multiple somatic complaints including symptoms referable to multiple organ systems, including neurologic, reproductive, gastrointestinal, and cardiopulmonary systems. Complaints are often offered in either a dramatic or vague fashion. Anxiety and depression are common, although not invariably present. The disorder typically begins before the age of 30 years and has a chronic, though fluctuating, course. These individuals seek medical attention from a variety of practitioners, take prescription medicines, and alter their usual pattern of living as a result of their symptoms. It is important to rule out the possibility of panic disorder as a cause of the patient's symptoms. Emergency management consists of avoiding unnecessary medical procedures, gentle confrontation of the patient, and referral to a primary care physician who is willing to see the patient for regular, but time-limited appointments. Many of these patients fail to benefit from psychotherapy; anxiolytics are rarely indicated for patients with this disorder.

b. **Pain disorder** is the DSM-IV name for what has often been referred to as *psychogenic pain.* This disorder is diagnosed when the patient is preoccupied with pain, but either no organic pathology or pathophysiologic mechanism can be uncovered after an appropriate evaluation or, when there is organic pathology, the complaint of pain or resulting social or occupational impairment is grossly in excess of what would be expected. Frequently, a temporal relationship can be established between an environmental stimulus associated with psychologic conflict and an exacerbation of the pain. This worsening may result in secondary gain (e.g., avoidance of a distressing situation or increased support from others). A variety of sensory and motor changes may be reported (e.g., paresthesias or muscle spasms), and disuse atrophy and related findings may be noted on examination. Despite extensive medical evaluations, many of these individuals persist in seeking medical attention; some insist on surgical cures. Requests for documentation of disability and analgesics are common; drug addiction frequently develops. In managing such patients it is important to look for, and treat, depression. Tricyclic antidepressants occasionally improve the symptoms even if the patient does not meet criteria for a major depressive episode. The physician should not prescribe narcotics for these patients.

c. **Conversion disorder** is diagnosed when a loss or alteration in function is suggestive of a physical disorder, but psychologic factors are judged to be etiologically related to the symptom because of a temporal relationship between a psychosocial stressor that is apparently related to a psychologic conflict or need and initiation or exacerbation of the symptom. The person is not conscious of intentionally producing the symptom. Most symptoms—for example, blindness, paralysis, seizure, amnesia, paresthesias—are suggestive of a neurologic disorder. However vomiting and pseudocyesis (false pregnancy) also occur. Typically, symptoms appear suddenly and arise in the setting of psychologic stress. Symptoms tend to involve a single system during any given episode, but may vary among episodes. The presence of "la belle indifference"—that is, an attitude conveying a lack of concern—is a frequent but not invariable feature of the disorder. More frequently, a prior history of conversion disorder or a family member with similar symptoms is found. Although most cases terminate abruptly and are usually of short duration, some individuals with the disorder have prolonged loss of function and develop serious medical complications such as contractures. A bona fide neurologic disorder (e.g., multiple sclerosis) may occasionally turn out to be the culprit in a patient thought to have this disorder. Because of their importance in the emergency department, conversion symptoms, and pseudoseizures in particular, are discussed in sec. **IV.C.**

d. Hypochondriasis. The predominant feature of this chronic disorder is the unrealistic interpretation of physical symptoms as abnormal. This leads to a preoccupation with the fear or belief that one has a serious illness. The disorder persists despite numerous medical evaluations and often causes impaired social and occupational functioning. Several organ systems may be the focus of the hypochondriac's concern although one system (e.g., the heart) may predominate. Although the intensity of complaints may be high, these individuals do not create or simulate the signs of a physical illness. They search out multiple medical opinions and often feel frustration and anger, as do their physicians, when treatment seems inadequate and complaints persist. Anxiety and depression commonly coexist with this disorder.

IV. Diagnosis and management of specific psychiatric problems frequently presenting with somatization in the emergency department

A. Malingering

1. Clinical features

a. Diagnosis rests on the voluntary production of symptoms (either somatic or psychologic) for the purpose of obtaining a goal that is understandable in terms of the individual's circumstances rather than in terms of his or her intrapsychic state (e.g., the individual seeks to avoid work or criminal prosecution, or seeks to obtain drugs or financial compensation).

b. Malingering is distinguished from factitious illness by the patient's motivation for the voluntary production of the symptoms—that is, in factitious disorders the production of symptoms is not for secondary gain but is meant to achieve the "sick" role. Although the production of symptoms in factitious disorders is under voluntary control, the general pattern of motivation often appears to be compulsive.

2. Clues to the diagnosis

a. Suspicion of the diagnosis is necessary if it is to be made. Those physicians who are all-trusting are prone to being used and manipulated by these patients.

b. Suspicion of malingering should be aroused when:

(1) The patient's symptoms fail to correlate with the physical findings or the amount of distress or disability reported.

(2) The patient fails to cooperate with diagnostic testing and treatment recommendations.

(3) The patient presents in the context of a medicolegal situation (i.e., when involved in litigation, worker's compensation, or disability hearings).

(4) The patient has a history of polysubstance abuse (especially with narcotics or sedative-hypnotic drugs).

(5) The patient responds to questions by providing approximate answers (e.g., "What color is the sky?" "Green"), a style of response sometimes associated with Ganser's syndrome.

3. Treatment. Malingering, although not a psychiatric disorder per se, reflects underlying psychopathology. It does not respond to psychologic interpretations, suggestion, or psychopharmacologic agents. The best outcome is obtained by excluding any treatable physical or psychiatric conditions and by refusing to contribute to the individual's quest to avoid responsibility. The findings should be explained to the individual in a straightforward fashion. Written statements, when provided at the request of the individual, should not distort the truth. Prescriptions that are not indicated should not be written.

B. Factitious illness (Munchausen's syndrome)

1. **Diagnosis** is based on three cardinal features.
   - a. The production of physical or psychologic symptoms that are apparently under the individual's voluntary control.
   - b. The signs and symptoms that are produced, simulated, or complained about are not explained by any other physical or mental disorder, although they may be superimposed on one.
   - c. The individual's goal is apparently to assume the patient role and is not otherwise understandable as a manifestation of secondary gain (as in malingering).
2. A **typical admission** has several characteristics:
   - a. The patient often arrives in the emergency department late at night or on a weekend.
   - b. He or she has an apparent acute illness or pain supported by a plausible and often dramatic case history.
   - c. The patient generally appeals to the qualities of nurturance and omnipotence in the physician in an attempt to convince him or her to provide treatment.
   - d. Use of extensive knowledge of medical jargon allows the patient to capitalize on any real organic disturbances and to make his or her case sound more interesting.
   - e. Demands by the patient for attention increase; irritation and anger develop when these demands are not met.
   - f. Complaints of misdiagnosis and mistreatment arise and are directed toward the staff.
   - g. The deception is often uncovered—for example, by the discovery of insulin-filled syringes in a patient's suitcase during his hospitalization for hypoglycemia.
   - h. The staff becomes angry and loses interest in the patient's medical issues. This results either in a swift discharge of the patient or the patient's storming out of the hospital. In either case, he or she is free until the next encounter with medical personnel.
   - i. The patient arrives at a nearby hospital with a similar presentation shortly after such a discharge.
3. **Clinical presentations vary.** Most cases resemble true medical emergencies. Well-known varieties are as follows:
   - a. **The acute abdominal type (laparotomaphilia migrans).** This type is the most common; many of these individuals have been operated on so frequently that abdominal symptoms may, in fact, be a consequence of intestinal obstruction secondary to adhesions.
   - b. **The hemorrhagic type (hemorrhagia histrionica).** These individuals have also been called hematemesis merchants or hemoptysis merchants based on their site of apparent bleeding.

c. **The neurologic type (neurologia diabolica),** often presenting with lo of consciousness, paroxysmal headache, or seizure.

d. **The dermatologic type (dermatitis autogenica),** frequently the resu of self-inflicted wounds or chemical abrasions.

e. **The febrile type (hyperpyrexia figmentatica).** These individuals ofte lose their fevers when thermometers are placed, monitored, and remove under observation.

f. **The endocrinologic type,** including those who present for evaluation hyperinsulinemia, hyperthyroidism, and hypoglycemia.

g. **The cardiac type,** including those individuals who complain of ches pain and arrhythmias.

h. **The hematologic type.** Profound anemias have been produced by su reptitious bloodletting and by complications of ingestion and sel administration of anticoagulants.

i. **Childhood type.** Children can be the victims of **Munchausen's syr drome by proxy**—that is, vehicles for parental psychopathology. Fc example, a mother may be administering thyroid medication to a chil without the knowledge of a physician.

4. **Diagnostic clues**

a. An acute, but not entirely convincing history—for example, a report profound bleeding but without tachycardia, orthostatic hypotension, c pallor.

b. A mixture of truculence and evasiveness in manner.

c. Numerous forms of identification—for example, hospital cards and ir surance forms.

d. A multiplicity of scars.

e. Evidence of addiction or multiple hospital admissions.

f. Pseudologia fantastica—that is, telling of tall tales.

g. Impostureship.

h. A masochistic acceptance of painful procedures.

i. Itinerant lives.

j. A facility with medical jargon.

k. A paucity of verifiable history.

l. An absence of close interpersonal relationships.

m. A history of having worked in a medically related field.

n. An early history of sadistic and rejecting parents, chronic illness, or a important relationship with a physician.

o. Personality disorders. Although a wide range of psychiatric diagnose have been associated with this syndrome, these individuals are usuall thought to have personality disorders.

5. Successful **treatment** of this syndrome is rare, and definitive managemen strategies are lacking. Early efforts were directed to help physicians avoi being duped rather than to help the patients. Recommendations have ir cluded:

a. Blacklisting such patients.

b. Individual and group psychotherapy directed at the masochistic chara ter of their relationships, their need for intimacy (even though it is entwined with pain), and their conflicts over dependency.

c. Behavior modification.

d. Prolonged inpatient psychiatric admission to combine several of the above interventions.

e. Education of caretakers. An awareness of the tendency of these patients to provoke anger and frustration is important to help minimize premature discharge.

f. Psychiatric consultation. If initiated early, such consultation may lead to a workable plan (via confrontation in a supportive context) before needless tests are ordered and a crisis arises.

C. **Conversion disorder.** Of the somatoform disorders, conversion disorder is the one most likely to present as a medical emergency.

1. **Diagnosis.** A sudden loss or alteration in physical functioning occurs and is usually suggestive of a neurologic disorder (e.g., blindess, paralysis, or seizures).

2. **Predisposing factors** may include:

   a. An antecedent physical disorder that provided the patient with a model for the symptoms.

   b. Exposure to other individuals with similar symptoms.

   c. Extreme psychologic or social stress.

3. **Mechanisms** for the development of symptoms are thought to involve primary and secondary gain.

   a. **Primary gain** is achieved by avoiding internal conflict (e.g., blindness) so that the individual avoids seeing something painful.

   b. **Secondary gain** is achieved by gaining environmental rewards—for example, a gathering of social supports that might not otherwise be available, such as blindness that leads to a reuniting of the patient's fragmented family.

4. Emergency treatment consists, initially, of utilizing the patient's suggestibility to try to relieve acute symptoms. If the patient is allowed a face-saving mechanism and it is suggested that the symptoms should resolve, improvement often will occur. Some clinicians have recommended hypnosis or an amobarbital interview (see Chap. 19, sec. **III.B.3.d**) for symptom reduction in patients who do not respond to suggestion alone. Occasionally it will be necessary to confront the patient directly. Following symptom reduction, crisis intervention as described in Chap. 2 may prove to be useful.

5. **Pseudoseizures** are clinically one of the most important forms of conversion disorder. (Another, psychogenic unresponsiveness, is discussed in Chap. 19, sec. **III.C.1.c.**)

   a. **Overview.** Alternative labels have been used frequently for this disorder; each label implies a different etiology.

      (1) Terms include: hysterical pseudoseizures, hysteroepilepsy (implying a relationship between hysteria and epilepsy), simulated epilepsy (suggesting a diagnosis of malingering), psychogenic seizures (a misleading term because true epileptic seizures can be precipitated by emotion), pseudoseizures, and pseudoepileptic seizures (probably the most accurate term because it is descriptive, but avoids invoking erroneous mechanisms of action).

(2) A patient may have both pseudoseizures and true epileptic seizures. Not all pseudoseizures are manifest by convulsive attacks; some may present with altered states of consciousness, pallor, muscle twitching, muscle weakness, or dissociated states. These episodes may be extraordinarily difficult to distinguish from simple and complex partial seizures.

b. Clinical manifestations of pseudoseizures

(1) Attacks may vary from one episode to the next, in contrast to epileptic seizures, which generally have stereotyped patterns.

(2) Generalized muscular rigidity is common, and convulsive movements may increase if restraint is applied. This is in contrast to the tonic-clonic phase of a true generalized seizure.

(3) Cyanosis is rare in pseudoseizures but almost invariably accompanies generalized tonic-clonic seizures).

(4) Reflexes are unchanged during or after a pseudoseizure, whereas with grand mal seizures, corneal reflexes are generally lost and the patient is unresponsive to painful stimuli.

(5) During a pseudoseizure patients usually resist attempts to open their eyes.

(6) Self-injury (e.g., tongue-biting) is commonly avoided, as is incontinence, in pseudoseizures.

(7) The level of consciousness may vary following a pseudoseizure. However, recollection of environmental events during the episode (if accompanied by bilateral convulsive movements) favors the diagnosis of pseudoseizure. The diagnosis cannot be made with certainty because some partial seizures of epileptic origin occur with a clear sensorium.

(8) Strong emotional stresses may precipitate both seizures and pseudoseizures; thus, one must be cautious about diagnosing an episode as a pseudoseizure on this basis.

(9) Headache frequently precedes pseudoseizures but is uncommon prior to epileptic seizures.

(10) Pseudoseizures do not occur during sleep but epileptic seizures do.

(11) Pseudoseizures may occur several times a day, a pattern that is uncommon in epilepsy.

(12) Descriptions of pseudoseizures are often vague and inconsistent.

(13) Electroencephalogram (EEG) tracings during an episode may be helpful in the diagnosis of pseudoseizures, but they are not conclusive. Paroxysmal abnormalities usually associated with epilepsy do not prove that any particular episode has an epileptic basis. Conversely, patients with pseudoseizures may have EEG abnormalities—for example, bursts of theta activity. Simultaneous EEG and videotaped recording may help establish the diagnosis and allow a more accurate assessment of movement artifacts. An attack with convulsive movements without EEG changes is unlikely. However, partial seizures frequently occur in the absence of EEG abnormalities.

c. Optimal management is guided by the correct diagnosis of pseudoseizures. Most patients are treated initially with anticonvulsant medications in the mistaken belief that the patient is experiencing epileptic seizures. If these patients are admitted to the hospital, the clinical pattern of seizures can be observed and EEG recordings (either via telemetry or with simultaneously videotaped recordings) can be arranged. If, after an extended period of observation, evidence in favor of an epileptic diagnosis is unconvincing, gradual withdrawal from anticonvulsants can be initiated. This evaluation should be accompanied by a psychiatric assessment that involves a discussion of the patient's symptoms and their relationship to current and past life events. Exploratory psychotherapy or use of hypnosis may lead to resolution of conflicts so that alternative means of dealing with stressful events can be employed. Strategies that foster strength and minimize the advantages of illness may include individual psychotherapy, family counseling, and behavior modification techniques.

Selected Readings

American Psychiatric Association Task Force on DSM-IV. *Diagnostic and Statistical Manual of Mental Disorders, Fourth Edition, Draft Criteria:* 3/1/93. Washington, D.C.: American Psychiatric Association.

Barsky, A. J. Somatoform Disorders. In S. E. Hyman and M. A. Jenike (eds.), *Manual of Clinical Problems in Psychiatry with Annotated Key References*. Boston: Little, Brown, 1990. Pp. 177–189.

Cramer, B., Gershberg, M. R., and Stern, M. Munchausen syndrome: Its relationship to malingering, hysteria and the physician-patient relationship. *Arch. Gen. Psychiatry* 24:573, 1971.

Fenton, G. W. Hysterical Alterations in Consciousness. In A. Roy (ed.), *Hysteria*. New York: Wiley, 1982. Pp. 229–246.

Kahan, B., and Yorker, B. C. Munchausen syndrome by proxy: Clinical review and legal issues. *Behav. Sci. Law* 9:73, 1991.

Stern, T. A. Munchausen's syndrome revisited. *Psychosomatics* 21:326, 1980.

Steven, H. Is it organic or functional: Is it hysteria or malingering? *Psychiatr. Clin. North Am.* 9:241, 1986.

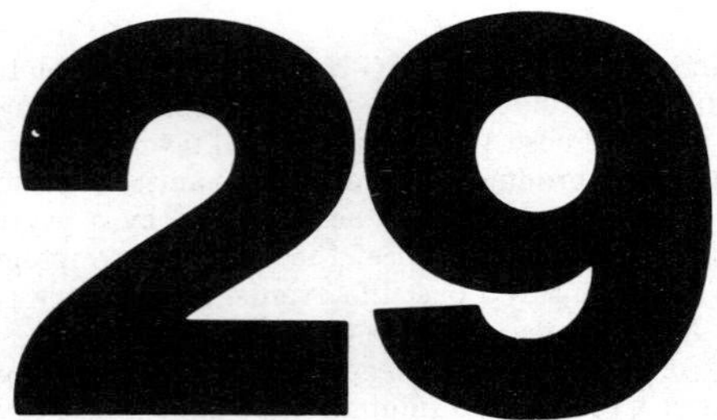

Disruptive Medica Patients

Steven E. Hyman
George E. Tesar

I. Some patients in the emergency department or on a medical or surgical floor ma behave in a disruptive manner that interferes with the delivery of medical care o endangers themselves or others.

A. Evaluation. The disruptive patient should be approached with an open mind.

1. Attention should be paid to vital signs, medical findings, and results of th mental status examination to rule out the possibility that the patient i experiencing acute psychosis (see Chap. 19) or delirium (see Chap. 23).

2. It should be recognized that **severe anxiety about illness may cause a individual to behave in a disruptive manner** that does not reflect thei usual manner of functioning.

3. **Misunderstandings or conflicts** between the patient and staff are mor likely when patients are anxious or irritable.

B. Approach to the patient. Especially if the patient is anxious, angry, or agitatec the approach should be calm and nonjudgmental. The physician should mak it clear that he or she wants to hear the patient's point of view and has the goa of making the patient's treatment as effective and easy as possible. Howeve if the patient's ongoing behavior is threatening to the safety of the patient o the staff, limits should be set firmly and physical restraints used if necessar The need for limits must be explained to the patient, but explanations shoul be brief, clear, and calmly given by the physician.

II. Specific situations

A. Patients who are delirious or anxious should be treated as described i Chap. 23.

B. Difficult personalities or personality disorders may introduce obstacles in th way of what should be the shared goal of the physician and patient—restorin the health of the latter.

1. Patients with borderline or similar personality disorders (see Chap. 2 may be demanding and manipulative. Such patients have primitive copin mechanisms that may create difficulties for the staff. For example, suc patients often idealize a small number of staff members (who often end u being "seduced" and manipulated) and devalue and detest the rest (so-calle *splitting*). This opens the staff to fruitless arguments about the best way t manage the patient; the idealized staff members may see the patient a basically good or "misunderstood," while the others see him or her as disrup tive. In the meantime the patient is able to "divide and conquer"—for exam ple, to obtain extra pain medication or otherwise bend the rules. It is there fore critical that the entire staff talk about any disagreements and decide o a treatment plan for the patient. Above all the staff must agree to maintai consistency among themselves. When clinicians interact with the patient they can acknowledge the difficulties that the patient is having but shoul not be seduced or badgered into bending the rules or making promises tha

are not normally made. Conversely, no matter how exasperating these patients may be, it is important not to show outright hostility or to act in a punitive manner. From a nonconfrontational stance the clinician may be able to point out to the patient what medical treatment is necessary and what the staff is trying to accomplish.

2. **Hostile patients** are extremely difficult to manage, in no small part because they arouse strong negative feelings in their caretakers. Patients are often hostile when they feel physically threatened or when they feel that their self-esteem is suffering. Focusing on complaints and on angry feelings serves the patient in that he or she does not have to face his or her fear or sense of loss of control. With extremely hostile or paranoid patients the best initial approach is nonconfrontational. The physician should make it clear that he or she wants to see the problem from the patient's point of view. It is useful to listen to the patient's angry complaints in as sympathetic a fashion as the physician can muster. It can be enlightening to ask whether the patient has had difficult experiences with physicians in the past or whether he or she has anger against physicians or hospitals because of experiences of a friend or family member. The physician should be willing to sympathize and to negotiate ways in which the current hospital admission can be more positive. As a degree of trust develops, the physician should explain to the patient how the medical staff has interpreted the patient's actions as a way of explaining their responses. The physician should not, however, put himself or herself in the position of undercutting other staff members or agreeing to things that are dangerous or countertherapeutic. Often when such patients feel they have at least one ally, their behavior improves.

3. **Rule violators** may harass physicians and nurses and threaten their own clinical care. Such individuals often have long-standing conflicts over dependency with the result that when put in a dependent situation, they fear that they will totally lose control. They often react maladaptively with hyperindependent behavior to try to reestablish control. The physician can cede control of some areas of the patient's care to the patient but should explain why other aspects cannot be considered discretionary—for example, "You can refuse your sleeping pill or your laxative if you like, but you really must take your antibiotic for your own safety." The patient can be asked further for advice on how he or she would like treatment to proceed.

C. **Patients who threaten to sign out against advice.** When called to see a patient threatening to sign out against advice the physician must rapidly make two inferences—whether signing out would constitute a serious medical danger to the patient and whether the patient is fully able to judge his or her situation or, alternatively, is psychotic, delirious, or demented.

1. If the patient is unable to make an informed judgment because of his or her mental state and if discharge would pose a serious threat to the patient's health or safety, the patient should be stopped from leaving, using restraint if necessary. A judicial determination of competency may be required to continue nonemergency treatments unless the patient changes his or her mind about complying with treatment (see Chap. 10). The examining physician should document the patient's inability to understand his or her medical condition and reasons for needing treatment and the risk to the patient if he or she left the hospital. Consultation with the hospital attorneys is prudent.

2. For patients who are not mentally impaired but whose signing out would entail a significant risk, the physician must do all he or she can to help the patient to stay. If it is determined that the patient is fleeing the hospital out of fear, he or she can usually be managed with reassurance and an anxiolytic as described in sec. **II.A.** Patients who want to sign out because

they feel misunderstood and maltreated are a more difficult problem. Often their anger with their physicians or nurses is long-standing and the decision to sign out is made because they feel that the situation is intolerable. It is usually most successful not to confront or lecture such patients, but to take their grievances seriously. The physician can offer to ally with the patient and can offer sympathy for what the patient has been through. Often some concession will have to be made to the patient to entice him or her to stay, which may restore his or her sense of control over the situation.

D. When **drug abusers** become medical patients special problems may arise. Patients may have withdrawal syndromes, may demand drugs, or may falsify symptoms to obtain drugs.

1. The management of **withdrawal syndromes** is presented in Chap. 30. It is important at all times to judge withdrawal by objective signs rather than subjective complaints.
2. It is important to judge whether it is clinically appropriate to withdraw a patient or whether the patient should be maintained on a drug, such as phenobarbital or methadone, during the course of his or her medical illness. For patients who are medically fragile the risk of withdrawal, e.g., from sedative-hypnotics, during the acute illness may outweigh any benefits. If patients are to be maintained, however, the maintenance dose should be based on objective findings. For narcotics and sedative-hypnotics the procedures for determination of a stabilization dose are outlined in Chap. 30.
3. When drug abusers, especially narcotic abusers, must be treated for pain (e.g., postoperatively), they may demand inappropriate amounts of medication or may become angry or demanding when the medications are tapered. Successful management requires that the patient's primary physician sets out guidelines for dosages that are clear to the patient. Other staff members must be consistent and must not supplement the medication. Patients often become quite skillful in trying to manipulate other physicians when the primary physician is out of the hospital.

Selected Readings

Cassem, N. H., and Hackett, T. P. Psychiatric consultation in a coronary care unit. *Ann. Intern. Med.* 75:9, 1971.

Cassem, N. H., and Hyman, S. E. Psychologic Management of Grief and Serious Illness. In E. Rubenstein and D. D. Federman (eds.), *Scientific American Medicine*. New York: Scientific American, 1987.

Groves, J. E. Taking care of the hateful patient. *N. Engl. J. Med.* 298:883, 1978.

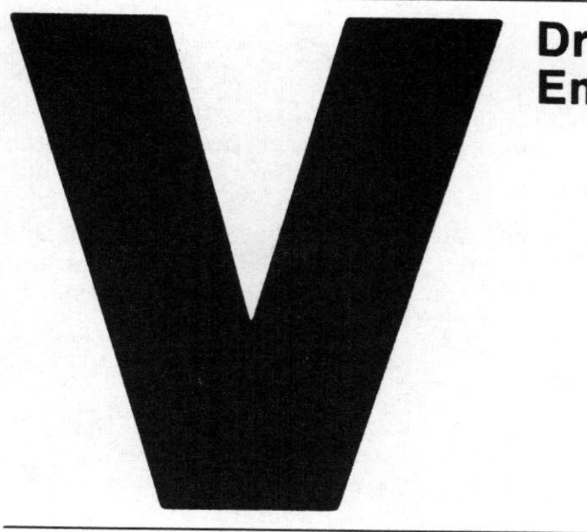

Drug Abuse Emergencies

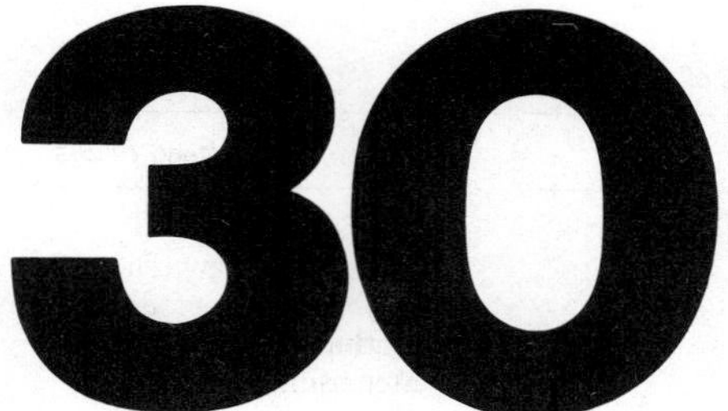

Intoxication and Withdrawal Syndromes

Roger D. Weiss
Shelly F. Greenfield
Steven M. Mirin

The emergency psychiatrist is frequently called on to evaluate a patient who may have developed complications of drug abuse. The manifestations of drug-related problems are protean; virtually all types of alteration in mood, perception, and cognition can be produced by abuse of psychoactive substances. Recognition of common intoxication and withdrawal syndromes is critical in formulating a differential diagnosis of psychiatric emergencies. The major drugs of abuse to be discussed include opioids, sedative-hypnotics, stimulants, hallucinogens, phencyclidine (PCP), and marijuana. Some of the more frequently abused drugs are listed in Table 30-1.

I. Opioids

A. General considerations. The most commonly abused opioid drugs are the semisynthetic derivatives of morphine, including heroin, hydromorphone (Dilaudid), and oxycodone (component of Percodan and of Percocet). Opioid abusers generally seek medical attention because of overdose (see Chap. 32), withdrawal, or medical or psychosocial complications related to drug use (e.g., HIV infection, hepatitis, or endocarditis).

B. Intoxication. Except in the case of overdose, patients rarely seek medical attention because of opioid intoxication. Symptoms include euphoria, mental clouding, a sense of tranquility, and drowsiness. Pupillary constriction is prominent; central respiratory depression is the major danger from an overdose.

C. Withdrawal

1. **Clinical manifestations.** Abstinence symptoms may occur as early as 6 hours after stopping heroin. Early symptoms include anxiety, insomnia, yawning, sweating, rhinorrhea, and lacrimation. As withdrawal progresses, dilated pupils, gooseflesh, and tremor may appear; the patient may complain of chills, anorexia, and cramps in the abdomen and legs. Eighteen to 24 hours after the last dose, blood pressure, pulse, respiratory rate, and temperature may rise, and the patient may experience nausea and vomiting. Diarrhea and dehydration sometimes occur after 24–36 hours. Peak symptoms occur 48–72 hours after the last dose, sometimes accompanied by leukocytosis, ketosis, and electrolyte imbalance. Most gross clinical symptoms disappear within 7–10 days. However, patients may complain of insomnia and malaise for days to weeks afterward.

2. **Treatment**

   a. **Methadone.** The crucial guiding principle in treating opioid withdrawal is to attend to objective clinical signs rather than symptoms. When signs of withdrawal occur (Table 30-2), oral administration of methadone 10 mg should reverse them. Methadone should be administered when two of the four criteria listed in Table 30-2 are fulfilled. The evaluation procedure should be repeated every 4 hours, and methadone adminis-

Table 30-1. Drugs of abuse

Drug class	Commonly abused drugs
Opioids	Heroin Hydromorphone (Dilaudid) Oxycodone (Percodan, Percocet) Methadone (Dolophine) Meperidine (Demerol)
Sedative-hypnotics	Benzodiazepines Barbiturates Methaqualone (Quaalude) Meprobamate (Miltown) Glutethimide (Doriden) Ethchlorvynol (Placidyl)
Central nervous system stimulants	Cocaine Amphetamine
Hallucinogens	LSD Mescaline Psilocybin MDMA ("ecstasy")
Arylcyclohexylamines	Phencyclidine (PCP, or "angel dust")
Cannabinoids	Marijuana Hashish

Table 30-2. Diagnosis and treatment of opioid withdrawal

Objective signs of opioid withdrawal
- Pulse 10 beats/min over baseline* or > 90 in the absence of history of tachycardia if baseline unknown
- Systolic blood pressure > 10 mm Hg over baseline or > 160/95 in the absence of known hypertension
- Dilated pupils
- Sweating, gooseflesh, rhinorrhea, or lacrimation

Treatment
- Administer methadone, 10 mg PO q4h prn, when two of the four criteria above are met; decrease by 5 mg/day to zero

**Baseline* refers to the patient's vital signs 1 hour after receiving 10 mg of methadone. For a patient who has received no methadone, these baseline vital signs should be estimated according to what one would expect from the patient's age, sex, and general health.

tered as often as necessary for 24 hours. Only rarely should a patient receive more than 40 mg of methadone during this period, unless he or she has been maintained on methadone at higher doses prior to the detoxification. The total dose of methadone administered during the first 24 hours (the stabilization dose) should be given the next day in two divided doses and should then be tapered by 5 mg/day, beginning with the morning dose, until the patient has been completely withdrawn. All methadone should be dispensed in crushed or liquid form and should be consumed under direct supervision in order to avoid illegal diversion of the drug onto the street. If there is mixed dependence on both opioid and sedative-hypnotics, the patient should be temporarily maintained on methadone and withdrawn from the sedative-hypnotics first.

b. Clonidine

(1) In the last several years, it has been noted that clonidine, an alpha-2-adrenergic agonist used to treat hypertension, could suppress or reverse the symptoms of opioid withdrawal. One advantage of clonidine is the fact that, unlike methadone, it has less (although some) abuse liability and is therefore not a controlled substance. Clonidine may be used either instead of or in addition to methadone during detoxification. Following a test dose of 0.025 or 0.05 mg, clonidine is usually initiated at a dose of 0.15–0.3 mg/day in three divided doses. The specific dose is adjusted to reduce withdrawal symptoms as much as possible without causing hypotension. The drug is usually withheld if a patient's blood pressure drops below 90/60 mm Hg. After stabilization on clonidine for between 4 (for short-acting opioids such as meperidine or heroin) and 14 days (for methadone), the drug is tapered over 4–6 days.

(2) Although clonidine offers some advantages over methadone, there are some patients who obtain very little symptomatic relief from clonidine; the high degree of sedation and hypotension produced makes it intolerable for some patients. In addition, the common complaint of insomnia in withdrawing opioid addicts is often not well controlled by clonidine. Also, certain medical conditions may preclude the use of clonidine; these include cardiac disorders or renal or metabolic diseases. Finally, the use of clonidine in the treatment of opioid withdrawal is not approved by the Food and Drug Administration at the time of this writing.

(3) In a number of studies, rapid withdrawal from opioids has been safely accomplished by precipitating withdrawal using low doses of naltrexone hydrochloride and treating the abstinence syndrome with clonidine. Although not standard therapy at this time, this approach holds promise for achieving rapid detoxification from opioids.

c. Several studies have demonstrated that **buprenorphine,** a mixed opioid agonist-antagonist, may block opioid withdrawal symptoms at low doses (2–4 mg/day). Further work with this drug is required before it can be recommended for widespread use.

II. Sedative-hypnotics

A. General considerations. Unlike the opioid addicts, a significant number of individuals dependent on sedative-hypnotics are not members of a drug-using subculture; rather, many of these patients have become addicted to these drugs as a result of a legitimate but misguided attempt to treat symptoms of insomnia or anxiety. A subgroup of sedative abusers are younger, abuse other drugs, and rely on illicit sources of supply. These patients are more likely to use drugs intravenously and to use extremely high doses (e.g., >100 mg diazepam/day).

B. Intoxication. Intoxication with sedative-hypnotics, by itself, rarely leads patients to seek medical attention except in the case of overdose (see Chap. 32, sec. **IV**), in which case respiratory depression is the primary danger. Nevertheless, individuals who have taken sedative-hypnotics may be disinhibited, belligerent, and at times, violent. Mild to moderate intoxication closely resembles alcoholic drunkenness without alcoholic breath. Slurred speech, lack of motor coordination, drowsiness, and slowed thinking are common symptoms. Nystagmus and ataxia are often seen on physical examination.

C. Withdrawal. The severity of the withdrawal syndrome from sedative-hypnotics depends on a number of factors, including the daily dose taken, the duration of use, the elimination half-life (e.g., long versus short half-life benzodiazepines), potency, and rate of taper (gradual versus abrupt). In some cases, withdrawal from sedative-hypnotics should be considered a medical emergency. It may lead to seizures, delirium, and in severe cases, death. For this reason, withdrawal from sedative-hypnotics should be carried out in a hospital setting when the daily dose taken is unknown (Table 30-3).

1. **Clinical manifestations.** Onset of withdrawal symptoms depends on the duration of action of the drug used. In the case of short-acting benzodiazepines or barbiturates, symptoms may appear 12–16 hours after the last dose; with a long-acting drug like diazepam, symptoms may not appear until as late as 7–10 days after the last dose. Early withdrawal symptoms include anxiety, restlessness, anorexia, nausea, and vomiting. Later, patients may complain of weakness and abdominal cramps and may develop tachycardia, postural hypotension, hyperreflexia, and a gross resting tremor that is most prominent in the upper extremities. Insomnia and nightmares frequently occur. Peak withdrawal symptoms from short-acting, sedative-hypnotics occur 1–3 days after the last dose; generalized seizures may occur within this period. About half of those patients who develop seizures will develop delirium characterized by disorientation, anxiety, and visual hallucinations.

Table 30-3. Diagnosis and treatment of sedative-hypnotic withdrawal

Clinical manifestations

Mild: agitation, anxiety, anorexia, nausea, vomiting, tachycardia, postural hypotension, hyperreflexia, tremor

Severe: seizures, delirium, hypothermia, cardiovascular collapse

Management

1. If total daily dose is known, the drug can be gradually tapered.
2. If total daily dose is unknown, there is significant morbidity and mortality associated with withdrawal, making hospitalization mandatory in most cases. Pentobarbital tolerance test and detoxification:

Day 1

When the patient is no longer intoxicated, give pentobarbital 200 mg PO.

If intoxication results (nystagmus, ataxia, or dysarthria), patient's 6-hour pentobarbital requirement is 100–200 mg. If patient *falls asleep,* he or she was probably not addicted.

If no intoxication, give an additional 100 mg PO q2h until intoxication develops.

Total dose required to produce intoxication is the patient's 6-hour requirement.

Multiply by 4 to calculate 24-hour pentobarbital requirement.

Phenobarbital substitution. After 24-hour pentobarbital requirement is calculated, substitute phenobarbital 30 mg for each 100 mg of pentobarbital. Give this amount of phenobarbital in three divided doses for 48 hours.

Day 2

Give 24-hour phenobarbital requirement as given on day 1.

Day 3 and thereafter

Subtract 30 mg/day of phenobarbital (beginning with the A.M. dose) from the total dose given on day 1 until the patient is detoxified. If signs of intoxication develop, eliminate a single dose and resume treatment 6–8 hours later. If signs of withdrawal develop, give 60–120 mg of phenobarbital PO or IM immediately.

Mixed opioid-sedative dependence. Maintain temporarily on methadone and withdraw the patient from sedatives first, then from methadone.

2. Treatment

a. **Gradual taper.** If the total daily dose of sedative-hypnotics is reliably known, it is often possible to taper the daily dose gradually. For example, gradual weekly reduction of long-term therapeutic doses of benzodiazepines by no more than 25% per week may result in a safe withdrawal (i.e., no precipitated seizures, psychosis, delirium) but will result in some mild to moderate withdrawal symptoms in 90% of patients who have had long-term use of both longer- and shorter-acting benzodiazepines. Withdrawal symptoms might include anxiety, insomnia, tremulousness, irritability, fatigue, lethargy, and dysphoria. There has been some preliminary evidence that pretreatment with carbamazepine at dosages of 200–800 mg qd may decrease withdrawal symptoms when a gradual taper is then undertaken. However, these data are somewhat controversial. The exact rate of weekly dose reduction must be determined according to the specific drug and the patient's symptoms. For example, the *Physician's Desk Reference* recommends that the daily dose of alprazolam be decreased by no more than 0.5 mg every 3 days to avoid withdrawal seizures. Since even this schedule is very uncomfortable for some long-term, high-dose users, some authors have recommended gradually switching from alprazolam to clonazepam and then tapering the patient off the latter drug. In a hospital setting, on the other hand, where frequent monitoring of vital signs and clinical status is possible, a considerably more rapid taper may be attempted.

b. When the dosage of drug is not known, or when the patient is dependent on several sedative-hypnotics simultaneously, a longer-acting drug to which the patient is cross-tolerant may be substituted for the drug(s) of abuse; the patient is then gradually withdrawn from the longer-acting drug. For the sedative-hypnotics, the drug of choice for this procedure is **phenobarbital.** To determine the initial dose of phenobarbital, a pentobarbital tolerance test is performed.

c. **Pentobarbital tolerance test.** When the patient is no longer intoxicated he or she is given pentobarbital 200 mg PO. One hour later he or she is examined for signs of sedative intoxication: nystagmus, slurred speech, ataxia, or sedation. Nystagmus on lateral gaze is often the earliest indicator of intoxication. If the patient is intoxicated after receiving 200 mg, he or she probably has been taking less than the equivalent of 800 mg of pentobarbital daily. Therefore he or she can be stabilized on a dose of 100–200 mg of pentobarbital every 6 hours (depending on the degree of intoxication). If the patient promptly falls asleep, it is likely that he or she has no tolerance to the drug and will not need detoxification. If the patient shows no response to 200 mg, it can be assumed that tolerance has been produced by daily use of an equivalent of more than 800 mg of pentobarbital. Therefore, the patient is given an additional 100 mg of pentobarbital every 2 hours until he or she becomes intoxicated, at which time the test is stopped. The maximum dose of pentobarbital that should be given is 500 mg. The total dose required to produce intoxication comprises the patient's 6-hour requirement of pentobarbital; this dose should be multiplied by 4 to calculate the patient's 24-hour pentobarbital requirement. Phenobarbital can then be substituted for pentobarbital by giving 30 mg of phenobarbital for each 100 mg of pentobarbital required. Over the next 2 days, the 24-hour phenobarbital requirement is given in three divided doses each day. Thereafter the dose is decreased by 30 mg/day until the patient is totally withdrawn. If signs of withdrawal emerge, an additional 60–120 mg of phenobarbital can be given immediately IM and the total daily dose of phenobarbital increased accordingly. Phenobarbital should not be administered in a dose exceeding 500 mg/day.

d. **Case example.** A patient is given 200 mg of pentobarbital and is examined 1 hour later. He shows no signs of intoxication. He is therefore given an additional 100 mg of pentobarbital and over the next 2 hours still has no response. He is given an additional 100 mg of pentobarbital and examined 1 hour after this third dose. At this time he displays nystagmus on lateral gaze. Because of this sign of pentobarbital intoxication, the test is stopped. His 6-hour pentobarbital requirement (the total amount necessary to cause intoxication) is 400 mg. His 24-hour pentobarbital requirement is 400 × 4 = 1600 mg. His 24-hour phenobarbital requirement is 30% of 1600 mg, or 480 mg. He is started on a regimen of phenobarbital 160 mg PO tid. Two days later the physician begins to taper the phenobarbital by 30 mg/day, beginning with the morning dose, until the patient has completed his detoxification.

e. **Mixed opioid-sedative dependence.** Simultaneous abuse of more than one class of psychoactive drug is common. Although there is no cross-tolerance between opioids and sedatives, the latter drugs may partially alleviate the symptoms of opioid withdrawal. Therefore, heroin addicts and patients on methadone maintenance may also abuse sedatives and alcohol. However, neither methadone nor heroin will prevent sedative withdrawal. If mixed opioid-sedative dependence is suspected, the clinician should determine the degree of sedative dependence using the pentobarbital tolerance test. Following this, the patient should be maintained on a dose of methadone sufficient to prevent symptoms of opioid withdrawal while gradually tapering the sedative. Assuming that the patient wishes to be detoxified from opioids, this procedure would then occur.

III. Central nervous system stimulants

A. Amphetamine

1. **General considerations.** Amphetamine and its related compounds are sympathomimetic agents that have both peripheral adrenergic as well as central stimulatory effects. The most commonly abused amphetamine is dextroamphetamine; other derivatives include methamphetamine, methylphenidate, phenmetrazine, and diethylpropion. A smokeable form of D-methamphetamine, known as "ice," has gained favor in the past several years, particularly in California and Hawaii.

2. **Intoxication.** Serious toxic reactions from acute ingestion of amphetamine occur primarily in infrequent users who ingest large doses (e.g., more than 60 mg/day). The intoxication syndrome is characterized by restlessness, irritability, tremor, confusion, talkativeness, anxiety, and lability of mood. Peripheral effects may include headache, chills, vomiting, drug mouth, and sweating. In severe cases, there may be auditory or visual hallucinations, seizures, and hyperpyrexia.

3. **Treatment** of acute amphetamine toxicity includes reducing central nervous system (CNS) irritability and autonomic nervous system hyperactivity, controlling psychotic symptoms, and promoting rapid excretion of the drug and its metabolites. Fevers of greater than 102°F should be treated vigorously. Seizures that may occur with amphetamine toxicity should be treated with diazepam 5–10 mg IV at a rate not exceeding 5 mg/minute. This can be repeated every 10 or 15 minutes as necessary, up to a total dose of 30 mg. CNS irritability can be further reduced by decreasing stimulation. Excretion of amphetamine can be enhanced by acidification of the urine. If there are no signs of liver or kidney failure, ammonium chloride 500 mg PO may be given every 3–4 hours. Psychotic symptoms may accompany acute amphetamine toxicity; these may be treated by a dopamine-blocking agent such as haloperidol. There is some evidence that chlorpromazine should not be used because it may slow the metabolism of amphetamine.

4. **Withdrawal.** Without treatment, symptoms of acute amphetamine toxicity will usually resolve within 1 week. The withdrawal period may be characterized by dysphoria, irritability, anxiety, fatigue, sleep disturbance, hyperphagia, psychomotor agitation, and rebound increase in rapid eye movement (REM) sleep. As recovery progresses, it is necessary to monitor the patient's level of depression and suicide potential. If depressive symptoms do not remit, antidepressant treatment should be considered.

B. Cocaine

1. **General considerations.** Cocaine, or benzoylmethylecgonine, is an alkaloid derived from the coca plant, *Erythroxylon coca*. Cocaine exerts stimulatory effects on the cerebral cortex and produces feelings of excitation, restlessness, euphoria, decreased social inhibitions, increased energy, and enhanced strength and mental ability. It also causes central and peripheral sympathomimetic effects such as vasoconstriction, tachycardia, increased blood pressure and temperature, and dilated pupils. Tolerance to the cardiovascular and behavioral effects of cocaine has been demonstrated.

2. **Forms of cocaine use.** Cocaine hydrochloride may be prepared as a powder and inhaled. A euphoric effect is produced in seconds to minutes, peaks in 10 minutes, and lasts 45–60 minutes or longer (Table 30-4). Cocaine hydrochloride may also be dissolved in water without heating it and then injected intravenously. This produces an effect within 15 seconds, peaking in 5 minutes, and lasting up to 15 minutes. Finally, cocaine may be smoked, most commonly in the form of alkaloidal (freebase) cocaine. Freebase ("crack") is prepared by adding a strong base, such as baking soda, to an aqueous solution of cocaine hydrochloride. Smoking cocaine produces an effect beginning in 6–12 seconds, peaking at 3–5 minutes, and lasting 10–20 minutes.

3. **Intoxication** (Table 30-5). There are three clinical phases in acute cocaine toxicity.

   a. The **first phase,** acute cocaine intoxication, is characterized by stimulation of the central nervous and cardiopulmonary systems. The patient feels the typical central stimulatory effects of euphoria, increased mental ability, and self-confidence. Peripheral effects include vasoconstriction and other symptoms of adrenergic stimulation, including an increase in blood pressure, pulse, and temperature. Pupils are often dilated. High doses of cocaine or amphetamine may lead to peculiar repetitive stereotyped behaviors, emotional lability, and paranoid psychosis with auditory, visual, or tactile hallucinations.

   b. In the **second phase,** there may be decreased responsiveness to all stimuli, increased deep tendon reflexes, incontinence, generalized seizures and status epilepticus, and malignant encephalopathy. Severe tachycardia, hypertension, and hyperthermia may be noted. Ventricular

Table 30-4. Time course of cocaine effects

Route of administration	Onset of mood change	Peak effects	Postdrug dysphoria
Intranasal (snorting)	Seconds–2 minutes	10 minutes	45–60 minutes
IV	Seconds	3–5 minutes	15 minutes
Smoking freebase or crack	Seconds	3–5 minutes	10–20 minutes

Table 30-5. Diagnosis and treatment of central nervous system (CNS) stimulant intoxication

Clinical manifestations
- Moderate: euphoria, restlessness, talkativeness, repetitive stereotyped behavior, bruxism, irritability, tremor, emotional lability
- Severe: tachycardia, hypertension, mydriasis, grand mal seizures, hyperthermia, paranoid delusions, hallucinations (auditory, visual, or tactile), ideas of reference, violent behavior

Treatment
- Reduce CNS irritability.
  - Treat high fevers vigorously with ice baths.
  - For seizures give diazepam 5–10 mg IV, injected no faster than 5 mg/minute.
- Decrease sympathetic nervous system overactivity.
  - Propranolol 1 mg IV injected slowly may be helpful for cocaine toxicity that has resulted in severe hypertension and tachycardia; up to 8 mg may be given, but very slowly. (There is some controversy regarding the effectiveness of this treatment and the possibility of causing increased hypertension). If there are no significant tachyarrhythmias, consider other treatments such as sedation, nitroprusside, or phentolamine.

Promote drug excretion.
- For amphetamine toxicity, acidify urine with ammonium chloride 500 mg PO q4h if renal and hepatic function are normal.

Decrease psychotic symptoms
- Haloperidol 5 mg may be given PO. Low-dose antipsychotics such as chlorpromazine should not be used in amphetamine toxicity, because it may slow metabolism of amphetamine.

---

dysrhythmias may produce a fall in blood pressure and pulse with peripheral cyanosis and rapid, irregular respirations.

c. The **third, or premorbid, phase** is characterized by flaccid paralysis of muscles, coma, fixed and dilated pupils, loss of reflexes, loss of vital support functions and paralysis of respiration. Cardiac arrest, ventricular fibrillation, and respiratory arrest at this phase may result in death.

4. Treatment

a. Patients with **phase I** acute cocaine intoxication may be safely observed and monitored in an emergency department until the symptoms abate. The major goals in the management of this phase of cocaine toxicity are the reduction of CNS irritability, sympathetic nervous system overactivity, and psychotic symptoms, while hastening the excretion of the drug. Diazepam or haloperidol is preferred for the treatment of agitation, but physical restraints may also be necessary.

b. For **more severe toxicity,** the goals of therapy are support of the respiratory system, control of hypertension, management of malignant cardiac dysrhythmias, correction of metabolic acidosis, and aggressive control of hyperthermia and seizure activity. Diazepam 5–10 mg IV injected at a rate not exceeding 5 mg/minute can be used to treat seizures. Care should be taken to protect the patient's airway, and resuscitation equipment should be available in case the diazepam causes respiratory depression or arrest. Metabolic acidosis is generally corrected by controlling seizures, agitation, and cardiovascular derangements; the role of sodium bicarbonate is unclear. Some clinicians advocate treating significant sympathetic nervous system hyperactivity with propranolol 1 mg IV, injected slowly every minute up to a total of 8 mg; however, beta blockers like propranolol must be used cautiously because of the possibility of worsened hypertension. In the absence of hemodynamically significant tachyarrhythmias, other therapeutic agents such as sedation, nitroprusside, or phentolamine may be used to control tachycardia and hypertension.

5. **Withdrawal.** Recent studies have not supported the earlier theory of a cocaine abstinence syndrome characterized by the three phases, "crash," "withdrawal," and "extinction." Instead it appears that abstinence symptoms following cessation of cocaine use in those with uncomplicated cocaine dependence are relatively mild and decrease steadily over the first month, without medical treatment. A number of different agents have been tried to treat cocaine craving, although there is, at this time, no generally agreed on medication for this purpose.

IV. Hallucinogens

A. General considerations.

The hallucinogens are a group of agents of similar structure that produce perceptual changes (primarily visual hallucinations and illusions) and enhanced awareness of internal and external stimuli. Pharmacologically, the commonly abused hallucinogenic substances can be divided into three major groups. The indolealkylamines include D-lysergic acid diethylamide (LSD), psilocybin, and dimethyltryptamine (DMT), which bear a structural resemblance to the neurotransmitter 5-hydroxytryptamine (serotonin). The phenylethylamines include mescaline and phenylisopropylamines such as 2,5-dimethoxy-4-methylamphetamine (DOM, "STP") and are structurally related to dopamine, norepinephrine, and the amphetamines. The "designer drugs," MDMA ("ecstasy") and MDEA ("eve"), are hallucinogens with some amphetamine-like sympathomimetic effects.

B. Intoxication

1. **Intoxication from LSD** may occur at doses as low as 50 μg. The drug is usually taken orally, either as part of a pill or dissolved on a piece of paper. Absorption from the gastrointestinal tract is good; the plasma half-life is 2–3 hours. Within an hour of ingestion, patients develop sympathomimetic effects, including an increase in pulse, body temperature, blood pressure, and pupil size. Two to 3 hours after ingestion, peak effects occur; visual illusions, wavelike perceptual changes, and emotional lability are the predominant symptoms. Patients may describe peculiar phenomena, called synesthesias, in which the boundaries between sensory perceptions become blurred; colors are "heard," noises "seen." Perception of time may be distorted, and depersonalization may occur. Drug effects begin to wane 4–6 hours after ingestion; after 8–12 hours most of the symptoms have cleared, although patients may describe feelings of psychic "numbness" for several days.

2. **Intoxication from MDMA or MDEA** produces an initial phase of disorientation. This is followed by a "rush," which may be accompanied by spasmodic jerking of the muscles and then a feeling of happy sociability. The effects wear off in 4–6 hours, and some users have reported subsequent confusion, anxiety, and depression.

3. While **death** from an overdose of LSD appears quite rare, ingestion of high levels of MDMA or MDEA might carry significantly higher risk of death from hyperthermia, cardiovascular collapse, and convulsions.

C. Adverse reactions (Table 30-6)

1. **Panic reaction or bad trip.** An episode of panic is by far the most common adverse reaction following the use of LSD or other hallucinogens. Factors

Table 30-6. Adverse reactions to hallucinogens

Reaction	Symptoms	Duration	Treatment
Panic or bad trip	Fear of going crazy; severe anxiety	2–24 hours	Reassurance. Call in friends if possible. Rarely, diazepam 10–30 mg PO. Avoid anticholinergic medications.
Delirium	Delusions, hallucinations, paranoia, agitation, confusion, inadvertent suicide attempts (e.g., trying to fly)	2–24 hours	Reassurance, support, protection of patient. Do not leave alone. Diazepam 15–30 mg PO initially, then 5–20 mg q4h if necessary
Drug-precipitated psychosis	Symptoms of mania, depression, or schizophrenia; usually disorder already present	Indefinite	Treatment appropriate to the underlying disorder
Recurrent drug experience or flashback	Emotional lability, perceptual distortions, depersonalization, often similar to prior drug experiences; may occur for months after last drug use	Seconds to hours	Reassurance

that influence the likelihood of a panic reaction include the setting in which the drug is taken, the dose and type of drug administered, and the user's expectations and level of emotional health. Those at high risk include inexperienced users who are isolated and anxious and users who have difficulty dealing with the loss of control and disorganizing effects these drugs produce. Taking the drugs in a familiar setting with supportive companions who are familiar with the drug decreases the likelihood of a bad trip. The most important treatment of a panic reaction is to support the patient. The patient should be reassured that he or she is not "going crazy" and that his or her mind will return to normal when the drug wears off. These patients should not be left alone. Soliciting the help of calm, supportive friends can be very effective. If support and reassurance are not sufficient and the patient is extremely agitated, diazepam 10–30 mg PO may be helpful. Medications with anticholinergic properties should be avoided because hallucinogens are often adulterated ("cut") with anticholinergic compounds before being sold on the street. In general, however, psychotropic medication is not necessary. Most panic reactions end within 24 hours as the hallucinogen is eliminated from the body.

2. **Delirium.** Some hallucinogen users experience an acute toxic confusional state characterized by hallucinations, delusions, agitation, disorientation, and paranoia. In this state, assaults and inadvertent suicide attempts may occur. Absence of a history of mental disorder and visual rather than auditory hallucinations suggest a diagnosis of toxic drug reaction rather than schizophrenia or mania. The major goal of treatment is to support the patient until the drug is eliminated. Psychotropic medications should be given with great caution so as not to confuse the clinical picture. If they are used, a drug with few anticholinergic side effects is preferable. Diazepam 15–30 mg PO, repeating 5–20 mg every 4 hours as needed, may be given. It may be best to avoid chlorpromazine or other antipsychotic drugs. Physical restraint may be necessary to prevent the patient from harming self or others. Untreated cases generally clear within 24 hours as the drug is metabolized and excreted.

3. **Drug-precipitated psychosis.** On occasion, patients who develop psychotic symptoms on hallucinogens continue to display these symptoms long after the drug is excreted. This may occur particularly in patients with underlying affective disorders or schizophrenia, some of whom use these drugs in the hope of achieving some kind of psychic reintegration. Treatment should include cautious use of neuroleptic drugs, lithium carbonate, or antidepressants, depending on the underlying disorder. When the patient's acute psychosis has subsided, attention should be focused on the reasons for drug use.

4. **Post-hallucinogen perception disorder ("flashbacks").** Patients may experience the spontaneous recurrence of drug effects a few days to several months after the last drug experience. These flashbacks may last a few seconds to several hours and may be precipitated by stress, use of other drugs such as marijuana or stimulants, and a number of other stimuli. The symptoms can sometimes be brought on by intention. The most frequent flashbacks are visual hallucinations, perceptions in the peripheral visual fields, flashes or trails of color, trailing color, positive afterimages, halos around objects, macropsia, and micropsia. Other symptoms include feelings of depersonalization, paresthesias, auditory trailing, and emotional lability. Approximately half of the people with this disorder experience remission within months; however, 50% may experience such symptoms for at least 5 years. In most cases, treatment consists of reassurance that the flashback will pass. For those individuals who continue to experience perceptual difficulties, there is no known treatment for this problem.

D. **Withdrawal.** Hallucinogens do not produce physical dependence or a withdrawal syndrome.

V. Phencyclidine

A. **General considerations.** Phencyclidine (PCP, or "angel dust"), an arylcyclohexylamine, was originally developed as a human anesthetic, but its use in humans was discontinued because it induced psychotic and hallucinatory reactions. It is now legally used only in veterinary medicine as a tranquilizer. In addition to the people who knowingly use PCP, others unknowingly take the drug in the form of adulterated marijuana, heroin, or LSD. Individuals who complain of adverse reactions to these drugs should, therefore, be examined for potential PCP toxicity as well. PCP poses a public health problem, since its use can predispose to accidents, violence, and suicide. Indeed, PCP-related deaths and emergencies have increased. Street samples of the drug have been shown to contain nearly 30 analogues of PCP, many of which are more potent than PCP itself. An individual who has used phencyclidine may experience stimulant, depressant, hallucinogenic, or analgesic effects, depending on the dose and mode of administration. Most often the drug is smoked with tobacco or marijuana, but it can be taken orally, intranasally, or intravenously. The serum half-life is about 45 minutes at low doses but may be as long as 3 days after an overdose because of sequestration in adipose tissue and the brain.

B. Intoxication (Table 30-7). At low doses of 5 mg or less, the effects of phencyclidine resemble intoxication with CNS depressants. Muscular incoordination and nystagmus are prominent. Patients may describe blurred vision and numbness in their extremities; they often appear to be staring blankly into space. At doses of 5–10 mg, slurred speech, nystagmus, ataxia, increased muscle tone, hyperreflexia, and catalepsy may be seen. Doses of 10–20 mg can produce psychosis and catatonia. An overdose of greater than 20 mg may lead to seizures, hypertensive crisis, respiratory depression, coma, and death. Subjectively PCP causes feelings of dissociation, perceptual distortions, and occasionally auditory or visual hallucinations. While some users become euphoric, feelings of anxiety and depression are quite common. In the emergency room setting, patients are generally brought in by others because of bizarre behavior. These patients may exhibit confusion and physical or verbal aggressiveness, which may progress from anger to violence. They may exhibit a variety of motor disturbances, including posturing or catatonia. Increased bronchial and salivary secretions are commonly seen, as are horizontal nystagmus, ataxia, slurred speech, and systolic hypertension. Any patient exhibiting bizarre behavior accompanied by hypertension, nystagmus, and drooling must be suspected of PCP intoxication. The effects of phencyclidine generally last 4–6 hours, often followed by amnesia for the period of intoxication.

C. Treatment for PCP intoxication. The two goals of treatment should be, first, to keep the patient and the staff safe while the drug is being excreted and, second,

Table 30-7. Diagnosis and treatment of reactions to phencyclidine (PCP)

Reaction	Clinical presentation	Treatment
Intoxication	Nystagmus, hypertension, drooling, ataxia, dysarthria, numbness, hyperreflexia, posturing, auditory or visual hallucinations, occasionally violence	Keep patient and staff safe. Use quiet room. Do not try to "talk patient down." Diazepam, 10–20 mg PO if necessary to calm patient. Use carefully. Monitor until vital signs stable and patient calm.
Psychosis	May last days to weeks, rarely for months. Usually three stages, each lasting 5 days: 1. Paranoia, delusions, hyperactivity, assaultiveness 2. Paranoia, restlessness; patient somewhat calmer 3. Gradual resolution of symptoms	Keep patient and staff safe. Use quiet room. Do not try to "talk patient down." Treat psychosis, e.g., use haloperidol cautiously at doses of 5 mg IM every hour as needed. Promote drug excretion. Acidify urine with ammonium chloride to pH < 5.

to treat any complications that may arise. Treatment differs from that for panic reactions from hallucinogens or marijuana since a patient on PCP may be made worse by trying to "talk him or her down." The patient should be placed in isolation in a quiet room to decrease the amount of external stimulation. If the patient is combative or self-destructive, restraints may be needed. Diazepam, 10–20 mg PO may be given if necessary to calm the patient. However, this should be done judiciously since the patient may have also ingested other drugs including CNS depressants. All patients should be monitored until their vital signs are stable and they are fully oriented and calm. Most patients improve within several hours after taking PCP.

D. **PCP-induced psychosis** (see Table 30-7). Some individuals who ingest PCP develop a psychotic reaction that may last for days or weeks. While this happens more often in individuals who have not used PCP previously, it may also occur in regular users. Patients with a past history of psychotic episodes are more vulnerable to this complication. The PCP-induced psychosis may be divided into three phases, each lasting about 5 days. During the initial phase, which is the most severe, the patient may be paranoid, delusional, hyperactive, and unpredictably assaultive. In the second phase, the patient begins to calm down and gain some control over behavior, although remaining paranoid and restless. The third phase consists of a gradual resolution of the symptoms, usually within 2–6 weeks. There are some individuals, however, who remain psychotic for months.

E. **Treatment of PCP-induced psychosis.** As in the treatment of simple PCP intoxication, the primary goal is to maintain the physical safety of the patient and those around him or her while attempting to decrease psychotic symptoms and hasten excretion of the drug. The patient should be hospitalized and placed in a quiet room with minimal sensory stimulation. Neuroleptic drugs with few anticholinergic effects, such as haloperidol, may be helpful, though many patients respond slowly. Haloperidol may be given 5 mg IM every hour as needed, but high doses should be avoided, because haloperidal may be associated with greater muscle damage in these patients. Low-potency neuroleptics such as chlorpromazine and thioridazine should not be given. If a chemical restraint is needed, it is probably best to use diazepam at a dose of 5–10 mg q4h. Since phencyclidine is a weak base with pK_a of about 8.5, the drug is more soluble in acidic aqueous solutions. Acidification of the urine may therefore speed excretion of the drug. This can be accomplished by administering ammonium chloride, 2.75 mEq/kg in 60 ml of saline solution every 6 hours through a nasogastric tube, along with IV ascorbic acid 2 gm in 500 ml of IV fluid every 6 hours. The urine pH should be kept below 5. Most patients improve after 2–3 weeks.

F. **Withdrawal.** Phencyclidine does not produce physical dependence or a withdrawal syndrome.

VI. Marijuana

A. **General considerations.** Marijuana, derived from the Indian hemp plant *Cannabis sativa,* has been used by over 60 million Americans, including 13% of those between the ages of 12 and 17. The drug is usually smoked but can be ingested orally as well. The major psychoactive component is Δ9-tetrahydrocannabinol (THC). After smoking marijuana, drug effects occur within seconds to minutes, peak in a half-hour, and disappear after approximately 3 hours. After oral administration, onset of action is slower, but the effects last for approximately 3–5 hours.

B. **Intoxication.** The major symptoms of marijuana intoxication include euphoria, relaxation, friendliness, and an alteration in the user's perception of time. The two most common physical signs are tachycardia and conjunctival injection.

There are several adverse reactions that may occur as a result of marijuana use and may prompt an individual to seek medical attention. These reactions are similar to those following hallucinogen use (see sec. **IV.C** and Table 30-6).

1. **Acute panic.** A panic reaction tends to occur in inexperienced users who find the loss of control of their thinking quite frightening. These individuals can be somewhat paranoid, and their thoughts may appear disconnected. Their most frequent fear is that they will "never come down." Treatment consists of reassuring the patient that he or she is not going crazy, that the symptoms have been caused by a strong dose of marijuana, and that they will disappear within several hours. Use of psychotropic medication is unnecessary.

2. **Delirium.** After a large dose of marijuana, patients may become confused and develop feelings of depersonalization and derealization, visual and auditory hallucinations, and paranoia. This syndrome is more common after marijuana is taken orally, perhaps because this may involve higher doses of THC. The treatment again consists of reassurance and close observation so that the patient does not cause harm to self or others.

3. **Recurrent drug experiences or flashbacks.** Though more common in hallucinogen users, flashbacks reminiscent of previous marijuana experiences can occur for up to several months after the last drug use. Patients should be reassured that these will eventually cease if they remain drug-free.

C. Withdrawal. Mild physical dependence has been described in individuals who have used the drug chronically in very high doses. Withdrawal symptoms may include irritability, insomnia, diaphoresis, nausea, and vomiting. No treatment is necessary.

VII. Further evaluation and follow-up treatment for drug abusers. No emergency evaluation of a drug abuser is complete without arranging for follow-up evaluation and treatment. Mere detoxification or emergency treatment of an acute drug reaction does not interrupt the course of the drug abuse problem itself. More definitive ongoing treatment is required, preferably in a setting specifically designed to evaluate and treat drug abuse problems.

Selected Readings

Charney, D. S., et al. Clonidine and naltrexone: A safe, effective, and rapid treatment of abrupt withdrawal from methadone therapy. *Arch. Gen. Psychiatry* 39: 1327, 1982.

Gorelick, D. A., Wilkins, J. N., and Wong, C. Diagnosis and Treatment of Chronic Phencyclidine (PCP) Abuse. In D. H. Clouet (ed.), *Phencyclidine: An Update*. NIDA Research Monograph 64, pp. 218–228, 1986.

Kosten, T. R., and Kleber, H. D. Buprenorphine detoxification from opioid dependence: A pilot study. *Life Sci.* 42:635, 1988.

Kosten, T. R., et al. Rapid detoxification from opioid dependence (Letter). *Arch. Gen. Psychiatry* 146:1349, 1989.

Mirin, S. M., Weiss, R. D., and Greenfield, S. F. Psychoactive Substance Use Disorders. In A. J. Gelenberg, E. L. Bassuk, and S. C. Schoonover (eds.), *A Practitioner's Guide to Psychoactive Drugs* (3rd ed.). New York: Plenum, 1991.

Savitt, D. L., Roberts, J. R., and Merigian, K. S. Psychoactive Drug Abuse. In P. Rosen et al. (eds.), *Emergency Medicine: Concepts and Clinical Practice*. St. Louis: Mosby, 1992. Pp. 2058–2066.

Schuckit, M. A. *Drug and Alcohol Abuse: A Clinical Guide to Diagnosis and Treatment* (3rd ed.). New York: Plenum, 1989.

Schweizer, E., et al. Long-term therapeutic use of benzodiazepines II: Effects of a gradual taper. *Arch Gen. Psychiatry* 47:908, 1990.

Schweizer, E., et al. Carbamazepine treatment in patients discontinuing long-term benzodiazepine therapy. *Arch. Gen. Psychiatry* 48:448, 1991.

Vassallo, S. Cocaine. In: J. E. Tintinalli (ed.), *Emergency Medicine: A Comprehensive Study Guide (3rd ed.)*. New York: McGraw-Hill, 1992. Pp. 579–581.

Weiss, R. D., Mirin, S. M., and Bartel, R. *Cocaine* (2nd ed.). Washington, D.C.: American Psychiatric Press, 1993.

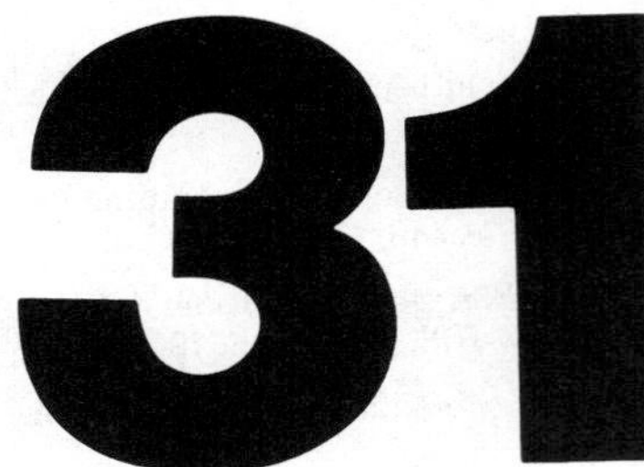

Alcohol-Related Emergencies

Steven E. Hyman

I. A substantial fraction of patients presenting for emergency treatment have alcohol-related problems, including alcohol intoxication and withdrawal, trauma, neurologic complaints, alcohol-related illnesses (such as gastrointestinal bleeding), and depression. In addition, alcohol is involved in at least 50% of fatalities from motor vehicle accidents and is a substantial risk factor in fatal injuries of all types (Anda et al., 1988). Alcohol use is involved in 67% of murders and 33% of suicides, and alcoholism is the **primary psychiatric diagnosis** in 25% of all suicides. Unfortunately, alcoholism is often denied by patients and missed by physicians. The emergency setting may be an ideal time to make the diagnosis and confront the patient with the results of his or her drinking. Therefore the physician must be ready to make the diagnosis and willing to intervene. This chapter focuses on alcohol-related problems that commonly present in the emergency department: intoxication, alcohol-related violence, alcohol withdrawal syndromes, the Wernicke-Korsakoff syndrome, alcoholic ketoacidosis, and toxic interactions of alcohol with disulfiram.

II. The evaluation of the alcohol abuser

A. In addition to determining the specifics of the episode that brought the patient to the emergency department and the relationship of alcohol abuse to the presenting problem, an attempt should be made to understand the patient's pattern of alcohol use and its overall impact on the patient's life. This information will help determine whether the patient is dependent on alcohol and therefore at risk for withdrawal; dependent alcoholics are more likely to have alcohol-related medical problems. It must be recalled, however, that alcohol-related problems are not limited to alcoholics with a high degree of dependence. Nondependent alcohol abusers may be responsible for nearly half of alcohol-related problems due to repeated episodes of intoxication associated with harmful or inappropriate behavior, such as drunk driving, alcohol-related violence, or drunkenness on the job. This latter group will not require detoxification but still require treatment for alcohol abuse.

B. Diagnosis. The clearest definition of alcoholism has been provided by the National Council on Alcoholism and Drug Dependence. Alcoholism is a primary, chronic disease with genetic, psychosocial, and environmental factors influencing its development and manifestations. The disease is often progressive and fatal. **It is characterized by impaired control over drinking, preoccupation with the drug alcohol, use of alcohol despite adverse consequences, and distortions in thinking, most notably denial.** Each of these symptoms may be continuous or periodic.

C. History. If the patient is intoxicated, a detailed history will only be obtainable after the patient has become sober. However, it is important to know about the presenting complaint and acute medical problems when the patient arrives, even if this history has to be obtained again later. For diagnosis, acute medical care, and treatment recommendations, the history should include the following items:

1. Why the patient came to the emergency room at the **present time.**
2. **The drinking history,** including:

a. The pattern of drinking (continuous, binging, or a binge superimposed on chronic use), number of drinking days per week, the amount consumed per drinking day, time and amount of the most recent consumption, and history of use of other drugs or nonbeverage alcohol.

b. Concern about drinking, attempts to control drinking, secretiveness about drinking (e.g., hiding bottles at home or in desk), and history of conflicts about drinking (e.g., with spouse, employers, parents).

3. **A history of physical symptoms directly related to alcohol abuse and withdrawal** including tremors, blackouts, withdrawal seizures, and other withdrawal symptoms.

4. **A medical history** including symptoms that are common sequelae of alcoholism (Table 31-1). It is also important to inquire about prescribed and over-the-counter medications because there may be significant interactions with alcohol (Table 31-2).

5. **Psychosocial problems** that might have resulted from alcoholism including family strife, job problems, financial and housing problems, drunk driving, alcohol-related violence, and arrests.

6. **A history of psychiatric symptoms**, especially depression and anxiety, which either may be causes or, more frequently, sequelae of alcoholism.

Table 31-1. Medical consequences of alcoholism important in emergency medicine

Neurologic and psychiatric
Coma, withdrawal syndromes, Wernicke-Korsakoff syndrome, cerebellar degeneration, hepatic encephalopathy, head injuries and subdural hematoma, depression, anxiety, sleep disorders
Gastrointestinal
Gastritis, esophagitis, ulcers, diarrhea, pancreatitis, hepatitis, cirrhosis and its complications (including esophageal varices)
Hematologic
Macrocytic anemias, thrombocytopenia, coagulopathies (due to decreased hepatic synthetic function)
Infectious
Increased risk of pneumococcal or *Klebsiella* pneumonia, tuberculosis, or aspiration pneumonia
Cardiovascular
Arrhythmias, cardiomyopathy
Metabolic
Hypoglycemia, ketoacidosis, hypomagnesemia, hypophosphatemia

Table 31-2. Significant drug interactions with alcohol

Synergistic central nervous system depressant effects with benzodiazepines, barbiturates and other sedative-hypnotics, antipsychotics, cyclic antidepressants, and opiates
Induction of hepatic enzymes decreasing the effectiveness of phenytoin (Dilantin), tricyclic antidepressants, anticoagulants
Potentiation of hypoglycemic effects of oral antidiabetic agents and insulin
Production of disulfiram-like reaction with metronidazole (Flagyl), griseofulvin, and occasionally oral antidiabetic agents

7. An evaluation of **suicide and violence potential.** Often patients who are profoundly depressed, suicidal or homicidal when intoxicated no longer harbor such feelings after they sober up. Patients who are suicidal only when drunk are not generally commitable to a mental hospital. However, if alcohol-associated dangerousness is a recurrent pattern, the need for treatment must be stressed to the patient.

D. **Physical examination** should include examination for injuries, ecchymoses, jaundice, hepatomegaly, gastrointestinal bleeding, and signs of chronic liver disease such as spider angiomata, testicular atrophy, gynecomastia, and asterixis. Neurologic examination should include tests for ataxia, nystagmus, ophthalmoplegia (signs of Wernicke's encephalopathy), and confusion.

E. **Laboratory tests** should include a urine screen for associated drug use, complete blood count (CBC) with platelet count, glucose, electrolytes, calcium, magnesium, and liver function tests. Albumin and prothrombin time can also be ordered as measures of hepatic synthetic function. A single **alcohol level** provides confirmation that a patient has been drinking but is not informative as to whether the level is on the way up or down. In addition, the significance of the level may be difficult to interpret in tolerant individuals.

1. In nontolerant individuals a level of 100 mg/dl usually results in intoxication and represents the legal level of intoxication in most states. Stupor is usually seen at levels above 300 mg/dl. Levels of 400–500 mg/dl are associated with unconsciousness, and levels above 500–800 mg/dl are associated with death.

2. Alcohol is metabolized at a rate of 7–10 gm/hour, which is about equal to one 1-oz drink of 86 proof per hour.

III. Intoxication

A. Signs of intoxication are disinhibition, slurred speech, ataxia, poor recent memory, poor judgment, and alcoholic breath. Behavioral tolerance develops with chronic alcohol abuse, so that signs of intoxication appear only at higher blood alcohol levels.

B. **The differential diagnosis** of alcohol intoxication includes:

1. Sedative-hypnotic intoxication.
2. Hypoglycemia.
3. Diabetic ketoacidosis.
4. Subdural hematoma; head injury.
5. Postictal states.
6. Hepatic encephalopathy.
7. Encephalitis.
8. Other causes of ataxia (e.g., multiple sclerosis, neurodegenerative disorders).

C. **Coma due to alcohol** should be treated in the same fashion as all drug-related comas, requiring protection of the airway, toxicologic screening for other ingested substances, and meticulous supportive care (see Chap. 32). As soon as blood samples have been drawn, thiamine 100 mg should be given IV as prophylaxis against Wernicke's encephalopathy, and 50 ml of 50% dextrose should be administered IV immediately thereafter because alcohol may cause hypoglycemia. Naloxone (Narcan) 0.01 mg/kg should be given because of the possibility of concomitant opiate use, which would potentiate alcohol-induced central nervous system (CNS) depression.

IV. Referral for treatment

A. When a diagnosis of alcoholism is made, it should be presented to the patient in a direct manner. The clinician's approach should be without chiding or blame. The clinician should focus on concern for the patient using the current admission and any alcohol-associated problems detected in the evaluation as concrete evidence for that concern. For patients with very severe loss of control over alcohol, potentially serious withdrawal symptoms, serious medical problems, or a history of prior outpatient treatment failures, inpatient treatment should be recommended. Otherwise, the option of inpatient or outpatient treatment (which might consist of Alcoholics Anonymous) should be offered to the patient.

B. Many patients will reject the diagnosis and refuse treatment. The clinician should emphasize the evidence that the patient has an alcohol problem and reiterate that alcoholism is a serious medical illness from which the patient is suffering and for which treatment can be very effective. Denying and defensive alcoholics frequently provoke anger in clinicians, but expression of anger is to be avoided. For patients who absolutely refuse treatment, the clinician should offer to be available or at least provide a referral number should the patient change his or her mind.

C. Patients who frequently return to the emergency department intoxicated, who refuse or fail follow-up treatment, and who abuse emergency services require clear limit setting, so long as serious medical problems have been attended to.

V. The belligerent drunk represents a serious problem in the emergency department. The patient's potential for violence must be taken seriously. Certain behavioral measures may help.

A. A show of force often proves calming. Security guards should be present before an attempt is made to interview the patient, although they can usually stand quietly to the side. The patient must not be baited in any way.

B. The interview should be conducted in a nonthreatening manner. The interviewer should be polite and address the patient by his or her proper name. No attempt should be made to reprimand the patient for his or her behavior.

C. An offer of food and a quiet comfortable environment is often helpful in calming the patient. Hot liquids that could be used as a weapon should not be given.

D. For belligerent, potentially violent patients, haloperidol (Haldol) 5 mg PO is often extremely effective. Liquid is preferable to tablets because of more rapid absorption. Low-potency neuroleptics such as chlorpromazine (Thorazine) or thioridazine (Mellaril) should not be given because of the risk of postural hypotension and because they lower the seizure threshold.

E. If the patient is actively violent, restraint and sedation will be necessary (see Chap. 5). Haloperidol 5 mg IM is usually effective in quieting patients in this circumstance. Occasionally a second dose will be needed in 30–60 minutes. Higher doses are almost never necessary. Chronic dosing is not indicated; the risk of side effects far outweighs any benefits. Neither haloperidol nor any other neuroleptic is effective as an agent for detoxification from alcohol.

VI. In tolerant individuals **alcohol withdrawal** can produce symptoms ranging from mild discomfort to a life-threatening delirium.

A. Tolerance to ethanol has two aspects, pharmacodynamic (end-organ effects) and pharmacokinetic (rates of metabolism and elimination).

1. Pharmacodynamic tolerance produces both neuronal adaptation, which predisposes to withdrawal symptoms ("physical dependence"), and behavioral tolerance.

a. Although relatively sustained alcohol levels are necessary for physical dependence to occur, the time course is shorter than most physicians realize and may take only weeks to several months in the most suscepti ble individuals.

b. The severity of the withdrawal syndrome usually reflects the intensity of drinking during the weeks just prior to cessation.

c. Withdrawal can occur with any substantial decline in blood alcohol levels; complete abstinence is not necessary. This may occur especially if an episode of binge drinking is superimposed on a pattern of lower level chronic abuse. Thus the suspicion of alcohol withdrawal must be kept in mind when the clinical syndrome is present even if the patient is still drinking or has measurable blood alcohol levels.

2. Pharmacokinetic tolerance results in an increased rate of metabolism.

3. Alcohol exhibits **cross-tolerance** with barbiturates, benzodiazepines, and other sedative-hypnotics such as meprobamate and chloral hydrate. Thus patients tolerant to alcohol will also be relatively tolerant to these other drugs and vice versa. The phenomenon of cross-tolerance is exploited in detoxification protocols; benzodiazepines can be used to safely withdraw a patient from alcohol. Drugs that do not exhibit cross-tolerance with ethanol such as neuroleptics or beta-adrenergic blockers, are not effective as sole agents of detoxification.

B. Abstinence may be due to a variery of factors including:

1. Intercurrent illness, especially gastritis with vomiting.

2. Medical intervention, especially admission to the hospital for an unrelated illness.

3. Lack of funds to buy alcohol.

4. A conscious attempt to decrease or stop alcohol intake.

C. Alcohol withdrawal syndromes may be divided into an early-onset, less severe syndrome, and delirium tremens, a severe syndrome usually of later onset that occurs in only a small percentage of patients. There is overlap in some of the symptoms that characterize these syndromes.

D. Although less severe than delirium tremens, **the early-onset withdrawal syndrome** can result in significant morbidity and discomfort. It usually begins within the first 24 hours of abstinence (90% of cases), often beginning within 6–8 hours of a substantial decline in blood alcohol levels. In a small number of cases the syndrome may begin later, rarely as late as 10 days after the last drink. Once begun, the syndrome varies markedly in duration and severity clearing in hours to up to 2 weeks. Only a few symptoms may be present, or the patient may exhibit the full syndrome.

1. Symptoms and signs

a. Autonomic overactivity

(1) Tachycardia.

(2) Hypertension.

(3) Diaphoresis.

(4) Tremor.

(5) Fever.

(6) Respiratory alkalosis.

b. Sleep disturbance

(1) Sleep latency insomnia.

(2) Increased rapid eye movement (REM) sleep.

(3) Decreased deep sleep (stages 3 and 4).

c. Gastrointestinal

(1) Anorexia.

(2) Nausea and vomiting.

d. Psychologic

(1) Agitation, anxiety.

(2) Restlessness.

(3) Irritability.

(4) Distractability, poor concentration.

(5) Impaired memory.

(6) Impaired judgment.

(7) Hallucinosis (may be calmly tolerated; often visual, but may affect all sensory modalities).

e. Generalized tonic-clonic **seizures.**

2. Treatment of the early-onset syndrome is most safely undertaken in a hospital because significant morbidity may occur.

a. Outpatient treatment may be necessary if resources are limited or if an offer of admission is refused.

(1) Outpatient treatment is contraindicated if the patient has fever above 101°F (38.3°C), seizures, signs of Wernicke-Korsakoff syndrome, inability to hold fluids, or a serious underlying medical disorder. Patients also should not be discharged if severely agitated, hallucinating, or demonstrating poor judgment or suicidality. Patients with a history of severe withdrawal syndromes should also be encouraged to remain in the hospital.

(2) Before discharge, the patient should receive a parenteral dose of thiamine 100 mg and a week's supply of thiamine (50 mg PO), multivitamins, and folate (1 mg PO). A 4-day supply of chlordiazepoxide (Librium) 25 mg qid (or the equivalent) should also be prescribed. If accompanied, a friend or relative can be asked to monitor the severity of symptoms. The patient should be instructed to return to the emergency department if serious withdrawal symptoms emerge. An appointment for outpatient alcohol treatment should also be made, and family members should be encouraged to ensure that the appointment is kept.

b. Inpatient treatment

(1) Thiamine 100 mg IV or IM should be given in the emergency department. The patient should receive 50–100 mg PO or IM daily thereafter. A daily multivitamin and folate should also be prescribed.

(2) Sedation provides symptomatic relief for the patient and makes management easier; it will treat agitation and decrease autonomic overactivity and may prevent progression to delirium tremens.

(a) Although many CNS depressant drugs have been used (including chloral hydrate and paraldehyde) the **benzodiazepines** are the agents of choice because of their safety, ease of administration, and lack of side effects. The major side effect is oversedation.

(b) For patients without significant liver disease, long-acting benzodiazepines, such as chlordiazepoxide or diazepam, have the advantage of requiring less frequent dosing (q4–6h rather than q2–4h) and providing a smoother decline in levels when being tapered. Patients who are elderly or who have significant liver disease as determined by decreased synthetic function (decreased albumin or prolonged prothrombin time) are most safely treated with one of the shorter-acting drugs that lack active metabolites, lorazepam or oxazepam (Serax).

(c) It it best to treat patients as needed (prn) rather than according to an arbitrary fixed dosage. Fixed dosage schedules commonly leave patients undertreated, although patients have widely varying requirements for benzodiazepines: Some patients may be oversedated by 100 mg/day of chlordiazepoxide; others will require more than 1000 mg/day (although total daily doses of more than 400 mg/day of chlordiazepoxide are needed only infrequently). Vital signs and mental status should be monitored every 2 hours, and the benzodiazepine given for objective signs of withdrawal.

(d) Depending on their estimated dosage requirements, patients may be started on 25–50 mg of chlordiazepoxide, 10–20 mg of diazepam, or 30–60 mg of oxazepam every 2 hours as needed. Doses can be subsequently adjusted as needed. Initially, close observation is needed. After the first day long-acting agents (e.g., chlordiazepoxide or diazepam) can usually be given in four daily doses. Once the patient has been stabilized (usually within 24 hours) the benzodiazepine dosage can be decreased by 20% per day for long-acting agents and by 10–20% per day for short-acting agents.

(e) Lorazepam or diazepam can be administered IM if necessary, if given in the well-perfused deltoid muscle, but they are less well absorbed from the gluteus maximus or vastus lateralis. (Lorazepam is more reliably absorbed than diazepam.) Chlordiazepoxide is poorly absorbed IM from any site and should not be given by this route.

(3) Fluid loss and electrolyte imbalances should be corrected. Especially if there is agitation, vomiting, or fever, fluid losses may be significant.

(4) Seizures almost always begin within 24 hours. Typically they are generalized tonic-clonic seizures. About a third of patients who develop seizures will have only one; two-thirds of patients will have multiple seizures, often closely spaced. Only about 2% of patients with seizures will develop status epilepticus, most representing epileptic patients who have discontinued their anticonvulsant medication (see Chap. 27).

(a) If seizures occur, anticonvulsants can be given, but prophylactic use of anticonvulsants may produce more risks than benefits. For severe or repeated seizures the patient can be treated with diazepam 5–10 mg or lorazepam 1–2 mg given slowly IV. This IV supplementation of benzodiazepines (assuming that the patient has already received one or more oral doses) usually terminates the seizures, although occasionally further IV doses are needed. Although it has been disputed, it appears that phenytoin is also effective in terminating seizures if given in a full loading dose of 15 mg/kg IV. The management of seizures is discussed in Chap. 27.

(b) If seizures begin later than 24 hours after the beginning of abstinence, if they continue for an extended period, if status epilepticus occurs, or if seizures are focal, a source other than withdrawal must be sought.

(c) For pure alcohol withdrawal seizures, long-term use of an anticonvulsant is not indicated.

E. Delirium tremens is a term best reserved for the severe, late-onset syndrome that occurs in a small minority of patients. Despite optimal therapy, delirium tremens results in mortality in 5–10% of cases.

1. Clinical manifestations. Most often there is no orderly progression of symptoms from early milder symptoms to delirium tremens. The syndrome may occur within 24–72 hours of abstinence. In 90% of patients who develop delirium tremens, it begins within 7 days. The syndrome is characterized by marked sympathetic overactivity, fever, hallucinosis, severe anxiety and agitation, confusion, fluctuating mental status, motor restlessness, and combativeness.

2. Death may result from volume depletion, electrolyte imbalance, infection, or cardiac arrhythmias. Unless proper precautions are taken to restrain patients, death may also result from suicide (e.g., while fleeing a frightening hallucination).

3. Treatment

a. An intensive care setting is preferable because of the need for frequent monitoring of vital signs and electrolytes and vigorous fluid replacement.

b. IV dextrose and saline should be given at a rate adequate to replace fluid losses (which are likely to be great in a febrile agitated patient) and maintain blood pressure. In cases of circulatory collapse, pressors may be needed.

c. Hyperthermia should be treated aggressively with acetaminophen 650 mg PO q4h for temperatures above 101°F and with cooling blankets for temperatures above 103.5°F.

d. Parenteral thiamine, 100 mg/day, should be continued, at least until a normal diet is resumed.

e. Sedation helps diminish autonomic symptoms and agitation. Parenteral administration is best because most patients will not be able to take anything by mouth. Diazepam 5–10 mg slowly IV can be given every 15–20 minutes until sedation is achieved. Repeat doses should be given as needed. More rapid dosing creates the risk of overdose because a repeat dose would be given before the peak effect of the prior dose is evident.

f. Seizures may be treated with IV supplementation of benzodiazepines or with phenytoin.

g. All severely agitated or combative patients should be restrained. Restraint should be carefully managed to avoid decubitus ulcers and nerve compression or traction injuries.

h. Infections, such as aspiration pneumonia, should be suspected and treated with appropriate antibiotics if present.

i. Reassurance and explanations to the patient are helpful.

VII. Wernicke-Korsakoff syndrome is caused by thiamine deficiency. It occurs most commonly in nutritionally deficient alcoholics but also occasionally in nonalcoholic patients. The acute stage of the syndrome, which often has a fairly abrupt onset, is referred to as Wernicke's encephalopathy.

A. Acute clinical manifestations. Any of the following may be the first to appear.

1. **Ocular findings.** One or all of the following may be present:
   - **a.** Nystagmus (horizontal and vertical).
   - **b.** Weakness or paralysis of the external rectus muscles.
   - **c.** Weakness or paralysis of conjugate gaze.
2. **Ataxia of stance and gait.**
3. **Mental status abnormalities**
   - **a.** Most common is a global confusional state; early symptoms include listlessness, inattentiveness, poor concentration, and an inability to sustain a conversation.
   - **b.** Drowsiness is common, but stupor or coma is rare.
   - **c.** Korsakoff's syndrome of anterograde and retrograde amnesia is occasionally present as the only manifestation of the Wernicke-Korsakoff syndrome.
   - **d.** Some patients will a have a superimposed alcohol withdrawal syndrome.

B. Korsakoff's psychosis is characterized by a striking inability to learn new information. In addition there is always some degree of retrograde amnesia. Confabulation is often, but not invariably, present early and is usually absent in the chronic state of the disease. Once Korsakoff's psychosis emerges, the prognosis for recovery is poor, with only 20% of patients making a substantial improvement.

C. Therapy consists of an adequate diet with supplementation of thiamine (100 mg daily). The ocular manifestations usually respond most readily, although often patients also become more alert and attentive. Administration of carbohydrates (including dextrose in IV solutions) prior to adequate repletion of thiamine probably worsens the clinical picture. Therefore it is prudent to give all patients who are potentially alcoholic or nutritionally deficient thiamine 100 mg IV prior to beginning other therapies.

VIII. The alcohol-Antabuse (disulfiram) syndrome. Disulfiram alters the intermediary metabolism of alcohol, resulting in markedly increased concentrations of acetaldehyde.

A. Clinical manifestations. Within 5–10 minutes of alcohol ingestion, facial flushing occurs. This is followed by marked systemic vasodilatation, often accompanied by a throbbing headache, nausea, vomiting, dry mouth, sweating, chest pain, hypotension, and even syncope. Often there is respiratory distress, vertigo, and confusion. Even with mild reactions, manifestations may last several hours. In severe reactions, there may be arrhythmias, shock, seizures, and death.

B. Treatment

1. Diphenhydramine (Benadryl) 50 mg IM or IV is symptomatically helpful.
2. **Hypotension** should be treated with IV saline. If shock is present it usually responds to vasopressors, such as ephedrine.
3. **Respiratory distress** often improves with administration of oxygen.
4. **Arrhythmias** should be treated if present; hypokalemia has been reported and should be corrected.

IX. Alcoholic ketoacidosis

A. Clinical manifestations. Occasionally alcoholic patients may present with a profound metabolic acidosis and its resulting symptoms (see Chap. 25). The diagnosis should be suspected if an anion gap acidosis is noted with only modest or absent hyperglycemia and no evidence for other ingestions or for sepsis. (Other causes of anion gap acidosis include salicylate toxicity; ethylene glycol, methanol, or paraldehyde ingestion; lactic acidosis; uremia; and diabetic ketoacidosis.) Urine and plasma ketones may be mostly in the form of beta-hydroxybutyrate and therefore not detected by routine laboratory tests.

1. The syndrome occurs in the setting of chronic alcoholism with superimposed starvation.
2. There may be superimposed withdrawal symptoms.
3. Frequent nausea, vomiting, and abdominal pain are present. An amylase should be checked to rule out pancreatitis.

B. Treatment

1. As always with malnourished alcoholics, thiamine 100 mg IV should be given first.
2. IV administration of glucose will suppress hepatic production of ketones.
3. Careful correction of dehydration and electrolyte abnormalities is necessary.
4. If a withdrawal syndrome is superimposed it should be treated.

Selected Readings

Anda, R. F., Williamson, D. F., and Remington, P. L. Alcohol and fatal injuries among U.S. adults. *J.A.M.A.* 260:2529, 1988.

Chang, G., and Astrachan, B. M. The emergency department surveillance of alcohol intoxication after motor vehicle accidents. *J.A.M.A.* 260:2533, 1988.

Cherness, M. E., Simon, R. P., and Greenberg, D. A. Ethanol and the nervous system. *N. Engl. J. Med.* 321:442, 1989.

Hyman, S. E., and Cassem, N. H. Alcoholism. In E. Rubenstein and D. Federman, (eds.), *Scientific American Medicine.* New York: Scientific American, 1993.

Victor, M. The Effects of Alcohol on the Nervous System. In J. H. Mendelson and N. K. Mello (eds.), *Medical Diagnosis and Treatment of Alcoholism.* New York: McGraw-Hill, 1992. P. 201.

Wrenn, K. D., et al. The syndrome of alcoholic ketoacidosis. *Am. J. Med.* 91:119, 1991.

32 Acute Drug Overdoses

Steven E. Hyman

I. **Drug overdoses are medical emergencies** that require the gamut of the emergency physician's skills. The cornerstone of treatment for most overdose patients is meticulous supportive care, which often requires treatment in an intensive care unit. If the patient is an IV drug abuser, management may be complicated by other illnesses, such as acquired immunodeficiency syndrome (AIDS), hepatitis, or acute bacterial infections. This chapter describes the **general approach to the overdose patient** and specific issues that arise in overdoses with **psychotropic drugs.** Overdoses with nonpsychotropic agents (such as aspirin and acetaminophen) are outside the scope of this manual.

II. Drug reactions and overdoses may present as central nervous system (CNS) excitation or depression, behavioral abnormality, or organ system malfunction. **The approach to the patient with a presumed overdose** depends on whether the patient is alert or alternatively showing signs of CNS depression or delirium.

A. When a toxic drug reaction or overdose is suspected, other causes of an intoxicated appearance or coma must be considered—for example, hypoglycemia, postictal states, postconcussive states, or delirium.

B. A major difficulty in approaching the overdose patient is that frequently the history obtained from the patient or accompanying individuals is unreliable. The overdose may be denied or minimized; if street drugs were involved, the purity of the drugs used is often unknown; and prior drug abuse, or psychiatric problems (including prior overdoses) may be denied. These problems may be exacerbated if the motivation for the overdose was manipulative. Thus the clinician must rely on his or her clinical judgment and the result of toxicologic tests. In no case, however, should the initial stages of treatment be delayed while awaiting results from a toxicology laboratory.

III. **Treatment of the overdosed patient who is alert**

A. Alert overdosed patients come to the emergency department for a variety of reasons that impact on the degree to which they cooperate with the treating physician. Some have taken an overdose in a suicide gesture or attempt and have changed their minds. Others have been discovered after an ingestion and are brought to the emergency department with varying degrees of aquiescence by family or police. Still others have accidentally overdosed while abusing drugs. Finally some are involved in a manipulative attempt to gain emergency treatment or to "deliver a message" to someone else. This last group is often the most difficult to treat both because they often refuse to cooperate with treatment, and because they frequently arouse antipathy and anger in the emergency department staff. Some of these will be emergency department "repeaters" with personality disorders (see Chap. 22).

1. Whatever the patient's degree of cooperation, no patient who has allegedly overdosed should be allowed to refuse emergency treatment; the overdose must be considered to be potentially lethal and therefore a true emergency. Treatment refusal must be considered to constitute a suicide attempt.

2. The physician is best served by remaining empathic but businesslike; both anger and rescue fantasies can interfere with optimal clinical care.

3. Physicians should be aware of hospital procedure for restraining and treating uncooperative suicidal patients.

B. Management (Table 32-1)

1. The physician should attempt to establish a rapport with the patient quickly and to gain the patient's cooperation. If there is good evidence of an overdose but the patient is uncooperative or dangerously delirious, restraints will be necessary (see Table 5-1).

2. Measure vital signs; observe for any injuries requiring emergency intervention.

3. Quickly attempt to gain further history from the patient; another staff member can try to gain corroborating data from those who accompanied the patient. It is important to ask for the drug and dose ingested. Ask if remaining pills were brought to the emergency department; these should be sent for analysis unless they are recognizable prescription drugs. It should be determined how much time has elapsed since the ingestion and whether vomiting has occurred.

4. Explain the necessary treatment to the patient in clear, simple terms; do not become engaged in arguments.

5. Note the patient's mental status and any obvious injuries. If the patient's mental status is deteriorating, follow the procedures below for treating a comatose patient.

6. Place a secure IV line (not in the antecubital fossa); draw blood samples for toxicologic analysis, complete blood count (CBC), glucose, and whatever other studies are clinically appropriate (e.g., electrolytes and renal function tests if lithium has been ingested).

7. If the patient may be alcoholic or is malnourished give thiamine 100 mg IV; if hypoglycemia is possible give 50 ml of 50% dextrose in water. If narcotics are involved, at least 0.01 mg/kg of naloxone (Narcan) should be

Table 32-1. Treatment of the overdose patient who is alert

1. Attempt to establish rapport quickly. If the patient is uncooperative, restrain.
2. Record vital signs.
3. If possible obtain a history from patient and any accompanying parties, including nature and dose of ingestion, time since ingestion, and whether vomiting has occurred. The history may not be reliable.
4. Explain the necessary treatment to the patient.
5. Note the patient's mental status. If loss of consciousness appears imminent, use procedures in Table 32-2.
6. Draw blood samples and place an IV line.
7. If appropriate give thiamine, 50% dextrose in water, and naloxone.
8. If appropriate initiate cardiac monitoring and obtain electrocardiogram.
9. Perform a quick physical examination including a check of gag reflex.
10. Induce emesis. Follow with activated charcoal.
11. Obtain a fuller history after emesis has subsided, including history of prior ingestions and psychiatric history, with special attention to suicidality.
12. Observe the patient or admit to hospital.

given. Any change in pupillary size or mental status should be noted and treatment with naloxone continued as indicated (see sec. **X.D**).

8. If appropriate (e.g., if cyclic antidepressants have been ingested), initiate cardiac monitoring.
9. Perform a quick physical examination. Listen to heart and lungs and examine for head trauma, injection sites, or other injuries. Perform a rapid neurologic assessment including a check of the gag reflex.
10. If the gag reflex is intact and unless the overdose is remote (more than 4 hours before) or involved a parenteral route, induce emesis. In alert patients induced emesis probably entails a lower risk of aspiration than gastric lavage. Emesis is contraindicated if the patient has ingested strong acids or alkalis, petroleum distillates, or sharp objects or if the patient has esophageal varices.
    a. **If the patient is cooperative,** give 30 ml of syrup of ipecac followed by several glasses of water. Vomiting should occur in 15–30 minutes. If no vomiting occurs the dose can be repeated in 30 minutes. Intractable vomiting is a rare complication; it can be treated with 10 mg IM of prochlorperazine (Compazine).
    b. **If the patient is uncooperative,** pass a nasogastric tube and check for placement by aspirating gastric contents and then pushing down 50 ml of air and listening over the stomach. Give 30 ml of ipecac through the tube followed by 100–200 ml of water, given slowly. Then remove the tube.
    c. If the patient begins to lose consciousness after ipecac is given but prior to completion of vomiting, place the patient in the left lateral decubitus position, intubate the patient with care not to induce vomiting, and then proceed with gastric lavage (see sec. **IV.B.11**).
    d. After emesis is complete (usually 45–60 minutes), give activated charcoal 50 gm in a slurry with tap water made up to 500 ml. This dose may be repeated after 30 minutes. Activated charcoal works by complexing with toxins in the gastrointestinal tract and preventing their subsequent absorption. Because charcoal might interfere with the action of ipecac most clinicians wait until vomiting is complete before administering charcoal.
11. Once the emergency has passed, a more complete history should be taken so that the appropriate disposition can be reached. In particular, the patient must be assessed for suicidality (see Chap. 4) and for the presence of major psychiatric disorders.
12. The patient should be medically stable before transfer to a psychiatric hospital or discharge is contemplated. Before transfer the results of the toxic screen should be known.

IV. Treatment of the overdosed patient who is stuporous or comatose

A. In these patients the diagnosis may be unclear. The physician must be alert for medical causes of stupor and coma other than overdoses. Continuing clinical assessment must proceed even while therapy is being given.

B. Management (Table 32-2)

1. Attention should first be given to the airway. If stuporous, the patient should be placed in the left lateral decubitus position to minimize the danger of aspiration. The oropharynx should be suctioned free of secretions or vomitus, and then the head positioned, and a cuffed endotracheal tube should be placed.
2. If the patient is ventilating poorly ($PCO_2 > 40$), ventilate and oxygenate

Table 32-2. Treatment of the overdose patient who is comatose

1. Clear the oropharynx of secretions or vomitus and place a cuffed endotracheal tube.
2. If breathing is poor, ventilate and oxygenate.
3. Obtain vital signs.
4. Place an IV line. Draw glucose and obtain complete blood count, electrolytes, calcium, blood urea nitrogen, creatinine, liver function tests, toxic screen, and arterial blood gases.
5. Give thiamine, an ampule of 50% dextrose in water, and naloxone.
6. Begin cardiac monitoring and obtain electrocardiogram.
7. If dangerous arrhythmias are present, place central line and treat. Treat hypotension, seizures, and other emergency conditions.
8. Perform quick physical examination of heart, lungs, and abdomen, and determine neurologic status. Examine for trauma.
9. Place Foley catheter.
10. Obtain history from accompanying parties.
11. Perform gastric lavage and then give charcoal if indicated.
12. Admit patient to an intensive care unit.

Unless aspiration pneumonia or other pulmonary compromise is suspected, FIO_2 need not be high. Overventilation and oxygenation may suppress spontaneous respiration and make neurologic evaluation more difficult. If personnel trained in intubation are not present, patients with depressed respiration should be treated with a bag and mask.

3. The vital signs must be determined including pulse rate, temperature, blood pressure, and estimation of jugular venous pressure. Note any obvious injuries. It is best to record vital signs, hourly urine output, relevant laboratory data—for example, electrolytes and arterial blood gases (ABGs)—and depth of coma on a flow sheet. In recording the depth of coma it is best to describe observations clearly, rather than simply recording terms such as "stuporous" or "obtunded."

4. Place a secure IV line. Draw blood for glucose, CBC, electrolytes, calcium, blood urea nitrogen (BUN), creatinine, liver function tests, toxic screen, and ABGs. Samples of urine and gastric aspirate should be collected later and also sent for toxicologic analysis.

5. Give 100 mg of thiamine, 50 ml of 50% dextrose in water, and at least 0.01 mg/kg of naloxone IV. If there is a response to naloxone, a repeat dose should be given.

6. Begin cardiac monitoring and obtain a full electrocardiogram (ECG) if possible.

7. Threatening **medical complications** must be attended to.

a. If dangerous **arrhythmias** are present they should be treated. This is best done with a central line in place.

b. If **hypotension** occurs, fluid repletion alone will usually correct it. Unless the central venous pressure (CVP) is elevated, 5% dextrose in normal saline can be given as a rapid IV bolus of 200–300 ml over 10–15 minutes and then infused at a rate of 150 ml/minute. Refractory hypotension or hypotension in the presence of congestive failure will require use of pressors.

c. If seizures develop:

(1) Lorazepam (Ativan) 1–2 mg or **diazepam** (Valium) 5–10 mg can be given slowly IV. Benzodiazepines should **never be given as a**

rapid IV bolus because of the risk of respiratory arrest. Either agent may be repeated every 10–15 minutes until seizures cease. Lorazepam is preferred because, despite its shorter elimination half-life, it has a much slower distribution phase than diazepam and thus produces a longer clinical effect in single-dose situations. (For a full discussion, see Arana and Hyman, 1991.)

(2) If a benzodiazepine fails, **phenytoin** (Dilantin) may be given. A full loading dose of 15 mg/kg is necessary for this agent to be effective. Phenytoin must be administered no more rapidly than 50 mg/minute through a freely running IV line. Overrapid loading will result in hypotension. During loading, blood pressure must be measured frequently. Because of its high pH, infiltration of phenytoin can cause severe tissue damage. Phenytoin precipitates if run with dextrose; thus saline alone must be used. (See Chap. 27 for a full discussion of this agent.)

8. A more detailed examination can now be performed including heart, lungs, abdomen, and neurologic status. Signs of trauma and self-injection should be looked for.

9. A Foley catheter should be placed, if not already done, and a specimen of urine obtained for toxicologic analysis.

10. A more detailed history should now be obtained from those who accompanied the patient. Any remaining pills that they have found should be identified or, if not identifiable, sent for toxicologic analysis.

11. Gastric lavage should be performed unless the overdose was parenteral. This maneuver is useful within 4 hours of an ingestion and longer if drugs with anticholinergic properties, e.g., tricyclic antidepressants, antihistamines, or thioridazine (Mellaril), were taken because such agents inhibit gastrointestinal motility. Lavage is contraindicated if strong acids, alkalis, petroleum distillates, or sharp objects were ingested.

a. The endotracheal tube must be secure.

b. A large-bore (preferably 40 F) orogastric tube (Ewald tube) should be placed, and the stomach lavaged with normal saline until clear. Gastric aspirate should be sent for toxicologic analysis.

c. Activated charcoal 50 gm in 500 ml of tap water can be given through the gastric tube.

12. The patient should be admitted to an intensive care unit (ICU).

C. Forced diuresis, hemodialysis, and hemoperfusion have potentially serious complications and should only be used if specifically indicated or if renal or hepatic failure makes metabolism of the offending agents impossible. They may also be tried if the patient deteriorates despite good conservative therapy. Perhaps the only drug that will frequently require dialysis is lithium.

V. Overdoses with barbiturates and other CNS depressants (sedative-hypnotics)

A. Sedative-hypnotics are a pharmacologically cross-reactive group of agents that includes the barbiturates, benzodiazepines, glutethimide (Doriden), chloral derivatives (Noctec, Beta-Chlor, and others), ethchlorvynol (Placidyl), meprobamate (Miltown, Equanil), methyprylon (Noludar), and methaqualone (see Appendixes III and IV). The sedative-hypnotics are commonly implicated in serious drug overdoses. Except for the benzodiazepines, all of these drugs can easily prove lethal in overdose, and all of them, including the benzodiazepines, can lead to fatal CNS depression if the overdose also involves alcohol or other drugs (e.g., tricyclic antidepressants). The CNS depressant drugs are prescribed as anxiolytics, hypnotics, anticonvulsants (phenobarbital), and muscle relaxants (diazepam). Given the ubiquity of anxiety and insomnia as medical complaints, these drugs are, as a group, among the most prescribed drugs in the United States. In addition, these drugs are commonly abused both alone or in combination with alcohol, narcotics, or psychostimulants. Given the relative safety of the benzodiazepines compared with the older sedative-hypnotics, most of the latter no longer have a rational use. Indeed the replacement of barbiturates and other similarly acting sedative-hypnotics by benzodiazepines in general practice has resulted in a sharp decrease in fatalities due to overdoses with "sleeping pills."

B. **Pharmacology.** All of these drugs appear to act as receptors for gamma-aminobutyric acid (GABA), the brain's major inhibitory neurotransmitter. In toxic doses they cause stupor, coma, apnea, and death by depressing brainstem arousal and respiratory centers. They are all able to induce tolerance if used over extended periods, thus making serum levels potentially difficult to correlate with the patient's clinical appearance. Tolerant individuals may develop a life-threatening withdrawal syndrome if not carefully detoxified after recovering from an overdose (see Chap. 30, sec. **III**).

C. **Manifestations of toxicity**

1. **Mild toxicity** may resemble drunkenness. Patients may exhibit ataxia, dysarthria, nystagmus, drowsiness, and mild confusion. Some individuals may become disinhibited and belligerent.
2. **Severe toxicity** results in stupor, coma, and respiratory depression, including apnea. Comatose patients may be unresponsive to deep pain, and deep tendon reflexes may be absent.

D. **Overdoses** may involve multiple drugs, making a variety of toxic effects possible. In addition to depression of arousal and respiration, CNS depressant drugs make patients vulnerable to a variety of complications.

1. **Aspiration penumonia.** The patient should be monitored for fever, leukocytosis, and purulent secretions even if an initial chest x ray is normal.
2. **Hypotension** is usually associated with dehydration and often correlates with the time elapsed before the patient was discovered and brought for medical attention. Expansion of capacitance vessels and capillary leak also occur and contribute to hypotension.
3. **Cardiac arrhythmias** may occur as a result of hypoxia and acidosis as well as concomitantly ingested drugs, such as tricyclic antidepressants.
4. **Erythematous and bullous skin lesions** are common at sites of pressure and at sites of nonsterile self-injection.
5. **Peripheral nerve injuries** due to compression or traction also occur.
6. Patients who have used **intravenous** drugs may have stigmata of nonsterile parenteral drug use, such as infected puncture sites, hepatitis, AIDS, and endocarditis.

E. **Therapy.** The general principles of overdose management, as described in secs. **III** and **IV,** should be followed. There are no specific antidotes for sedative-hypnotic overdose; thus treatment consists of good supportive care. The older practice of administration of CNS stimulants to these patients is dangerous and has no place in therapy.

1. There is evidence that repeated doses of activated charcoal via nasogastric tube will markedly shorten the duration of coma in phenobarbital overdoses (e.g., a slurry of 50 gm of activated charcoal q4h for six doses).
2. In addition, forced diuresis with urine alkalinization will speed the excretion of phenobarbital, but not of other barbiturates. Sodium bicarbonate can be given IV in doses that keep the urine strongly alkaline. This can be done with or without a forced diuresis of saline at 200 ml/hour. Because of

the volume load, this treatment should not be attempted in elderly patients or if the CVP is high.

3. Overdoses of **bromides** (now extremely rare) should be treated with a forced saline diuresis unless there are cardiac contraindications.

4. Forced diuresis is not effective in overdose of drugs with little renal excretion, such as short- and intermediate-acting barbiturates.

5. **Glutethimide (Doriden)** overdose may be particularly difficult to treat because of its tendency to cause hypotension and because of episodic absorption of the drug, which may continue for days and cause unexpected relapses. In these patients premature extubation should be avoided. Glutethimide is often abused in combination with codeine ("loads"), especially when heroin is scarce.

6. Patients who are **tolerant to sedative-hypnotics** may develop a withdrawal syndrome characterized by agitation, delirium, seizures, and, occasionally, death. Given the high risk of severe morbidity from this withdrawal syndrome, it is good practice to examine the patient for sedative-hypnotic tolerance once he or she is clearly awake and alert, and especially if showing any signs of withdrawal, such as anxiety, restlessness, nausea, tremor, or tachycardia. The method of testing for tolerance is the **pentobarbital tolerance test.** This test and procedures for withdrawing the patient safely are outlined in Chap. 30, sec. **II.C.** The test, rather than the history, should be relied on, because many patients will deny drug addiction. Once the withdrawal procedure is begun in tolerant patients, transfer to a psychiatric hospital or specialized detoxification facility can be arranged depending on the patient's psychiatric needs. It is crucial, however, that testing for tolerance and administration of the calculated stabilization dose be done promptly when the patient is alert because the withdrawal syndrome may be very difficult to treat once it begins.

F. Prevention of sedative-hypnotic abuse and overdose depends, in part, on good prescribing habits by physicians. In general there is no reason to prescribe nonbenzodiazepine drugs for anxiety or insomnia. Benzodiazepines should only be prescribed for good indications.

VI. Overdoses with tricyclic and other cyclic antidepressants

A. A major difficulty in treating depression is that the commonly prescribed drugs, the cyclic antidepressants, have among the lowest toxic to therapeutic ratios in medicine. Thus the depressed patient, with increased suicidal risk, is often armed with drugs that can easily prove lethal if taken in overdose. Although most patients who overdose with these drugs do not develop serious toxicity, a substantial minority develop significant morbidity or die. Indeed cyclic antidepressants have consistently ranked among the leading causes of fatal overdoses in recent years. Most of the patients who die do so prior to reaching an emergency room.

B. Pharmacology. Blood and tissue levels of cyclic antidepressants correlate poorly with oral dose, probably because of variable absorption and metabolic rates. Once absorbed, however, they achieve a high degree of protein and tissue binding (which makes dialysis worthless as a treatment for overdose). Acute doses of more than 1.0 gm are often extremely toxic and may be fatal. The toxicity of these drugs results from their anticholinergic (antimuscarinic) properties, their anti–alpha-adrenergic properties, their quinidine-like effects on the heart, and their proconvulsant effects. Death may result from cardiac arrhythmias, hypotension, or uncontrollable seizures. Given the frequency and potential severity of cyclic antidepressant overdoses, many different methods have been tested for predicting which overdose patients are at risk for serious morbidity. Unfortunately, none have proved to be ideal.

1. Because these agents circulate at very low levels—that is, in the nanogram per milliliter range, many toxicology laboratories are extremely inaccurate in determining serum levels. Since, in addition, patients have widely differing tolerances to high levels, serum level alone is not an adequate predictor of potential morbidity. In general, levels greater than 1000 ng/ml represent a serious overdose.

2. Some investigators (Boehnert and Lovejoy, 1985) have argued that a QRS duration of greater than or equal to 0.10 second is a better predictor of serious arrhythmias and seizures than serum drug level. A subsequent study (Foulke and Albertson, 1987) failed to replicate this result. Thus, at present, a normal QRS interval cannot be used by itself to suggest that an individual patient is "safe"; patients who have overdosed on cyclic antidepressants must be observed for an extended period before discharge is contemplated.

C. Manifestations of toxicity

1. Even at therapeutic levels, cyclic antidepressants commonly produce toxic side effects. These may include anticholinergic effects, orthostatic hypotension, tachycardia, ECG changes, and sedation (see Chap. 24, sec. **III**).

2. **Acute overdose.** Signs and symptoms of overdose develop rapidly. Almost all of the severe symptomatology is present within 24 hours. Indeed, serious sequelae (such as arrhythmias and seizures) most often manifest during the first few hours that the patient is in the emergency department.

   a. **Anticholinergic effects** are prominent and severe, including dry mucous membranes, warm dry skin, mydriasis, blurred vision, decreased bowel motility, and urinary retention.

   b. **CNS depression** commonly occurs, ranging from drowsiness to coma. Alternatively the patient may be agitated or delirious. The CNS depressant effects of tricyclics are potentiated by concomitantly ingested alcohol, benzodiazepines, and other sedative-hypnotics. Mixed ingestions of this sort are common, and the physician should be alert for them; in the case of mixed ingestions, respiratory depression or arrest is more likely.

   c. **Cardiovascular toxicity** presents a particular danger. (Table 32-3). Hypotension often occurs, even with the patient supine. A wide variety of arrhythmias may develop including supraventricular tachycardias, ventricular tachycardia or fibrillation, and varying degrees of heart block, including complete heart block.

   d. **Seizures** commonly occur early in the course.

Table 32-3. Cardiac toxicity of tricyclic and tetracyclic antidepressant overdose

Hemodynamic
Hypotension
Myocardial depression
Rhythm disturbance
Sinus tachycardia
Supraventricular and ventricular tachyarrhythmias
Prolongation of PR, QRS, and QT intervals
Bundle branch block
Second- and third-degree block
Sudden death

3. Relative toxicities

a. All of the cyclic antidepressants appear to have the same propensities to cause serious cardiac toxicity. The newer atypical drugs fluoxetine (Prozac), sertraline (Zoloft), paroxetine (Paxil), bupropion (Wellbutrin), and trazodone (Desyrel) have less cardiac toxicity than the cyclic compounds. For reasons that are unclear, a recent series found that desipramine caused death more frequently when used in overdose than other cyclic compounds (Kapur et al., 1992).

b. The newer agents amoxapine and maprotiline appear to have a greater propensity than the older drugs to cause seizures. In particular, there have been reports of increased frequency of status epilepticus and mortality with amoxapine. Therefore, it may be prudent to treat amoxapine-induced seizures more aggressively than otherwise (e.g., earlier intubation; preparedness to utilize general anesthesia if benzodiazepines and phenytoin fail to control seizures).

c. Fluoxetine, sertraline, paroxetine, bupropion, and trazodone appear to be safer than the cyclic antidepressants in overdose.

D. Therapy

1. Basic management follows the general principles for all drug overdoses enumerated above. In addition:

a. A toxic screen should be ordered, not only for antidepressant levels but also to look for other ingested agents. As described in sec. **VI.B,** cyclic antidepressant levels should be interpreted with caution.

b. Because bowel motility may be slowed by the anticholinergic properties of cyclic antidepressants, it is worth inducing emesis or performing gastric lavage at later times than for most other overdoses.

c. Since it appears that enterohepatic circulation contributes to the long half-life of cyclic antidepressants, repeat dosing with charcoal may be helpful. It has been reported (Swartz and Sherman, 1984) that an initial slurry of 50 gm of charcoal followed by repeat doses of 20–25 gm via nasogastric tube, given as frequently as possible without regurgitation through the tube, markedly increased the clearance of the drug.

d. It has been recommended that protein binding of these drugs be increased by administering sodium bicarbonate as a continuous IV infusion to maintain the arterial blood pH at 7.5 (Haddad and Winchester, 1983). There is no convincing evidence at present that this maneuver improves outcome.

2. Management of cardiovascular toxicity

a. Hypotension. In addition to the anti–alpha-adrenergic properties of cyclic antidepressants, volume depletion may be quite severe if the patient was unconscious for some time before being brought for emergency treatment. Administration of fluids is the first step in the treatment of hypotension. In refractory hypotension, or if heart failure is present, pressors (e.g., dopamine) will be required.

b. Cardiac arrhythmias. Patients who have overdosed on cyclic antidepressants are best followed with continuous cardiac monitoring. Although most dangerous arrhythmias make their appearance during the first 24 hours, there are case reports of arrhythmias and sudden death as late as a week after the overdose, even with nontoxic serum levels. This rare and unpredictable complication may be due to concentration of tricyclics by the myocardium, but this explanation is only speculative at present.

(1) Basic management. If arrhythmias are present, blood gases should be checked. Correction of acidosis with sodium bicarbonate is critical for successful treatment of arrhythmias.

(2) **Supraventricular tachycardia.** Sinus tachycardia usually requires no treatment. Supraventricular tachycardias contributing to myocardial ischemia or hypotension should be treated with DC cardioversion. Digoxin should be avoided because it might precipitate heart block. Propranolol appears to be safe in treating recurrent supraventricular tachycardias.

(3) **Ventricular tachyarrhythmias.** Cardioversion is the treatment of choice for ventricular tachycardia or fibrillation. A loading dose of lidocaine followed by a drip of 2 mg/minute may prevent recurrence. Higher doses of lidocaine may increase the likelihood of seizures. If lidocaine fails to prevent further arrhythmias, bretylium is probably the next agent of choice. Since the cyclic antidepressants act like class I antiarrhythmics, quinidine, procainamide, and disopyramide are likely to worsen the picture and should be avoided. Like class I antiarrhythmics, cyclic antidepressants may prolong the QT interval and predispose to **torsades de pointes** ventricular tachycardia, an electrocardiographically disorganized-appearing rhythm in which the axis of the QRS complex twists about the isoelectric point. It is important to recognize this rhythm because it is best treated by overdrive pacing or isoproterenol, which decrease the QT interval and interrupt the reentrant tachyarrhythmia. Agents such as lidocaine, which do not delay repolarization, may also be helpful.

(4) **Heart block.** Second- and third-degree heart block should be managed by insertion of a temporary pacemaker.

(5) **Physostigmine.** Some clinicians have advocated the use of the tertiary amine anticholinesterase physostigmine in the treatment of arrhythmias due to cyclic antidepressant toxicity. Since the serious cyclic antidepressant–induced cardiac arrhythmias are due to the quinidine-like effects of these compounds rather than to their anticholinergic effects, it is not surprising that there is no convincing evidence that physostigmine is effective. Given, in addition, its potential toxicities (see Table 24-2), **physostigmine should not be used for this indication.**

(6) **Phenytoin.** Based on the idea that phenytoin may improve cardiac conduction velocity and on anecdotal case reports, some clinicians have advocated phenytoin as the treatment of choice for tricyclic-induced arrhythmias; the evidence for its utility is not convincing and is not supported by animal studies (Mayron and Ruiz, 1986). In addition, IV loading of phenytoin must be slow and can have adverse effects on blood pressure.

3. Management of CNS toxicity

a. **Delirium.** For a patient whose delirium is so severe that it is significantly contributing to his or her morbidity (e.g., uncontrollable agitation despite low doses of lorazepam or diazepam), administration of physostigmine salicylate may be considered. Given the toxicity of this agent, including its propensity to cause seizures, the indications would have to be extremely compelling before it was used. Physostigmine is given IV in doses of 1–2 mg over 2–3 minutes. If there is no response the dose can be repeated in 20–30 minutes. If a good response occurs, the lowest effective dose can be repeated as the last wears off (approximately 30 minutes). Should a toxic response to physostigmine occur, it can be reversed by atropine sulfate 0.5 mg per milligram of physostigmine given. Given the dangers of this agent, it should never be given as a continuous IV infusion or without constant observation.

b. **Seizures.** Care must be taken to protect the airway and to protect the patient from injury. The general management of grand mal seizures is reviewed in Chap. 27, sec. **II.A.** For seizures due to cyclic antidepressant overdose the first-line drugs are the benzodiazepines, lorazepam or diazepam, or the anticonvulsant phenytoin.

(1) **Lorazepam** 1–2 mg or **diazepam** 5–10 mg can be given slowly IV (see sec. **IV.B.7.c.(1)**).

(2) Alternatively, a full loading dose of **phenytoin** 15 mg/kg can be given, but no more rapidly than 50 mg/minute (see sec. **IV.B.7.c.(2)** or Chap. 27).

4. **Forced diuresis and dialysis** are of no value because of protein and tissue binding of tricyclics. **Hemoperfusion** may have value when arrhythmias or seizures cannot be controlled by any other means, but its use must still be considered experimental. It is not without risk because of the need for heparinization and cannulation of major vessels.

E. Prevention. Given the indications for which cyclic antidepressants are prescribed, there is always some risk of overdose. That risk is not a reason to withhold what may be lifesaving therapy, and if the physician observes certain precautions, the risk can be minimized. The physician should not prescribe these drugs to an unknown patient who has been seen in an emergency evaluation. If, after a more extended evaluation, the patient is found to be trustworthy and not acutely suicidal, cyclics should be prescribed if indicated. Initially it is prudent to prescribe small supplies. If the physician does not trust the patient even with a 1-week supply, a responsible family member can be asked to supervise the medication. When the patient's risk of suicide is high (see Chap. 4), inpatient treatment will be necessary. For highly suicidal, impulsive, or disorganized patients, the atypical drugs, fluoxetine, sertraline, paroxetine, bupropion, and trazodone are safer alternatives to cyclic antidepressants.

VII. Monoamine oxidase inhibitors (MAOIs) are effective in treating panic disorder, atypical depression, and some major depressions unresponsive to cyclic compounds. However, MAOIs are extremely dangerous in overdose; suicidal patients may also exploit the interactions of MAOIs with sympathomimetic compounds in foods and drugs. A discussion of sympathomimetic crises resulting from these interactions is given in Chap. 24, sec. **V.** This section focuses on the dangers of overdose alone.

A. Pharmacology. MAOIs are rapidly absorbed from the gastrointestinal tract. Although the therapeutic mechanism of action of these agents is unknown, they are known to inhibit the enzyme monoamine oxidase (MAO), thus interfering with metabolism of dopamine, norepinephrine, epinephrine, and serotonin, and of other amines, such as tyramine, that are contained in foods. Their serum half-life is brief, but their inhibitory effects on MAO are long-lived. Because they are present at very low concentrations, they are difficult to measure in serum; there are no robust data on therapeutic or toxic serum levels.

B. Manifestations of toxicity may appear slowly, often taking up to 12 hours to appear and 24 hours to reach their peak. Thus even if patients appear clinically well in the emergency department, they should be admitted for observation after any significant overdose. A death has been reported with as little as 170 mg of tranylcypromine; acute ingestions of more than 2 mg/kg of an MAOI should be considered potentially dangerous, although given the small number of cases currently in the literature, it is difficult to be confident in that figure. Indeed, many clinicians are currently prescribing up to 90 mg/day of phenelzine or tranylcypromine, equivalent to nearly 1.3 mg/kg in a 70-kg man. Syndromes similar to overdose have also been reported in patients taking MAOIs together with cyclic antidepressants in "therapeutic" dosages. The symptoms of toxicity are reviewed in Table 32-4. After an asymptomatic period, symptoms of CNS and autonomic excitation usually occur. These may produce complications such as rhabdomyolysis contributing to renal failure. This phase may then be followed by CNS depression and cardiovascular collapse. Death may occur early

Table 32-4. Symptoms and signs of overdose with monoamine oxidase inhibitors

Mild
Flushing, diaphoresis, slight fever, tachycardia, headache, drowsiness or excitation, irritability, hyperreflexia, tremor, salivation, mydriasis, nystagmus
Moderate
Delirium (with hallucinations, confusion), fever, chills, fasciculations, myoclonus, tachycardia, hypertension
Severe
Delirium, rigidity, opisthotonus, high fevers, seizures, coma, decorticate or decerebrate posturing, pulmonary edema, rhabdomyolysis, renal failure, hemolysis, coagulopathy, bradycardia, death

from seizures or arrhythmias or later from asystole, arrhythmias, hypotension, or renal failure. Hemolysis and a coagulopathy also may occur and may contribute to morbidity and mortality.

C. **Treatment** should begin with the usual steps, including gastric emptying and charcoal. Even if asymptomatic, patients should be closely monitored for at least 24 hours. Obviously, an MAO diet (see Table 32-4) should be maintained. Throughout treatment, narcotics should be avoided, especially meperidine (Demerol), because of their potential adverse interaction with MAOIs (see Chap. 24). With the emergence of symptoms, the cornerstone of treatment is meticulous supportive care.

1. **CNS excitation and neuromuscular irritability** can be treated with small doses of lorazepam or diazepam IV. These agents should not be used excessively, however, because they may potentiate later CNS depression. If multiple doses are to be used, lorazepam is preferred because of its shorter half-life. Neuroleptics, especially low-potency agents such as chlorpromazine (Thorazine), should be avoided because they can produce or worsen hypotension.

2. **Seizures** may be treated with lorazepam 1–2 mg or diazepam 5–10 mg given slowly IV and repeated every 10–15 minutes as needed. Alternatively, a full loading dose of phenytoin can be administered (see sec. **IV.B.7.c.(2)**).

3. **Respiratory.** Impairment of respiration may occur because of rigidity of the chest wall musculature. In addition, there is a risk of aspiration due to seizures and impaired level of consciousness. Thus intubation and ventilation may be necessary. Severe rigidity or neuromuscular irritability may require the use of a paralyzing agent such as pancuronium.

4. **Fever** may be severe and should be treated agressively with acetaminophen, sponge baths, or hypothermia blankets depending on the severity. Aspirin should not be used because it might worsen any coagulopathy that emerges.

5. **Hypotension** should be treated initially with volume expansion. If vasopressors are required because of refractory hypotension, they should be used cautiously because they might precipitate a hypertensive crisis. There are no clear guidelines as to which would be safest. Directly acting agents, such as norepinephrine, may be preferable to indirectly acting agents (Linden et al., 1984).

6. **Hypertension** is best treated with phentolamine 5 mg IV, repeated as necessary, or with sodium nitroprusside. Use of the latter agent requires continuous blood pressure monitoring.

7. **Ventricular arrhythmias** can be safely treated with lidocaine. Bretylium should be avoided because of its adrenergic effects.

8. **Severe muscular irritability and rigidity** may contribute to fever, a hypermetabolic state, and rhabdomyolysis. There are now several case reports (Kaplan et al., 1986; Verrilli et al., 1987) of successful use of dantrolene sodium, a directly acting muscle relaxant to treat these problems. A dosage of 2.5 mg/kg IV q6h for 24 hours was used successfully in one case; it is prudent to continue therapy with lower doses for several days afterward.

9. **Other treatments** that have been recommended include forced diuresis with alkalinization of the urine. The evidence for effectiveness in acute situations is not convincing. Dopamine agonists, such as bromocriptine, should probably be avoided because of the risk of precipitating a hypertensive crisis.

VIII. Overdoses with lithium

A. Overdoses with lithium or accidental lithium poisoning because of sodium depletion, dehydration, or renal compromise are medical emergencies that may lead to death or permanent neurologic impairment. Treatment of lithium poisoning requires careful clinical management because symptoms and signs may initially be divergent from serum levels. In addition, even in acute overdosage, symptoms may take up to 48 hours to be fully apparent.

B. Pharmacology. Lithium is well absorbed from the gastrointestinal tract, is distributed throughout total body water, and is excreted almost entirely by the kidneys.

1. The therapeutic range for lithium is a serum level of 0.5–1.2 mEq/liter. The level at which toxicity occurs is widely variable. Some patients will have toxic side effects even at stable, low therapeutic levels (see Chap. 24, sec. **VI**).

2. In general, more serious toxic symptoms may occur at levels above 2.0, and life-threatening toxicity may occur at levels above 4.0 mEq/liter. The severity and reversibility of toxic symptoms is related both to **the serum level and the duration of high levels.** Thus prompt treatment is critical.

3. Since standard lithium levels represent trough levels, usually measured 12 hours after the last oral dose, levels measured in an emergency situation must be interpreted accordingly—that is, the closer the level is drawn to the most recent dose, the higher it will be.

4. Renal absorption of lithium is competitive with sodium; thus sodium depletion elevates the lithium level and may produce intoxication. The renal effects of thiazide diuretics and nonsteroidal anti-inflammatory agents may also result in serious lithium intoxication.

C. Manifestations of significant toxicity

1. **Neurologic** symptoms include neuromuscular irritability or flaccidity, ataxia, dysarthria, coarse tremor, confusion, delirium, hallucinations, seizures, stupor, coma, and death.

2. **Systemic** symptoms include nausea, vomiting, and diarrhea.

3. **Permanent neurologic sequelae** have been reported from poisoning with lithium alone (e.g., Apte and Langston, 1983). These include impairment of memory and severe cerebellar degeneration.

D. Therapy is predicted on removing lithium from the body as rapidly as possible to avert permanent neurologic sequelae or death.

1. If the intoxication represents an overdose, the basic principles of overdose management should be followed, as outlined in secs. **III** and **IV**, including evacuation of the gastrointestinal tract and measurement of a toxic screen.

Because lithium levels in gastric juice appear to be high, some clinicians recommend continuous gastric aspiration. If the intoxication is due to dehydration, on the other hand, induction of emesis, with further loss of electrolytes, is likely to be counterproductive.

2. While no randomized studies have been performed, there is enough anecdotal evidence of catastrophic results with conservative management to recommend early dialysis for serious poisoning that does not respond rapidly to saline diuresis. Hemodialysis is most effective, but in institutions where it is unavailable, peritoneal dialysis can be relied on. Levels may rise again several hours after a dialysis treatment as lithium reequilibrates from the tissues, so frequent levels are recommended. A reasonable treatment goal is a lithium level of 1.0 mEq/liter or less 6 hours after dialysis. The guidelines proposed by Thomsen and Schou (1975) and Schou (1980) for treatment of serious lithium intoxication are recommended here, with modification.

   a. If the lithium level is less than 3 mEq/liter and signs of intoxication are mild, supportive therapy alone is indicated, as long as urine output is adequate. Fluid and electrolyte abnormalities should be corrected, and normal saline administered at a rate of 100–200 ml/hour unless there is heart failure.

   b. If the lithium level is greater than 3 mEq/liter and signs of intoxication are severe, dialysis should be instituted if the level does not respond within a few hours to saline diuresis at a rate of 250 ml/hour.

   c. If the lithium level is above 4 mEq/liter and does not respond within a few hours to saline diuresis at a rate of 250 ml/hour, dialysis should be instituted as rapidly as possible regardless of the patient's clinical appearance.

IX. Overdoses with neuroleptic drugs

A. Although the neuroleptic drugs have many troublesome toxicities that occur with therapeutic use, they have little potential for causing death if taken in overdose. The most serious complications are usually coma and hypotension, both of which should respond to good supportive care. Rarely, lethal cardiac arrhythmias may occur, probably most commonly with the newly approved agent pimozide (Orap) and also with the older agent thioridazine (Mellaril) (Wilson and Weiler, 1984). In particular, these agents may prolong the QT interval and precipitate torsades de pointes ventricular tachycardia.

B. **Pharmacology and manifestations of toxicity** depend on the neuroleptic involved.

   1. **Aliphatic and piperidine phenothiazines** (e.g., chlorpromazine and thioridazine) produce CNS depression. Coma may result after 3–4 gm of chlorpromazine. These drugs also lower the seizure threshold markedly, and thioridazine has potent anticholinergic effects. In addition, these drugs have potent anti–alpha-adrenergic effects and may cause significant hypotension. Like all neuroleptics these drugs may produce hypothermia or hyperthermia. As mentioned above, cardiac manifestations occur infrequently, but may include QT prolongation and ventricular tachyarrhythmias especially with thioridazine.

   2. **Higher-potency neuroleptics** such as the piperazine phenothiazines (e.g., perphenazine, fluphenazine) and the butyrophenones (e.g., haloperidol) can produce either CNS depression or CNS excitation with agitation, delirium, and severe extrapyramidal effects such as muscular rigidity, tremor, or catatonic symptoms. Temperature regulation may also be impaired. Cardiac arrhythmias are rare but have been reported.

C. **Management.** The general principles of overdose management should be followed. Specific measures are as follows:

1. Attempts at **induced emesis** may be hampered by the antiemetic properties of neuroleptics.

2. If **CNS depression** is present, supportive measures should be instituted. **CNS excitation** can be treated with low doses of lorazepam or diazepam.

3. **Hypotension** that does not respond to volume expansion will respond to vasopressors such as norepinephrine (Levophed) or phenylephrine (Neo-Synephrine). Beta-agonists should be avoided because they may worsen vasodilation.

4. **Hypothermia** has been reported and should be treated with slow warming. Fluids given to hypothermic patients should be warmed.

5. **High fever** should be treated with antipyretics and, if necessary, ice baths.

6. **Severe extrapyramidal effects** should be treated with diphenhydramine (Benadryl) 50 mg IM or IV or benztropine (Cogentin) 2 mg IM or IV.

7. Because **cardiac arrhythmias** occur, cardiac monitoring is necessary. Ventricular tachyarrhythmias may be treated with lidocaine or bretylium. DC cardioversion is the treatment for life-threatening tachyarrhythmias. Torsades de pointes ventricular tachycardia, as may occur with pimozide or thioridazine, is best managed with isoproterenol or overdrive pacing.

8. Forced diuresis or dialysis is not helpful.

X. Overdoses with opioids

A. Overdoses with opioids most frequently involve heroin and are usually accidental, rather than the result of a suicide attempt, although the possibility of suicidality should not be ignored. Heroin-related deaths may occur:

1. When individuals unwittingly obtain heroin that is purer than usual.

2. In inexperienced users who have little tolerance and are poor judges of dose.

3. In experienced users after even brief periods of abstinence because tolerance quickly recedes, especially tolerance to respiratory depression.

4. With mixed overdoses. Opioids may act synergistically with other CNS depressants to produce a lethal overdose.

B. **Pharmacology.** The opioid drugs of abuse include heroin, morphine, codeine, hydromorphone (Dilaudid), oxycodone (component of Percodan and of Percocet), meperidine (Demerol), methadone, and pentazocine (Talwin). Individuals who abuse opiates IV usually use heroin but also use morphine and meperidine and will solubilize and inject pills of oxycodone and hydromorphone in times of shortage. Heroin may also be absorbed intranasally; other compounds are used orally. The danger of overdose lies in CNS depression with resulting coma, respiratory depression, and apnea. When death occurs it is usually due to respiratory depression.

C. **Manifestations of toxicity.** The typical opioid overdose patient presents with a depressed level of consciousness, pupillary constriction, and depressed respiration.

1. **On examination** respirations are slow or absent. Blood pressure and pulse are usually normal, although in a minority of cases there is hypotension and tachycardia. Temperature is usually normal, although rarely hypothermia is noted. Fever suggests the presence of an infection (most often as a result of nonsterile parenteral drug use). The patient is stuporous or comatose. Pupils are tightly constricted (tolerance to miosis does not normally occur). The skin may be cyanotic and may reveal injection sites and track marks (although there may be few such stigmata on examination of the inexperienced user). The presence of an abnormal chest finding should alert

the physician to the possibility of noncardiogenic pulmonary edema (which may be present in half of all heroin overdoses) or of bacterial pneumonia.

2. The **laboratory results** are usually unrevealing. A toxic screen should be sent to discover exactly which drugs have been ingested or injected. Arterial blood gases including pH are useful in judging the severity of the respiratory depression.

D. Therapy. As always, the basics of care of the stuporous or comatose patient with a suspected drug overdose must be followed, starting with attention to the airway and respiratory support if needed. Blood pressure in opioid overdoses usually responds to correction of hypoxia and moderate fluid replacement. In addition, the following specific measures should be instituted.

1. In suspected opioid overdose, **naloxone,** a pure opioid antagonist, should be given IV. The dose is 2 mg (5 ampules) as an IV bolus. For overdoses with pentazocine (Talwin) or propoxyphene (Darvon), much larger doses (up to 20 times greater) are needed. Naloxone does not completely reverse the toxic effects of buprenorphine. This agent will reverse coma and respiratory depression. It is safest to put the patient in restraints prior to giving naloxone.

   a. In using naloxone it must be recalled that its half-life is shorter than that of most abused opioids, including heroin; thus the patient requires frequent observation (at least every 15 minutes) for 4–8 hours depending on the size and nature of the overdose. Commonly patients will begin to show signs of drowsiness again within 45 minutes. Because of the short half-life of the drug some clinicians advocate the use of a **naloxone drip** after the initial IV bolus doses. Four mg of naloxone (10 ampules) can be added to 1 liter of 5% dextrose in water, and run at a rate of 100 ml/hour. However, given the risk of IV infiltration, the use of a drip should not be an excuse for less frequent observation of the patient.

   b. Once awake, if the patient gives a history of addiction to opioids, doses of naloxone should be kept to the minimum necessary. This is because the antagonist may cause "precipitated withdrawal," an acute and severe withdrawal syndrome. This is extremely uncomfortable, and, although not usually physically dangerous, can cause the patient to become disruptive and uncooperative. Treatment for precipitated withdrawal consists of reassurance that when the naloxone wears off, symptoms will improve. Except for precipitated withdrawal, there are essentially no side effects to naloxone.

2. Pulmonary edema is a serious complication of heroin overdose. Patients with this complication have mortality rates of about 20%. Heroin-induced pulmonary edema is not due to fluid overload but presumably to pulmonary capillary leakiness. The treatment is therefore not digitalis and diuretics but intubation, with adequate oxygenation (with FIO_2 to be determined by ABGs) and, if necessary, positive end-expiratory pressure (PEEP).

3. **Aspiration pneumonia** should be treated with appropriate antibiotics.

4. **Other sources of fever** in these patients may include endocarditis, meningitis, and cellulitis because of nonsterile injections. There may also be infected pressure bullae if the patient was in a coma for an extended period prior to emergency treatment. The possibility of AIDS or hepatitis must also not be overlooked (and requires care in the handling of blood specimens).

E. Prevention of recurrence is difficult; often the best chance for treatment of the underlying drug addiction is transfer of the patient, once medically stable, to an inpatient drug treatment facility. Unfortunately, most of the individuals who present with heroin overdoses will lack health insurance or interest in treatment. Thus referral to local public drug treatment programs, including methadone maintenance programs, may be the only alternative.

XI. Overdoses with cocaine and amphetamine

A. Cocaine and amphetamine are **psychostimulant** drugs that enhance the actions of norepinephrine, serotonin, and dopamine in the nervous system. Cocaine acts predominantly by inhibiting the reuptake transporters for these three neurotransmitters, thus prolonging their life in synapses; amphetamine acts predominantly by causing release of these three neurotransmitters.

B. Patterns of use (see Chap. 30).

1. **Cocaine** as the hydrochloride salt is generally used intranasally (snorting) or intravenously. Cocaine freebase (including "crack") is smoked, a method of use that produces high blood levels as rapidly as intravenous use. Most cocaine overdoses occur following intravenous use or smoking. However, lethal overdoses have also occurred when drug couriers swallow condoms filled with large amounts of cocaine and a condom bursts.

2. **Amphetamines** include racemic amphetamine sulfate (Benzedrine and others), dextroamphetamine (Dexedrine and others), and methamphetamine (Methedrine). Methamphetamine is the most potent and potentially toxic form of amphetamine. Amphetamine is taken orally, intravenously, or smoked ("ice"). Although ingestion of 20–25 mg/kg is potentially lethal to a drug-naive individual, tolerance to very high doses is observed in addicts.

C. Manifestations of psychostimulant toxicity

1. **Mild toxicity** includes tachycardia, palpitations, mild hypertension, slight fever, slight tachypnea, dry mouth, hyperactivity, agitation, mild paranoia, and anxiety (which may reach the level of panic).

2. **Severe toxicity** includes serious tachyarrhythmias, which may be life-threatening, marked hypertension (strokes have been reported), high fever, seizures, delirium, paranoia, psychosis, coma, and cardiovascular collapse.

D. Therapy

1. The general principles of overdose management should be followed. If the overdose occurred by ingestion, induced vomiting followed by charcoal administration is indicated.

2. Amphetamine is a weak base; for amphetamine, forced diuresis with acidification of the urine will hasten renal excretion.

3. **Seizures** should be treated with diazepam or lorazepam administered IV. For seizures that are unresponsive or recur, a full loading dose of phenytoin should be given.

4. **Hyperpyrexia** can be treated with chlorpromazine 10 mg IM q6h; if severe, cooling blankets should be used as well.

5. **Tachyarrhythmias** caused by cocaine and amphetamine often respond to propranolol IV in 1 mg doses up to 0.1 mg/kg.

6. Severe **hypertension** should be treated with phentolamine or nitroprusside.

7. Extreme **agitation** should be treated with a benzodiazepine (e.g., lorazepam 1–2 mg PO or IM q1–2 h) as needed. Significant **paranoia or psychotic symptoms** that interfere with treatment can be treated with haloperidol 5 mg PO (as a liquid) or IM. As the patient's medical condition allows, a quiet, low-stimulation environment will help minimize agitation.

Suggested Readings

GENERAL

Arana, G. W., and Hyman, S. E. Handbook of Psychiatric Drug Therapy (2nd ed.). Boston: Little, Brown, 1991.

Freedman, G. E., Pasternak, S., and Krenzelok, E. P. A clinical trial using syrup of ipecac and activated charcoal concurrently. *Ann. Emerg. Med.* 16:164, 1987.

Levy, G. Gastrointestinal clearance of drugs with activated charcoal. *N. Engl. J. Med.* 307:676, 1982.

OVERDOSES WITH SPECIFIC PSYCHOTROPIC DRUGS

Sedative-Hypnotic Overdoses

Goldberg, M. J., and Berlinger, W. G. Treatment of phenobarbital overdose with activated charcoal. *J.A.M.A.* 247:2400, 1982.

Tricyclic Overdoses

Biggs, J. T., et al. Tricyclic antidepressant overdose: Incidence of symptoms. *J.A.M.A.* 238:135, 1977.

Boehnert, M. T., and Lovejoy, F. H. Value of the QRS duration versus the serum drug level in predicting seizures and ventricular arrhythmias after an acute overdose of tricyclic antidepressants. *N. Engl. J. Med.* 313:474, 1985.

Foulke, G. E., and Albertson, T. E. QRS interval in tricyclic antidepressant overdosage: Inaccuracy as a toxicity indicator in emergency settings. *Ann. Emerg. Med.* 16:160, 1987.

Haddad, L. M., and Winchester, J. F. *Clinical Management of Poisoning and Drug Overdose.* Philadelphia: Saunders, 1983. P. 359.

Hermann, H. C., Kaplan, L. M., and Bierer, B. E. QT prolongation and torsades de pointes ventricular tachycardia produced by the tetracyclic antidepressant agent maprotiline. *Am. J. Cardiol.* 51:904, 1983.

Kapur, S., Mleczkowski, T., and Mann, J. J. Antidepressant medications and relative risk of suicide attempt and suicide. *J.A.M.A.* 268:3441, 1992.

Litovitz, T. L., and Troutman, W. G. Amoxapine overdosage: Seizures and fatalities. *J.A.M.A.* 250:1069, 1983.

Marshall, J. B., and Forker, A. D. Cardiovascular effects of tricyclic antidepressant drugs: Therapeutic usage, overdose, and management of complications. *Am. Heart J.* 163:401, 1982.

Mayron, R., and Ruiz, E. Phenytoin: Does it reverse tricyclic-antidepressant-induced cardiac conduction abnormalities? *Ann. Emerg. Med.* 15:876, 1986.

Swartz, C. M., and Sherman, A. The treatment of tricyclic antidepressant overdose with repeated charcoal. *J. Clin. Psychopharmacol.* 4:336, 1984.

Wedin, G. P., et al. Relative toxicity of cyclic antidepressants. *Ann. Emerg. Med.* 15:797, 1986.

Monoamine Oxidase Inhibitors

Kaplan, R. F., et al. Phenelzine overdose treated with dantrolene sodium. *J.A.M.A.* 255:642, 1986.

Linden, C. H., Rumack, B. H., and Strehlke, C. Monoamine oxidase inhibitor overdose. *Ann. Emerg. Med.* 13:1137, 1984.

Verrilli, M. R., et al. Phenelzine toxicity responsive to dantrolene. *Neurology* 37:865, 1987.

Lithium Overdoses

Apte, S. N., and Langston, J. W. Permanent neurological deficits due to lithium toxicity. *Ann. Neurol.* 13:453, 1983.

Jefferson, J. W., and Greist, J. H. Lithium intoxication. *Psychiatry Ann.* 8:458, 1978.

Schou, M. The Recognition and Management of Lithium Intoxication. In F. N Johnson (ed.), *Handbook of Lithium Therapy*. Lancaster, England: MTP Press, 1980.

Thomsen, K., and Schou, M. The Treatment of Lithium Poisoning. In F. N. Johnson (ed.), *Lithium Research and Therapy*. New York: Academic Press, 1975.

Neuroleptics

Baldessarini, R. J. *Chemotherapy in Psychiatry* (2nd ed.). Cambridge: Harvard University Press, 1985.

Wilson, W. H., and Weiler, S. J. Case report of phenothiazine-induced torsades de pointes. *Am. J. Psychiatry* 141:1265, 1984.

Opiate Overdoses

Greene, M. H., and Dupont, R. L. The Treatment of Acute Heroin Toxicity. In P. G Bourne (ed.), *Acute Drug Abuse Emergencies*. New York: Academic Press, 1976.

Appendixes

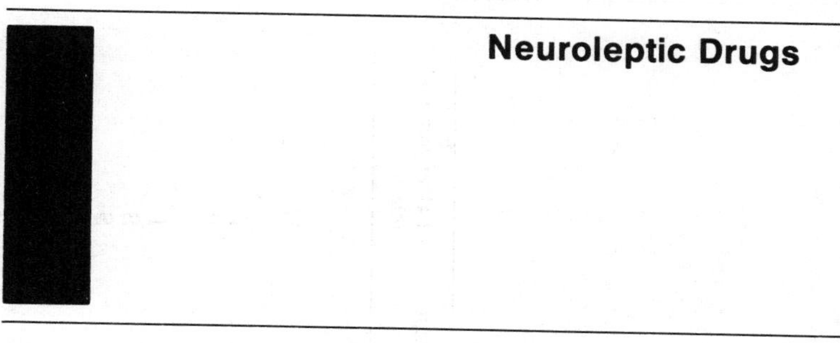

Neuroleptic Drugs

Drug	Approximate dose equivalent (mg)	Sedative effect	Hypotensive effect	Anticholinergic effect	Extrapyramidal effect
Phenothiazines					
Aliphatic					
Chlorpromazine (Thorazine)	100	S	S	I	W
Piperidine					
Mesoridazine (Serentil)	50	S	W	I	I
Thioridazine (Mellaril)	100	S	S	S	W
Piperazine					
Acetophenazine (Tindal)	20	I	W	W	I
Fluphenazine[a] (Prolixin, Permitil)	2	I	W	W	S
Perphenazine (Trilafon)	8	W	W	W	S
Trifluoperazine (Stelazine)	5	I	W	W	S
Thioxanthines					
Aliphatic					
Chlorprothixene (Taractan)	75	S	S	S	W
Piperazine					
Thiothixene (Navane)	5	W	W	W	S

Dibenzazepine					
Loxapine (Loxitane, Daxolin)	10	I	I	I	S
Clozapine (Clozaril)[b]	NA	S	S	W	W
Butyrophenones					
Haloperidol[a] (Haldol)	2	W	W	W	S
Droperidol[c] (Inapsine)	1	W	W	W	S
Indolone					
Molindone (Moban)	10	I	W	I	I
Diphenylbutylpiperidine					
Pimozide (Orap)	1	W	W	W	S

S = strong; I = intermediate; W = weak; NA = not available.

[a]Fluphenazine is available as the decanoate and enanthate esters at 25 mg/ml. Haloperidol is available as the decanoate ester at 50 mg/ml. The dosage equivalents are not directly comparable to those of the standard unesterified preparations.

[b]Clozapine is classified as an atypical antipsychotic drug because unlike classical antipsychotic drugs, it has a relatively low affinity for dopamine D_2 receptors and a high affinity for limbically located D_4 receptors. Its greater activity at limbic rather than striatal dopamine receptors may explain its relative freedom from extrapyramidal side effects.

[c]Available for injection only.

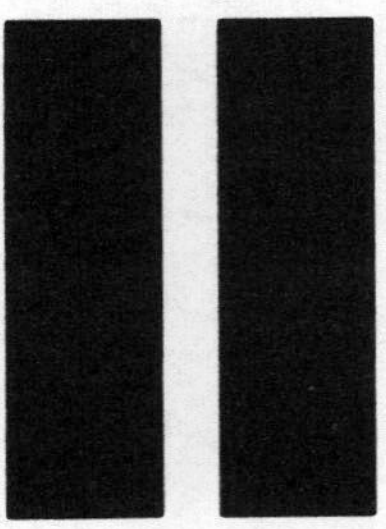

Antidepressant Drugs

Drug	Usual daily dose (mg/day)	Sedative effects	Anticholinergic effects	Half-life (hr)	Therapeutic plasma levels[a] (ng/ml)
Tricyclic and similar agents[b]					
Amitriptyline[c] (Elavil, Endep)	75–300	S	S	22–26	
Desipramine (Norpramin, Pertofrane)	75–300	W	W		150–300
Doxepin (Adapin, Sinequan)	75–300	S	S		100–250[d]
Imipramine[c] (Janimine, Tofranil)	75–300	I	I	30	150–250[d]
Nortriptyline (Pamelor)	30–150	W	W	26	50–150
Protriptyline (Vivactil)	15–60	W	S		
Trimipramine (Surmontil)	75–300	S	I		50–200
Amoxapine (Asendin)	75–300	W	W	30	
Maprotiline (Ludiomil)	75–200[e]	I	W	51	180–450
Atypical agent[b]					
Trazodone	150–400	S	W	3–9	800–1600
Monoamine oxidase inhibitors					
Isocarboxacid (Marplan)	20–50	W	W		
Phenelzine (Nardil)	30–60	W	I[f]		
Tranylcypromine (Parnate)	20–50	W	W		
Serotonin-specific reuptake inhibitors					
Fluoxetine[g] (Prozac)	20–80	W	W	7–9 days	
Paroxetine[g] (Paxil)	20	W	W	21	
Sertraline (Zoloft)	50–200	W	W	26	

I = intermediate; S = strong; W = weak.

[a] Plasma levels may not reflect tissue levels. Their use is controversial.

[b] Elderly patients require lower than usual doses of these drugs.

[c] Available also in injectable form.

[d] Parent drug plus *N*-desmethyl metabolite.

[e] Because of risk of seizures, this is the maximum dose.

[f] No anticholinergic effect in vitro.

[g] Inhibits the hepatic metabolism of some drugs (e.g., tricyclic antidepressants, anticonvulsants).

Benzodiazepines

Drug	Approximate dose equivalent (mg)	Onset of effect	Half-l (hr)
Alprazolam (Xanax)	0.5	F–I	6–20
Chlordiazepoxide (Librium)	25	F	30–10
Clonazepam (Klonopin)	0.25	I	20–40
Clorazepate (Tranxene)	7.5	F	30–10
Diazepam (Valium)	5	F	30–10
Estazolam (ProSom)	1	I	10–24
Flurazepam (Dalmane)	30	I	50–10
Halazepam (Paxipam)	20	I	30–10
Lorazepam (Ativan)	1	I	10–20
Oxazepam (Serax)	15	S	5–21
Prazepam (Centrax)	10	SL	30–10
Quazepam (Doral)	15	I	40–80
Temazepam (Restoril)	30	I	9.5–12
Triazolam (Halcion)	0.25	I	1.7–3.

F = fast; I = intermediate; S = slow; SL = slowest.

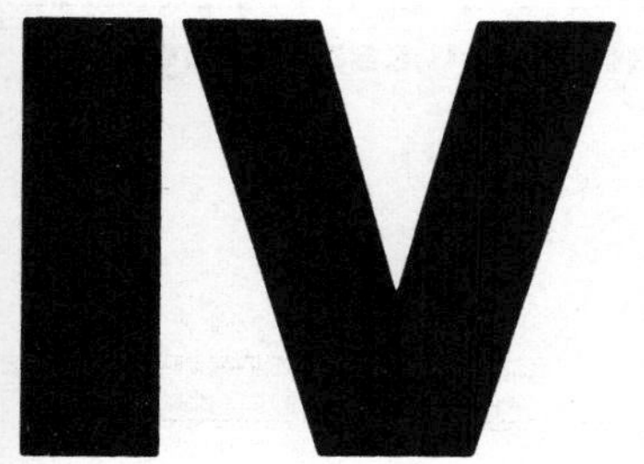

Nonbenzodiazepine Sedative-Hypnotics

Drug	Daily dose range	Initial dose for sleep
Barbiturates		
Short-acting		
Secobarbital[a] (Seconal)		100 mg
Pentobarbital[a] (Nembutal)		100 mg
Intermediate-acting		
Amobarbital[a] (Amytal)		100 mg
Butabarbital[a] (Butisol)		100 mg
Long-acting		
Phenobarbital (Luminal)	45–300 mg	
Propanediols		
Meprobamate[a] (Equanil, Miltown)	1.2–1.6 gm	
Antihistamines		
Hydroxyzine[b] (Atarax, Vistaril)	30–200 mg	
Promethazine[b] (Phenergan)	50–200 mg	
Diphenhydramine[b] (Benadryl)	25–100 mg	50 mg
Chloral derivatives		
Chloral hydrate (Noctec)		1.0 gm
Piperidinedione derivatives		
Glutethimide[a] (Doriden)		500 mg
Methyprylon[a] (Noludar)		300 mg
Acetylinic alcohols		
Ethchlorvynol[a] (Placidyl)		750 mg
Atypical anxiolytics		
Buspirone (Buspar)	20–30 mg	

[a]High abuse potential; little rational use.
[b]Strongly anticholinergic.

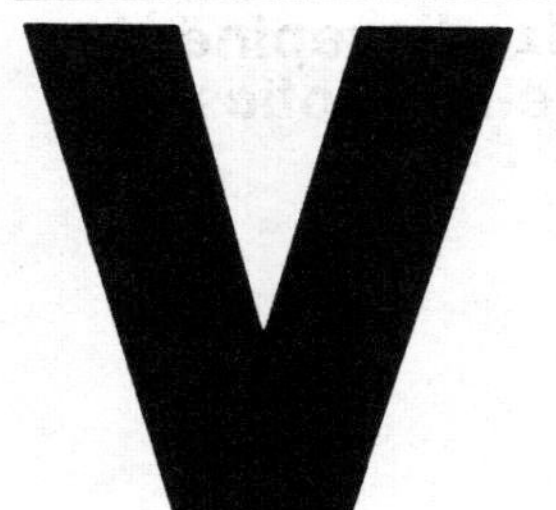

Anticonvulsant Drugs

Drug	Initial dose (adult)	Maintenance dose (adult)	Time to steady state	Therapeutic levels (μg/ml)
Valproic acid (Depakene)	250 mg/day	20 mg/kg/day (1200–1400 mg/day) tid dosing	1.5–3 days	50–120
Phenytoin (Dilantin) Intravenous	Loading doses: 15 mg/kg at rate < 50 mg/minute	4–8 mg/kg/day (300–400 mg/day) qd or bid dosing		10–20
Oral	300–400 mg every 2–4 hours for three doses		5–10 days for oral	
Carbamazepine (Tegretol)	200 mg/day	1000–1200 mg/day bid or tid dosing	3 days	4–12; 8–12 for mania
Phenobarbital (Luminal, others)	30–60 mg/day	2–4 mg/kg/day (150–250 mg/day) qd dosing	2–3 weeks	10–40
Primidone (Mysoline)	50–125 mg/day	10 mg/kg/day (600–700 mg/day) bid dosing	Primidone 1–3 days; PEMA 2.5 days; phenobarbital 2–3 weeks	Primidone, 4–12; phenobarbital, 10–40
Ethosuximide (Zarontin)	250 mg/day	15–40 mg/kg	12 days	40–100

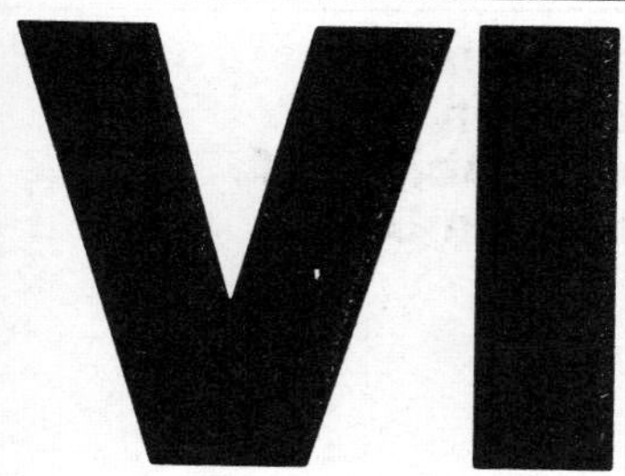

VI Antiparkinsonian Drugs

Drug	Usual dosage for drug-induced extrapyramidal symptoms
Anticholinergic drugs	
Benztropine (Cogentin)	1–4 mg qd–bid
Biperiden (Akineton)	2 mg qd–bid
Procyclidine (Kemadrin)	2.5–5.0 mg tid–qid
Trihexyphenidyl (Artane, Tremin)	1–5 mg tid
Antihistamines	
Diphenhydramine (Benadryl)	25 mg tid–qid
Dopamine-releasing	
Amantadine (Symmetrel)	100 mg bid–tid

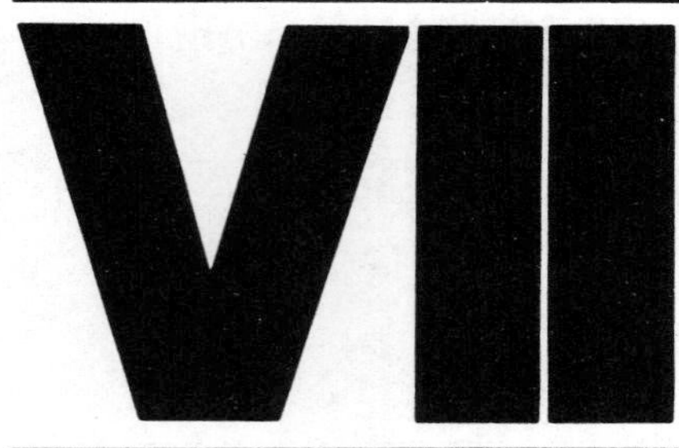

Approximate Duration of Detectability of Drugs in Urine

Drug	Retention tir
Amphetamine and methamphetamine	48 hours
Barbiturates	
Short-acting (e.g., secobarbital, pentobarbital)	24 hours
Intermediate-acting (e.g., amobarbital, butabarbital, butalbital)	48–72 hours
Long-acting (e.g., phenobarbital)	2–3 weeks
Benzodiazepines (at therapeutic doses)	3 days
Cannabinoids	
Moderate smoker (4 times/week)	3 days
Daily smoker	10 days
Daily heavy smoker	3–4 weeks
Cocaine	6–8 hours
Cocaine metabolites	2–4 days
Ethyl alcohol	7–12 hours
Methaqualone	7 days
Narcotics	
Codeine	48 hours
Heroin (as morphine)	36–72 hours
Hydrocodone	24 hours
Hydromorphone	48 hours
Methadone	3 days
Morphine	48–72 hours
Oxycodone	24 hours
Propoxyphene	6–48 hours
Phencyclidine	8 days

Index

Index

The abbreviations *f* and *t* stand for figure and table, respectively.

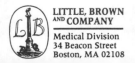